T0074942

Traumatic Brain Injury

This new book from leading neurosurgeon and author Gary E. Kraus is an account of traumatic brain injury (TBI) from the time a brain-injured patient arrives in the emergency department through to the wide range of clinical outcomes of such an injury. Written with the voice of experience, the author examines causation of TBI, the patient's stay in the neurointensive care unit and the many neurological assessments and tests that inform of the outcomes that the patient and their families will encounter.

A wide range of medical professionals will benefit from Dr. Kraus' acute insights into TBI including neurosurgical residents, neurosurgeons with a subspecialist interest in neurotrauma, neurologists managing patients post-TBI, neurointensivists, neuropsychologists, researchers and scientists involved in clinical trials in TBI, and those with a specialist interest in neurorehabilitation.

Traumatic Brain Injury

A Neurosurgeon's Perspective

Gary E. Kraus, MD, FAANS, CLCP
Kraus TBI, Brain & Spine Institute
Neurosurgery, PA
Houston, Texas

CRC Press
Taylor & Francis Group
Boca Raton London New York

CRC Press is an imprint of the
Taylor & Francis Group, an **informa** business

First edition published 2023
by CRC Press
6000 Broken Sound Parkway NW, Suite 300, Boca Raton, FL 33487-2742
and by CRC Press
4 Park Square, Milton Park, Abingdon, Oxon, OX14 4RN

CRC Press is an imprint of Taylor & Francis Group, LLC

ISBN: 9781032406589 (hbk)
ISBN: 9781032394893 (pbk)
ISBN: 9781003354154 (ebk)

DOI: 10.1201/9781003354154

Typeset in Minion Pro
by KnowledgeWorks Global Ltd.

This book is dedicated to the patients that I have cared for, who have taught me so much about life, medicine, courage and humanity.

Contents

Foreword

Gary E. Kraus, who did a fellowship with me 29 years ago, has written an exhaustive book on traumatic head injury. Many books have been published on this topic as it is a malady that, as neurosurgeons, we treat far too frequently. What sets this excellent volume apart from its competition is that Dr. Kraus has interspersed personal vignettes with the factual data that makes up our knowledge of head injury.

His attention to detail provides a dazzling display of statistical data so critical to decision-making. He says it as it is, the devastating effects of head injury, whether mild or severe. He emphasizes the need for speed in removal of expanding blood clots on the brain and covers the myriad consequences that a patient and his/her loved ones must deal with in the aftermath of a head injury. His points are presented factually, but also with empathy and understanding.

I found this book easy to read, appreciating how the data was presented in a cogent and absorbable manner while providing an authoritative compendium on traumatic brain injury (TBI), from philosophy to sports-related TBI, from anatomy to understanding consciousness, from imaging to socioeconomic consequences, and so on.

Initially, I thought it is a terrific read for trainees and neurosurgeons dealing with this too frequent entity, however, upon reflection, I believe it deserves a much wider readership: certainly all the caretakers involved with these patients from rehabilitation physicians and staff, to the psychologists and psychiatrists dealing with head injury, the nurses that wish to be enlightened, and the various consultants called in to help manage these complex patients.

But, additionally, patients and their families can peruse the pages to better understand what happened to them or their loved ones. Understanding the injury can help with treatment and enlightenment to adjust to the new reality that exists after head trauma. By realizing a patient and their family are not alone, that mild or debilitating consequences of head injury are all too common, can help to reach acceptance.

There is much in this book that will attract the neurosurgical trauma expert while also being a reference book for the patient and family. I am delighted to recommend this well-written volume on head trauma with enthusiasm and without reservation. Well done, Dr. Kraus!

Robert F. Spetzler, MD
Emeritus CEO and President
Barrow Neurological Institute
Phoenix, Arizona, USA

Preface

The brain is the only organ in the body which, if transplanted, would benefit the donor, and not the recipient.

—Gary E. Kraus

(.... Hypothetical, to emphasize that the brain, and not the body, is the essence of who we are.)

As a neurosurgeon, I have treated many patients who have had the unfortunate experience of having suffered a traumatic brain injury. A momentary brain injury can have ramifications that last a lifetime.

To talk about brain injury, one must first have a basic understanding of the normally functioning brain. Studying its anatomy on a macroscopic and microscopic level is one side of the puzzle, while understanding its function and how it relates to consciousness and the essence of who we are, is another. To attempt to close this elusive chasm requires mastery and cooperation of multiple disciplines that are vast and divergent, ranging from biology, neuroanatomy, psychology, and biochemistry, to physics, mathematics, big data, and computer science, as well as to philosophy and religion. Perhaps the answer lies somewhere in this panoply of fields of study, or possibly the absolute truth lies in recesses to which humankind has limited or no access.

Unfortunately, things in the brain do go awry as a result of trauma or other pathologies such as tumors, vascular disease, infections, and degenerative processes. Learning about brain function has also been achieved in these instances, when changes in function may be attributed to alterations in anatomical structure.

Although I am a neurosurgeon, medicine was the one field I knew I didn't want to go into when I was an adolescent. My mother passed away when I was 15 years old after having been very ill with emphysema for three years prior to that. I had been in enough ambulances, hospitals, and ICUs.

My interest in science started at a very early age and was fostered by discussions my father had with me about Einstein and other areas of science when we went for walks. I attended Stuyvesant High School, a public high school in New York City, which is geared to students who are interested in science and math. While I was in high school, I became interested in computers and wrote code in Fortran for playing games. It was at Stuyvesant when my geometry teacher Ms. Selma Landsberg introduced me to the book *Flatland* (391), which describes a two-dimensional world, the significance of which is discussed later in this book. I subsequently attended college at Rensselaer Polytechnic Institute and received a B.S. degree in Physics with studies in Electrical Engineering and Psychology as well. During the summer between my first and second years of college, I worked at a job in Manhattan in New York City, but found myself getting home too late in the evening to do activities I enjoyed, such as playing tennis in the nearby city park. I thought about volunteering in a hospital. The first hospital (close to where I lived) I called told me that they already had candy stripers and didn't need my services. The second hospital (also close to where I lived) wanted me to work in the supply room, but I declined that position. The third hospital, which was located in Manhattan and a distance from where I lived, told me they have an opening, but it would be in the same ICU where my mother had passed away and had in fact spent a good portion of the last three years of her life. I was initially anxious about doing this, but I showed up at the volunteer office. They gave me a volunteer coat and I proceeded to the ICU. My fear was replaced with a compassion for the patients whom I was allowed to visit.

Returning to college, I knew that I was interested in medicine. During two summers in college, I worked in the laboratory of Dr. Jonathan C. Newell, a professor of biomedical engineering and pulmonary physiology who inspired me to do research. I researched electrical modeling of analog pressure and flow systems by means of a technique known as Fast Fourier transforms. While I continued on with my studies in Physics and Electrical Engineering, I also applied to medical school.

For three summers, at the end of college and during my first two years of medical school, I worked at IBM doing research and development in computer hardware and software. I worked on hardware for the mainframe 3081 computer, and I also worked on software design for handwriting recognition at the IBM Thomas J. Watson Research Center.

During medical school at State University of New York at Stony Brook, I realized that medicine was the right field for me. In selecting which medical school to attend, I inquired about what pulmonary research the schools did, as I thought I wanted to go into pulmonary medicine. It was during medical school that I became fascinated with the nervous system and I knew that I had found a field that would intrigue and fulfill me for a lifetime. I decided to go into neurosurgery.

I did run into a health problem while in medical school, as I had encountered periodic bouts of spontaneous supraventricular tachycardia, which eventually subsided on their own. I was diagnosed with Wolff-Parkinson-White syndrome (extra electrical conducting pathway in the heart) and ended up having a cardiac electrophysiological study. I was started on quinidine, which created a profound, how do I say, urgent need to visit the restroom. I knew that if I wanted to go into neurosurgery, frequent restroom breaks were not compatible with long surgeries. I also knew that if I didn't take the medication, I might run the risk of having a tachycardia during a long neurosurgical procedure and I never wanted to encounter that risk. At the age of 24, I decided to have an open cardiac surgery procedure to divide the extra electrical conducting bundles of Kent. The surgery went beautifully and after I completed medical school, I entered neurosurgery residency at St. Louis University School of Medicine, St. Louis, and trained under Dr. Kenneth R. Smith. Dr. Smith instilled in me the passion always to be intellectually honest and devoted, and hold the health and safety of the patient above all else. Despite long and intense hours in the operating room, neuro-ICU, floors and emergency room, I thoroughly enjoyed the training and experience.

After residency, I completed a fellowship in Neurovascular and Skull Base Surgery under Dr. Robert F. Spetzler, at Barrow Neurological Institute in Phoenix, AZ. This was a training that would further transform my surgical skills and shape my life. Dr. Spetzler is a truly incredible person on many levels. Not only is he one of — if not the best — neurosurgeon in the world, his profound respect for understanding and protecting the brain, his constant quest to aim for perfection in the operating room, and his courage to perform the most complex operations that few other neurosurgeons would be willing to touch, along with his great leadership abilities and incredible kindness and compassion as a person, have left an indelible impression on me.

In the operating room, Dr. Spetzler ensured that every measure was taken to protect the brain during a surgery. The special suction tips that Dr. Spetzler designed are an extension of a surgeon's hand and enable a neurosurgeon to avoid inadvertently harming delicate brain tissue or nerves. In the operating room, every patient was strategically positioned so that surgical exposure was easiest, and that gravity assisted in brain dissection, with minimal use of retraction, again protecting the brain. One of the most complex pathologies a neurosurgeon will encounter are blood vessel malformations in the brain known as arteriovenous malformations (AVMs). Through Dr. Spetzler's immense neurosurgical experience and research into these challenging lesions, the Spetzler-Martin grading system for classifying these was born, is used throughout the world, and has remained the standard for all neurosurgeons. This grading system, along with the microsurgical teachings of Dr. Spetzler, have helped to determine which lesions can and can't be treated safely, always with the goal of protecting brain tissue and function. Dr. Spetzler has performed more than 6,400 aneurysm surgeries and has pioneered and mastered the technique of deep hypothermic circulatory arrest (cardiac standstill) for complex basilar artery aneurysms, always with the goal of protection and preservation of brain tissue and function. In addition, Dr. Spetzler has published a countless number of academic papers and books describing the numerous procedures and techniques he has taught the world, tackling the most difficult lesions including giant intracranial aneurysms, arteriovenous malformations, cavernomas, brain tumors and skull base tumors, and spinal AVMs. Dr. Spetzler has also invented and designed numerous neurosurgical instruments that are being used in operating rooms throughout the world on a daily basis.

As neuroanatomy is the basis of neurosurgery, my interest in neuroanatomy led me to co-author a textbook *Microsurgical Anatomy of the Brain: A Stereo Atlas.* (314) The function behind the brain represents who we are as people, our personalities, social interactions, creativity, memory and so forth. Two novels which I co-authored, *Body Trade* (251) and the sequel *Unexpected: Body Trade 2* (250), delve into this topic and upon brain injury and the theoretical topic of brain transplantation.

To gaze upon the splendor of the brain is an experience filled with awe, certainly when one is able to admire its intricacy that has been designed with perfection beyond human understanding, but also when one ponders the vast array of function, which is incomprehensible.

Traumatic brain injury is very prevalent in modern society. Its visible and invisible impacts on individuals and those around them can be devastating. For a long time, mild traumatic brain injury and its long-term impact has been under-recognized. This book reviews the past, present, and possible future in the evaluation and treatment of traumatic brain injury.

Due in part to exponential growth in technology and communications, understanding of the brain and its injured state is growing at an unprecedented rate, with more advances made in the last century than in the previous 5,000 years. We are at the cusp of breakthroughs in transcranial stimulation, neural modulation, neural plasticity, stem cells, and other treatments of brain injury. If this knowledge can ultimately be transformed into significantly enhancing and improving the lives of those who have suffered a traumatic brain injury, the journey will have accomplished its purpose.

Gary E. Kraus, MD, FAANS, CLCP
Houston, Texas
September 2022

Acknowledgments

Writing a book requires assimilation of knowledge and experiences acquired during life.

My mentors have had a significant influence on my life. Dr. Jonathan C. Newell helped to kindle my interests in medical research. Dr. Kenneth R. Smith and Dr. Richard D. Bucholz taught me the skills of becoming a neurosurgeon. Dr. Robert F. Spetzler has had a profound impact on my life, further refining my skills and serving as a mentor on methods to approach and tackle challenging problems, both in the operating room and in leadership. I consider Dr. Spetzler to be one of, if not the best neurosurgeon in the world to tackle the most complex lesions in the brain, and I am grateful to have had the opportunity to train under him. Dr. Simon Horenstein shared his vast knowledge of neuroanatomy during Saturday morning conferences, which were always very educational and stimulating.

I would like to acknowledge my most caring and supportive family Audrey Carr, Tom Carr, Brendan Carr, Dr. Daniel Carr (also a neurosurgeon), and Dr. Michelle Carr (a neuroscientist specializing in dream engineering). My parents Gusti and John Kraus who instilled in me the desire to be passionate about what I do, and help others.

My neurosurgery partner, friend and colleague Dr. Masaki Oishi, who has had countless discussions with me about neurosurgery, and ways to improve patient care. My office staff Patsy Chavez, Maria Cortez, Elvia Rodriguez, and Julio Ramirez, who have been with me for many years and have strived in every way they can to improve the lives of our patients.

My wonderful friends who have discussed the book with me, listened to my ideas on this subject or otherwise significantly contributed to my thoughts, ideas, and knowledge over the years. They include Veronica Soltys, Rhodalyn Suarez, Rahul Dhawan, Sayeeda Kurlawala, Punit Shah, Mario Chavez, Dr. Jin Zhou, Thomas George, Carolyn Crump, Paul Popp, Pamela Novick, Drew Skally, Edye Leuin, Dave Ziegler, Anil Patel, Dr. Subbarao Kala, Gerry Szkotnicki, Louis Kokernak, Terry Arnold, Gary Savage, Fred Bucholz, Julian Martinez, and Dr. Lori Noaker.

I would like to express my gratitude and appreciation to several individuals for their input, communications, or contributions of several images used in this book: Dr. Brian L. Edlow, Massachusetts General Hospital, Harvard Medical School; Dr. Bruce Rosen, Massachusetts General Hospital, Harvard Medical School; Dr. Arthur W. Toga (Director), Sidney Taiko Sheehan (Communications Manager), and Jim Stanis (Medical Illustrator), who are all with the USC Mark and Mary Stevens Neuroimaging and Informatics Institute; Dr. Ryan Seiji Kitagawa, Director of Neurotrauma at University of Texas Health Sciences Center at Houston; Dr. David S. Levey, diagnostic radiology and nuclear medicine. I would also like to thank my friend Dr. Jaimie M. Henderson, Stanford University, for his input and discussions.

I would also like to acknowledge and thank the publishing house Taylor & Francis, Routledge, and CRC Press and their outstanding publishers and editors. It is a pleasure working with Miranda Bromage, Jacob Jewitt-Jalland, Leanne Hinves, Kyle Meyer, Misbah Sabri and Amanda Cortright on this project. I am also grateful to Dr. V. Robert May, who has offered guidance and suggestions, and without whom I would not have written this book.

I would like to also thank the patients who have entrusted me with their lives. Their wisdom, insight, patience, and courage in dealing with some of the most difficult nervous system diseases imaginable is extraordinary. Although we always strive for an excellent outcome, there are some illnesses in which that is regrettably not possible. I have learned greatly from the patients I have treated, and I am grateful for them having the confidence in me to care for them to the best of my ability.

I also acknowledge Mango, who for many hours while I was writing this book, sat on the chair next to me while looking out the window, gazing at the same world I was, but likely noticing, perceiving, and analyzing the world from a completely different perspective.

There are many others who have had an instrumental role in shaping my life and thoughts, and many who I have lost touch with over the years — I am grateful and thankful to them as well.

Introduction

If the human brain were so simple that we could understand it, we would be so simple that we couldn't.

—Emerson Pugh

The human brain, which is who we in essence are, is at the core of our existence and awareness as we know it. Understanding the human brain and its impact on our daily existence has challenged society since the dawn of civilization. As a neurosurgeon, I have been fortunate to have had patients entrust me with their care as I treat them for disorders of the brain and spine.

The almost unfathomable coalescence of neurons, glial cells, blood vessels, and much more, all coordinating in a most incredibly harmonious and synergistic manner to create the brain means that although much has been learned, there is still an enormous amount to be learned. In the relentless quest of physicians, psychologists, and medical scientists to understand the human body, the brain remains the most elusive of structures. With advances in science and technology, significant progress has been made in unraveling the mysteries of the brain, yet only the surface has been scratched. Understanding the brain requires expertise from a variety of fields, including medicine (neurosurgery, neurology, neuroradiology, psychiatry), neuropsychology, neuroanatomy, physics, mathematics/big data/computer science, philosophy, and religion. (**Figure I.1**).

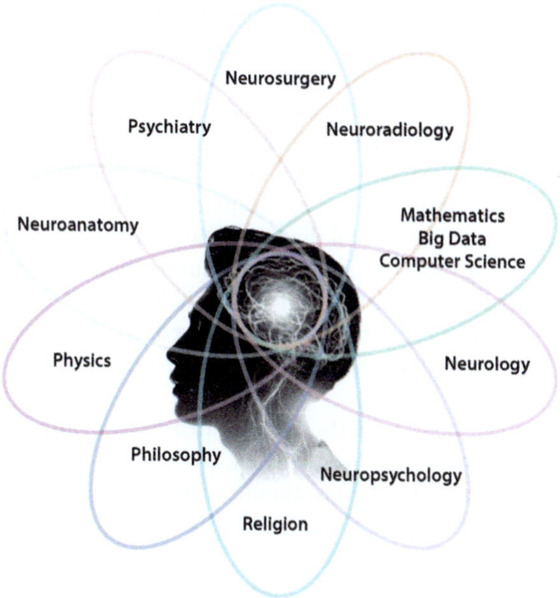

Figure I.1 Venn diagram showing the intersection of domains required to increase knowledge of the brain: neurosurgery, neuroradiology, mathematics/big data/computer science, neurology, neuropsychology, religion, philosophy, physics, neuroanatomy, and psychiatry.

Ultimately, our quest to understand the brain and do our best to help treat patients depends not only on merging data from these diverse fields, but also on our ability to constantly shift our analysis and questions from the microscopic to the macroscopic, and to each level in-between, grasping both the big and the small picture. Analogously, the earth appears very differently when viewed from 60,000 feet of altitude than it does when one is standing on the ground, but the ability to see the earth from both vantage points, and at intervening levels, provides insights not apparent at only one level. Similarly, the ability to evaluate a patient's neurological status, study advanced imaging of the brain, and review critical and pertinent anatomic features while correlating function with structure, will ultimately serve to further our understanding of the brain and to better evaluate and treat patients.

Traumatic brain injury (TBI) remains a significant challenge for the world. Although the consequences of severe TBI are typically immediately apparent and often devastating, mild TBI, which is the most frequently encountered, may also have tremendous life-long implications for a patient, but these injuries and their sequelae are often under-recognized or un-recognized, and under-treated or untreated. In some cases, even significant brain damage may go un-diagnosed (chapter 3).

The way that things are named is important and has consequences. The Meriam-Webster online dictionary defines "mild" as an adjective meaning: "gentle in nature or behavior; moderate in action or effect; not sharp, spicy or bitter; not being or involving what is extreme; not severe."(661) While this term may be appropriate to describe many things that are encountered on a daily basis (such as the spiciness of food or severity of weather patterns), when used to describe brain injury, it may lead to the misperception that an individual who has suffered a mild TBI will have "mild" consequences, and will not suffer long-lasting and severe difficulties. As will be discussed in this book, that is not necessarily the case.

People are often capable of recognizing differences in another person's behavior. These differences may be due to a TBI, mental illness, substance abuse, etc. With advances in science, technology, and medical imaging applied to the study of brain anatomy, in addition to advances in methods of evaluation of cognition and psychological function in a person who has suffered a TBI, the goal of matching structure and function of the brain is constantly evolving and improving. The intersection of the medical specialties that evaluate structure with those that evaluate function allows for anatomical and chemical biomarkers, which are greatly improving our ability to recognize, diagnose, and treat TBI as well as predict future needs and likely required care of a person who has suffered a TBI. TBI is not an isolated event, but rather a chronic disease and potentially the beginning of life-altering changes for the patient and all those around them. With advances in understanding and diagnosis, as well as novel treatments, a goal of better outcomes for patients appears to be on the horizon.

We live in a very exciting time. Advances in neuroscience made in the past century have exceeded what has been learned during the previous 5,000 years. This tremendous explosion of knowledge is shedding light on TBI in a way not possible before. Historically, TBI — especially mild TBI — was difficult to evaluate, as imaging studies were often completely "normal" despite obvious changes in a patient's behavior. With the advent of advanced imaging, it is now possible for medical providers to essentially perform noninvasive "in vivo" dissections of the injured brain of a patient. Imaging studies now allow for the analysis of subtle traces of parenchymal blood, cortical injuries, white-matter tract injuries, and changes in volume of different regions of the brain. This technology has been combined with brain parcellation atlases as well as functional imaging studies to provide understanding of brain function at a level not imaginable in the past.

The diagnosis of TBI is a clinical determination. To properly assess, diagnose, and ultimately treat patients with TBI to the best of our ability as physicians, an assemblage of critical information from vastly different clinical domains is needed by the clinician, who will then attempt to put together all of the pieces to arrive at an accurate diagnosis and understanding of a patient's pathology.

The pertinent domains required to fully understand and diagnose a TBI patient include:

- Evaluation of the patient's history, including family members, friends, and co-workers, to understand more about the injury, physical and cognitive changes the patient has suffered, and their impact on a patient's ability to function in the family, work, and social setting.

- A thorough physical examination and assessment of the patient, including neurosurgical, neurological, neuropsychological, cognitive and psychiatric evaluations: Even the most subtle agnosias (see Chapter 7) may be recognized with a detailed evaluation in which the appropriate questions are asked.
- Evaluation of conventional and advanced imaging techniques: Thorough understanding and detailed analysis of advanced imaging techniques allow a clinician to gain knowledge about even subtle changes to the white-matter connecting fibers/fasciculi within the brain, cortical brain regions, changes in brain volume, and traces of "microbleeds" within the brain parenchyma.
- Detailed understanding of neuroanatomy, white-matter connecting tracts and fasciculi, cortical regions, neurofunction associated with cortical regions and connectomes (lesion network mapping), and how these relate with and impact each other and how they correlate with the specific clinical findings of a patient.
- Assemblage of all the above information by the clinician, who will take time to review all the data and attempt to formulate a diagnosis in which anatomical changes may be related to functional changes, resulting in a consistent diagnosis. The clinician must also be cognizant of the fact that any clinical, radiological, or other biomarker findings which may be identified are likely the "tip of the iceberg."
- This information and diagnosis can be implemented to design a personalized treatment plan for a patient, with future assessments determining the success of treatments.

This detailed approach to formulating diagnoses will help to longitudinally evaluate results of personalized treatment plans for patients. It will also help with studying and implementing future therapeutic options for patients suffering from a TBI. The knowledge gained is vital to anticipating a TBI patient's future medical needs for both treatment purposes as well as anticipation of potential complications and co-morbidities which may arise. A life care plan for a patient will incorporate this information which is critical for addressing the future needs of a patient.

The future for the treatment of TBI looks very encouraging. With currently available objective tools that can help to assess treatment modalities, as well as advances in stem cells, neural plasticity, and other areas of research, great strides of advances in all arenas of the care of TBI look extremely promising.

1

Experience as a neurosurgeon

Nothing ever built arose to touch the skies unless some man dreamed that it should, some man believed that it could, and some man willed that it must.

—Charles Kettering

As a neurosurgeon, I have on many occasions had the experience of being called into the emergency department of a hospital at all hours of the day and night to take care of patients who have suffered a traumatic brain injury (TBI) and multiple traumas to their body. I have pushed my way through a barrage of medical personnel surrounding a patient who had suffered a major trauma and who had just been transported by a helicopter or ambulance, still strapped to a spine board with a hard collar on the neck and an endotracheal tube protecting the lungs. Surrounding the patient were doctors, nurses, respiratory therapists, and X-ray technicians trying to assess and stabilize the patient's condition, looking for better intravenous access, compressing an Ambu bag to deliver oxygen into the patient's lungs, getting a "stat" lateral "C" (cervical spine) X-ray to rule out a fracture, monitoring vital signs, and getting a Foley catheter into the bladder. Yet, I pushed my way through this multitude of people who were trying to save the patient's life so that I could perform my role as a neurosurgeon. I made my way to the patient's head and tried to start my neurological assessment, often beginning in the emergency department, but sometimes continuing as I ran with the patient traveling on a gurney en route to the computed tomography (CT) scanner for a view of the brain. Frequently, we would go straight from the CT room to the operating room, where I might perform an emergency craniotomy to evacuate a hematoma in an attempt to save the patient's life. The goal was to have the elapsed time from when the patient first arrived at the emergency room to when I actually made an incision in the skin on the scalp, and subsequently opened the skull and decompressed the brain, be as brief as possible. Time is of the essence, as an expanding hematoma around or in the brain, resulting in a shift of the brain from one side to the other, is a severe insult to and is extremely poorly tolerated by the brain for

DOI: 10.1201/9781003354154-1

more than a short while before a deteriorating cascade of events occurs, with increasing intracranial pressure (ICP) building, increasing brain shift worsening, and subsequent death or otherwise extreme neurological damage imminent. Despite such swift measures, the outcome is often very poor, and even if the patient survives, they are often left with severe impairment and permanent deficits for life.

In the operating room, I have rushed to first open the scalp with a large flap, cut open a large segment of bone, then widely open the dura mater to expose a very swollen and tense brain. If the patient suffered a subdural hematoma, I would immediately see a large amount of mixed clotted and fresh blood pouring out of the brain, and I would use copious amounts of irrigation to try to wash out any clot that remained beneath the far reaches of the skull. If there were a severely contused frontal or temporal lobe, I may have had to remove a portion of brain tissue and try to stop all active bleeding. After adequately decompressing the brain and achieving hemostasis, I would repair the dura, replace and secure the bone flap, close the scalp, insert an ICP monitor in the brain, apply the wound dressing, and re-evaluate the patient shortly thereafter in the neuro-intensive care unit. The patient would have an ICP monitor and often a ventricular catheter in the brain, which allowed for the drainage of cerebrospinal fluid (CSF) to help manage ICP.

Meeting with the family after the surgery was difficult, as I had to explain what happened, and what measures we were taking to try to save the patient's life, as well as possible and probable future outcomes.

From the time a brain-injured patient arrives in the emergency department, whether or not they undergo a craniotomy, and throughout their stay in the neuro-intensive care unit, I have, on many occasions, gone through the neurological assessments and tests to confirm brain death if the patient's neurological condition had severely deteriorated. As a neurosurgeon, my role in the treatment of patients has been to assess TBI in the acute, subacute, and chronic setting, and treat patients for their TBI to the best of my ability. In the acute phase, this often involves assessing patients in a hospital emergency department, making rapid assessments to save a patient's life, and helping manage their postoperative care. In the subacute and chronic phases, this requires taking care of issues that had arisen after the patient was stabilized from their initial injury, as well as issues that may have arisen weeks or months after the injury. My interactions would frequently require the input of and coordination with other medical specialists such as intensive care physicians, anesthesiologists, neurologists, radiologists, physiatrists, neuropsychologists, orthopedic surgeons, as well as occupational and physical therapists, respiratory therapists, nutritionists, orthotists, and other medical experts.

Eventually, in the chronic phase of recovery from a TBI, determinations regarding the future care of a patient will need to be assessed. This may include likely future medical treatments, anticipated complications, future therapy, medications, and other adaptive changes to their surroundings, such as modifications to living arrangements, attendant care, day-to-day environmental needs (eating utensils, raised toilet seats, etc.), and modification to the architecture of their living spaces (widened doorways, bathrooms, ramps, etc.).

Much of the assessment involves trying to determine the condition of an individual who has suffered a TBI, on both a qualitative and quantitative basis, for current and future care. To accomplish this, we must do our best to understand the functioning of the injured brain and determine what types of deficits an individual with a TBI has. As we attempt to understand the functioning of the brain in an individual who has suffered a TBI, we must try to understand both the "structure" or anatomy and the "function" of the injured brain, which are extremely interrelated, as structure may impact function, and function may reflect structure.

THROUGH THE OPERATING MICROSCOPE: A NEUROSURGEON'S VIEW

To attempt to appreciate the almost unimaginable complexity and delicacy of the brain, it is helpful to look at the brain through a microscope from the perspective of neurosurgeon. A textbook that I co-authored, *Microsurgical Anatomy of the Brain: A Stereo Atlas* (Kraus & Bailey), contains three-dimensional (3-D) photographs taken through the operating microscope (the textbook comes with 32 View-Master Reels and a 3-D viewer), depicting the surgical approaches to the brain that a neurosurgeon typically utilizes. Shown in **Figure 1.1** is a two-dimensional (2-D) photograph of the undersurface of the right side of the brain (in a cadaver specimen in which the arteries have been injected with a red latex dye and the veins with blue latex) in an approach known as the pterional approach. (314) In **Figure 1.2**, a 2-D photograph shows the back of

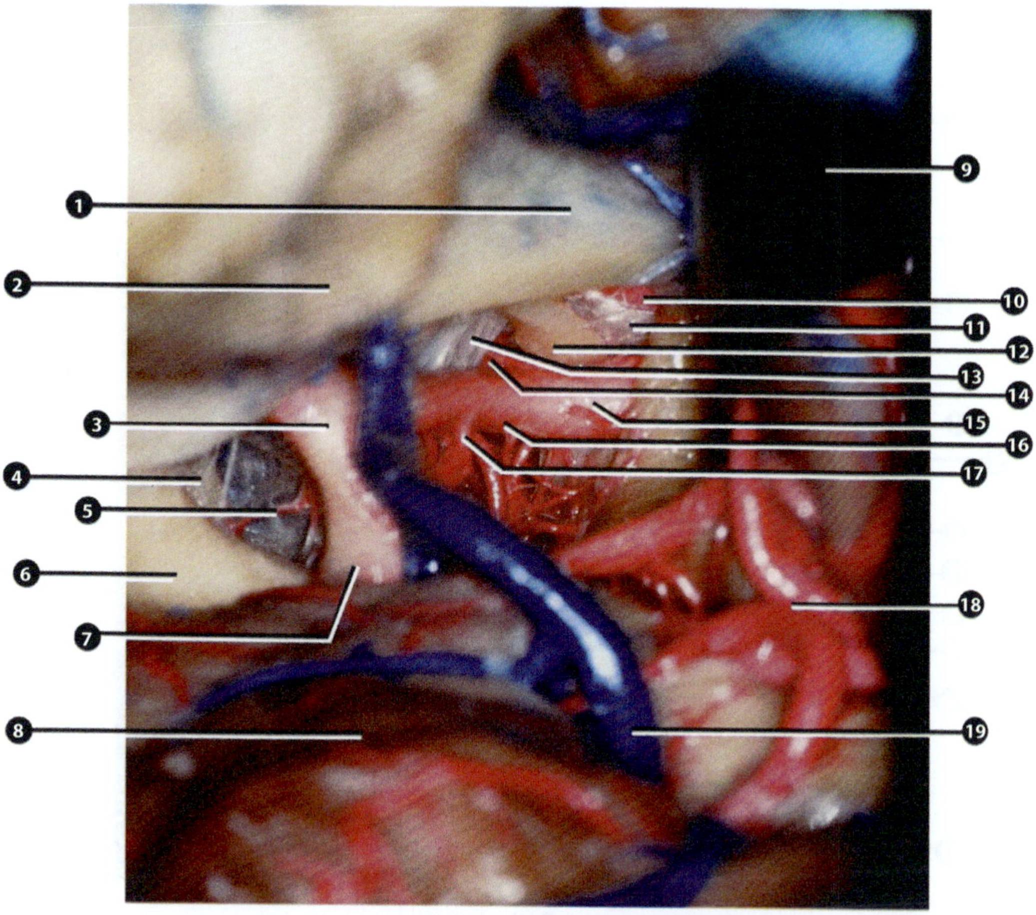

Base of Frontal/Temporal Lobes
Anterior incisural space; right pterional approach

1. Tentorium
2. Lesser wing of sphenoid
3. Right internal carotid artery
4. Pituitary stalk
5. Superior hypophyseal artery
6. Right optic nerve
7. A1 portion of right anterior cerebral artery
8. Right frontal lobe
9. Retractor on temporal lobe
10. Superior cerebellar artery
11. Interpeduncular cistern
12. Third cranial nerve
13. Liliequist's membrane
14. P1 portion of right posterior cerebral artery
15. P2 portion of right posterior cerebral artery
16. Right posterior communicating artery
17. Anterior thalamoperforating arteries
18. M3 branch of middle cerebral artery
19. Superficial sylvian vein

Figure 1.1 Right anterior skull base in a cadaver specimen, showing the region between the right temporal lobe (seen on the right) and the right frontal lobe (seen on the left). (Adapted from Kraus, Bailey, *Microsurgical Anatomy of the Brain: A Stereo Atlas*, (314) with permission Wolters Kluwer.) Arteries and veins have been injected with red and blue latex dye, respectively.

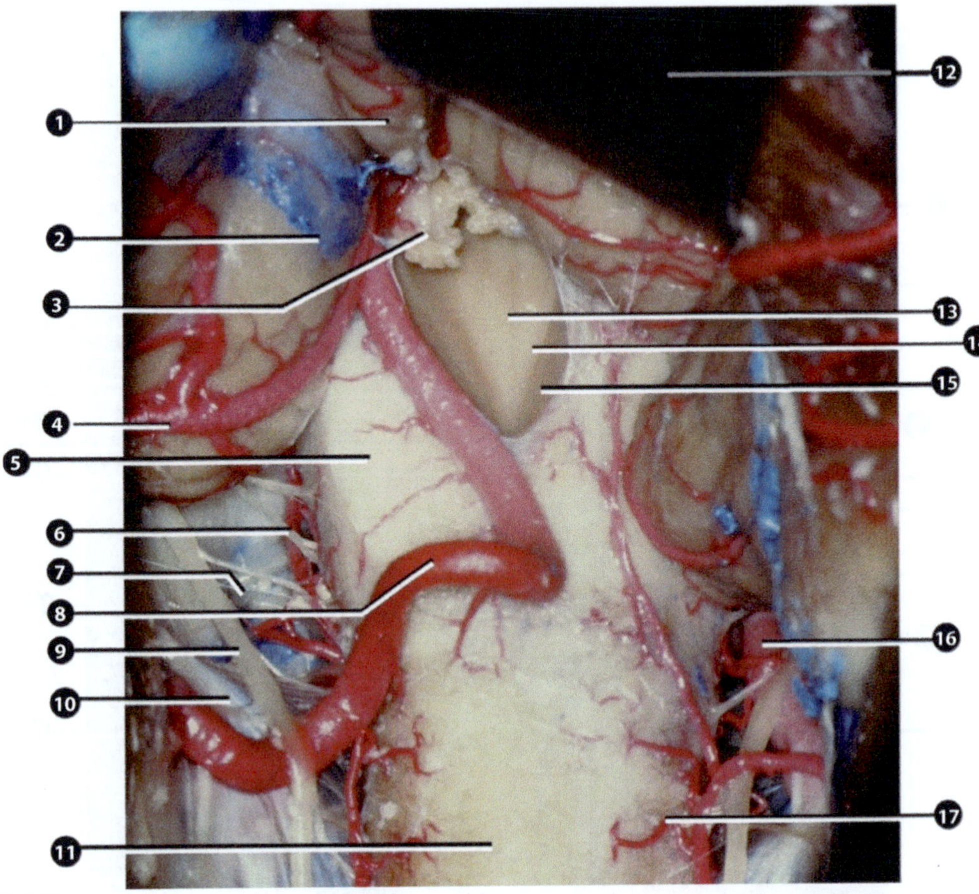

Brainstem
Foramen of Magendie; midline suboccipital approach

1. Uvula
2. Tonsil
3. Choroid plexus of fourth ventricle protruding through foramen of Magendie
4. Tonsillar artery
5. Medulla
6. Medullary rootlet of cranial nerve eleven
7. Cranial nerve twelve entering hypoglossal canal
8. Left posterior inferior cerebellar artery
9. Left cranial nerve eleven (spinal portion)
10. Dentate ligament
11. Spinal cord
12. Retractor under right tonsil
13. Median sulcus
14. Hypoglossal triangle
15. Vagal triangle
16. Right vertebral artery
17. Posterior spinal artery

Figure 1.2 Posterior aspect of cervical spinal cord entering the brainstem (medulla oblongata portion) in a cadaver specimen. (Adapted from Kraus, Bailey, *Microsurgical Anatomy of the Brain: A Stereo Atlas*, (314) with permission Wolters Kluwer.) Inferior skull at foramen magnum and upper cervical lamina have been removed. Arteries and veins have been injected with red and blue latex dye, respectively.

the brain with the cerebellum being lifted, exposing the dorsal aspect of the brainstem (medulla oblongata (medulla) portion) with the cervical spinal cord entering it from below. (314)

Figure 1.1 shows the undersurface of the right-hand side of the brain after dissecting the Sylvian fissure, with the right frontal lobe on the left side of the image and the right temporal lobe on the right side, through what is known as the pterional approach. Among the important structures we see are the right internal carotid artery (supplying blood to a large portion of the right cerebral hemisphere), the right optic nerve (sending visual information from the right eye to the brain), the right cranial nerve III (oculomotor nerve controlling a portion of the movement of the right eye), the pituitary stalk (connecting the pituitary gland with the hypothalamus, which can be injured during a TBI), the posterior cerebral artery (supplying blood to the posterior portion of the cerebral hemispheres and other regions), the region anterior to the brainstem, and the tentorium (a dural membrane separating the upper and lower portions of the brain, medial to which the uncal portion of the temporal lobe can herniate, pressing on the third cranial nerve and causing the ipsilateral pupil to dilate). The delicate and dense interweaving of critical structures at the base of the brain is evident, as are the small perforating arteries that are visualized, supplying blood to the thalamus. While thalamoperforating arteries, such as those seen in **Figure 1.1**, can be 0.41–4.71 mm in diameter, the arteriole diameters progressively decrease as the vasculature bifurcates to eventually reach neurons, the size of which are measured in terms of microns (roughly 1/25,000th of an inch). (1)

Figure 1.2 shows a photograph after a midline suboccipital approach (a portion of the skull over the posterior fossa foramen magnum region is removed) and cervical laminectomy have been performed. The cerebellum has been elevated (retractor under right tonsil) to show the dorsal aspect of the brainstem (region of medulla) as the cervical spinal cord ascends through the foramen magnum to merge with it. Again, extremely small arteries are seen, which enter and supply the upper cervical spinal cord and brainstem. The fine and delicate spinal portion of the left cranial nerve XI (spinal portion of the accessory nerve controlling the sternocleidomastoid and trapezius muscles) and left cranial nerve XII (hypoglossal nerve controlling ipsilateral tongue movement) are visualized. Seen on the dorsal surface of the medulla oblongata, the lowest portion of the brainstem, are the vagal trigone (region of vagal nuclei that control cardiac and other vital functions) and the hypoglossal trigone (region of nucleus of cranial nerve XII). Deep within the brainstem are critical structures, which, among serving many other vital life sustaining functions, keep an individual awake instead of being in a coma. Also, the vital and life-sustaining pathways connecting the brain with the body pass through this narrow but critical region.

HUMAN BRAIN METRICS

The importance of the brain may be well recognized and emphasized by the fact that even though its weight (~1,400 grams, ~3 pounds) represents about 2% of a person's body weight, it still receives roughly 20% of the blood pumped out of the heart, with the other 80% going to the remainder of the body. While there is debate about the actual number, it has been estimated that there are about 86 billion to 100 billion neurons within the human brain, about 100 billion or less glial cells (older studies suggested that there are about 1 trillion glial cells within the human brain), 164 trillion to 200 trillion connections or synapses with each neuron having thousands of synapses, and the brain having an estimated processing speed of roughly 52 quadrillion (52,000 trillion) bits per second. Conduction velocities of axons can range from a couple of feet per second to 650 feet per second. There is good reason to believe that brain function happens mostly in a parallel manner, as individual neurons are likely too slow to allow brain function to operate in a serial manner. There are more than 100,000 neurons and 900 million synaptic connections per cubic millimeter of brain tissue. There are hundreds of different types of neurons (perhaps more than 1,000), with roughly 20 different types of ganglion cells in the retina alone. Gary Marcus stated, "it is doubtful that evolution would sustain such diversity if each type of neuron were essentially doing the same type of thing." There are more than 100 cortical areas in the human brain, interconnected by a tremendous number of connections, with hundreds of types of neurons and immense molecular complexity within individual cells and synapses. Neurons combine individually weak signals from synapses of thousands of other neurons and these connections can be shaped by experience to change their strength through synaptic plasticity in addition to being influenced by the chemicals in which they are bathed, called neuromodulators. The total surface area of the human brain (both hemispheres) is approximately 1,570 cm^2, with about 70% located within the sulci. About 20–25% of the neocortex is involved with vision. White matter comprises about 50% of the human brain volume. The brain has both myelinated and unmyelinated axons, and the total myelinated fiber length in a 20-year-old male brain (if laid out end-to-end) is estimated to be about 109,000 miles. The glial cells (astrocytes and oligodendrocytes) insulate the axons and significantly increase transmission speed of nerve impulses, and, because they contain a fatty substance called myelin, the tissue is known as white matter, which lies deep to the gray matter. White matter also contains microglia. Despite its extreme complexity, the brain is a delicate system; if proper cells aren't connected in the right way, mental/cognitive and other issues will result. (2, 247, 252, 253, 289, 313, 385, 402–406, 479, 526)

BRAIN STRUCTURE AND FUNCTION

Brain structure may be evaluated through advanced imaging studies of the brain, which look at *in vivo* anatomy. Despite the most modern imaging techniques, the level of resolution in a patient is not sufficient to see down to the level of the neuron (as opposed to histologic [*in vitro*] examination under the microscope in the laboratory). As technology improves, significant insight is being gained into the evaluation of structures and their relationships to function. Among these advances, diffusion tensor imaging (DTI), segmental volume analysis of the brain, positron emission tomography (PET), functional magnetic resonance imaging (MRI), magnetoencephalography, and other technologies may provide additional information about both structure and function of the brain.

In addition to clinical evaluation (history, physical examination, etc.) of a patient who has suffered a brain injury, much information about functioning ability will be gleaned by talking with the patient's family, friends, employers, etc., about performance at work, in the family setting, in social settings, and in various other environments. Information about performance in various settings will help provide an understanding as to a patient's ability to function in different settings and under different levels of stress. There may be deficiencies in their functioning that might not be elucidated in an office evaluation and may only be revealed in certain situations that have not been tested.

To gain an understanding of how a person is affected when there is damage to the brain, it is important to understand the functioning of the brain when everything is working properly. Function of the brain can start to be appreciated by recognizing its anatomy and function, its capability of memory across the five body senses (sight, sound, touch, taste, and smell) and more, its processing speed, its higher executive functioning, memory, learning, social cognition, language skills, its intricate pathways interconnecting structure and function of different parts of the brain, the redundancy of the pathways of the brain that attempt to compensate for neurological damage, and much more.

FORCES OF BRAIN INJURY AND CONSEQUENCES OF TBI

During a head injury, the brain may sustain force vectors of translation, rotation, acceleration and deceleration, compression, tension, and shearing, as well as blast induced forces, and coup (trauma to the brain under the location of impact on the skull) and contra coup (trauma to the brain in a location remote to or on the opposite side of the head from the region of impact to the skull) injuries. Many factors play a role in the functional outcome an injured patient may experience, including the severity (force of impact) and location of the injury (which side of the head was struck and with what vector of force), the type of force (blunt or penetrating injury, blast injury, etc.), and the patient's age and pre-injury health. These injuries may result in cortical contusions, intracerebral hematomas, subdural hematomas, and epidural hematomas, as well as diffuse axonal injury (DAI)/traumatic axonal injury (TAI). Nondepressed and depressed skull fractures may occur.

Every TBI is unique. While an acute epidural hematoma may be life-threatening, its prompt removal may result in the patient having an excellent outcome. However, a DAI in the brain may not show hemorrhage on an initial CT scan of the brain, and subsequent MRI of the brain may appear normal, but the lifelong consequences and disability to a patient might be significant. A brain injury can instantly change a person's life and their ability to care for themselves and interact with others. It can also change the lives of all those around the patient, who interact with them on a personal or professional level. The consequences of a brain injury may be temporary or permanent. TBI is one of the largest causes of disability and death. On many occasions, the sequelae a patient may experience after suffering a TBI are significant, with severe and obvious physical and cognitive findings. As an example, a patient may experience varying degrees of paresis or paralysis, difficulty speaking and understanding (Broca's and Wernicke's aphasia), significant cognitive and psychiatric concerns, and many other issues. Awareness of the consequences of a mild TBI may be low, possibly because changes may at times be subtle and may chronically evolve, which may not be apparent to observers or to the patient themselves. In addition, many individuals who have suffered a mild TBI may not seek medical care.

Patients who have suffered moderate and severe traumatic brain injuries will show more obvious clinical findings than those who have suffered a mild TBI, in whom objective findings might not readily be seen. Most likely, many of those patients who are felt to be "normal" may in fact have unrecognized and undiagnosed pathology, both in structure and in function. If a patient sustains a TBI and their relatives state that since the injury, the individual is "just not right" or "there is something different about them, but I just can't put my finger on it," and despite this all objective imaging studies, neuropsychological tests, and other evaluations are normal, it may be more likely that medicine and science have not properly evaluated and diagnosed what is wrong, rather than there actually being nothing wrong.

COMPLICATIONS AND COMORBIDITIES OF TBI

Eventual TBI comorbidities may include neurological disorders, sleep disorders, neurodegenerative diseases, Alzheimer's disease, Parkinson's disease, epilepsy, depression, amyotrophic lateral sclerosis (ALS), dementia, endocrine disorders, spasticity, psychiatric disorders, chronic traumatic encephalopathy (CTE), sexual dysfunction, incontinence, musculoskeletal disorders, metabolic dysfunction and many others, as well as an acceleration of the aging process. For these reasons, TBI may be considered a silent epidemic as well as a chronic disease, which is a risk factor for future neurological and psychiatric illness, epilepsy, neurodegenerative disease, and a cascade of other negative events that may act synergistically with each other. TBI has dramatic consequences and impact on injured patients, as well as their families, caretakers, and society as a whole. (3, 4, 47, 179, 254)

NEUROSURGICAL PROCEDURES: AVOIDING IATROGENIC BRAIN INJURY

The subject of brain injury is close to the heart of every neurosurgeon. Not only does a neurosurgeon treat patients who have a TBI as being the reason for their hospital admission, but in addition, every neurosurgical procedure performed has the potential to cause iatrogenic trauma or injury to the brain. Opening the skull to resect a brain tumor or clip an aneurysm that is located within the deep recesses of the brain necessarily exposes the surrounding brain tissue to potential harm. One of the most important tenets of operating on the brain, which is paramount during every brain operation, is to at all times take every possible measure to protect normal brain, which may inadvertently be subject to trauma due to its proximity to the target pathology or which may be harmed during circumnavigation of that tissue during the neurosurgical approach to a deeper region of the brain. Techniques to minimize injury to the normal brain include the use of the stereo operating microscope, proper handling of brain tissue with appropriate techniques and the use of microsurgical instruments, detailed knowledge of the cisterns (subarachnoid pockets of CSF) that are external to the brain parenchyma and provide passage corridors to deep portions of the brain, intraoperative drainage of CSF to "relax" the brain, opening the fissures of the brain widely to let the lobes and gyri of the brain separate easily (thus providing deeper exposure while minimizing the peril of retraction), and strategically positioning the patient properly to let gravity assist with the gentle and progressive separation of the more superficial regions of the brain to access the deep ones. In addition, medications, anesthetic techniques, and electrical monitoring of brain activity and function are critical.

Despite taking all possible measures to protect the normal brain, it is frequently necessary to cut into and enter normal brain parenchyma to access the target pathology. Although every measure is made to minimize harm to the patient, using the most sophisticated intraoperative navigation techniques and possibly adding functional mapping, normal brain tissue will be impacted. Neurosurgeons have for decades strived to avoid eloquent (such as motor or sensory regions, speech, comprehension, and visual areas) portions of the brain and instead go through or, if necessary, remove relatively silent areas of the brain. To save or vastly improve a patient's life and treat the offending pathology, this entry into the normal brain is often necessary, as the anticipated benefits of this surgery outweigh the risks.

Dr. Robert Spetzler, in a seminal paper published in 1986, introduced a grading system for one of the most difficult neurosurgical lesions encountered in the human brain, cerebral arteriovenous malformations (AVMs). The goal of the grading system was to predict the risk of morbidity and mortality associated with neurosurgical operative treatment of an AVM. With this grading system, an AVM could be assigned a grade from I to V based on the size of the AVM, its pattern of venous drainage, and the eloquence of adjacent brain tissue. Grade VI lesions were considered essentially inoperable. Dr. Spetzler stated "surgical removal of an AVM is indicated if the risk of operation is less than the risk determined by the natural history of the AVM." (350) This grading system was updated by Dr. Spetzler in 2011 based on additional clinical data. (351) This grading system, as well as the countless extremely innovative and very insightful surgical techniques and approaches that Dr. Spetzler has taught the world of neurosurgery, has tremendously improved the safety and outcomes of neurosurgical procedures on the most complex intracranial and spinal pathologies and have been used to address all areas of intracranial surgery including neurovascular surgery and skull base surgery. (353, 357, 388)

CEREBRAL ARCHITECTURE, NEURAL NETWORKS, AND ASSEMBLIES

Theories about brain functioning are evolving. Traditionally, it had been felt that a particular function of the brain resides within a focal region of the brain, and that this neural hub provides executive function or cognitive control, with perception, cognition, and action being discrete functions of the human brain. A growing body of data suggest that instead of having a single neural apex to act as an executive, the brain is organized into modules, themselves functioning in parallel rather than in a simple progression. This represents an organizational and functional structure of the brain that is an interaction of neuronal assemblies without the need for a central controller. This is consistent with the understanding that many functions of the brain defy the simple classification as perception, cognition, or action. (348) As neurons are connected into circuits, this circuit activity drives perception, thought, and action. Complexity theory and network science show that the global outcomes cannot be reduced to simple causes, but rather the functioning of the network exceeds the functioning of its individual elements. In fact, the concept of "emergence" is introduced, and is the realization that the collective interactions of complex networked systems allow for new properties that do not exist at lower levels of organization. (396) Relating to consciousness, Christof Koch, a neurophysiologist and computational neuroscientist who performed research at the California Institute of Technology for over 25 years, stated "phenomenal consciousness is a property of an integrated system of causally interacting parts. Yet consciousness also has surprisingly local aspects. . . .small chunks of the cerebral cortex are responsible for specific conscious actions." (529)

The growing volume of big data in neuroscience emphasizes the need for theoretical ideas that can unify the understanding of brain structure and function. Network neuroscience may provide a common conceptual framework and toolset with which to do so, connecting theoretical approaches such as dynamical systems, neural coding, and statistical physics. (344) The concept of a networking approach of cerebral function has been described as a result of additional knowledge and insight of the brain connectome gained by combining multimodal data from anatomic dissections, lesion studies, neuroimaging, electrophysiological mapping methods, and computational modeling. This networking theory may provide for interindividual anatomo-functional variations and neuroplastic phenomena, which go beyond apparent limitations of the white matter connectivity, possibly explaining how the brain can adapt to the environment, with potential implications for TBI. (345) Concepts of small world networks, local connectivity, long-distance connectivity, hierarchical modularity, interconnected hubs, rich clubs, connectivity backbones, and centrality have been used in analyzing neurological disorders. (325, 346) It is quite possible that the brain may be organized and respond through distributed networks rather than localized regions. Disconnections in these networks may have significant impacts, and a variety of disconnection phenomena and disconnection syndromes may arise. When brain connectivity in patients with schizophrenia is compared with healthy controls, an association is found between clinical symptoms and impaired functional coupling between the parietal and frontal regions of the brain, possibly due to connection problems in long-distance interregional projections. In a similar manner, beyond diagnosis of conditions of the brain, it may be possible that new treatments and rehabilitative therapies may be aimed at attempting to restore a disrupted network into a functional state. (396)

The cerebral cortex may function partly in a hierarchical array of feature detectors, progressing initially from bottom-up sensory information to higher-level abstract concepts. Low-level detectors may perceive edges and other simple shapes, with this information sent to nodes of the brain that detect complex stimuli such as faces, objects, and letters. The fundamental question remains as to how the brain encodes and stores memories, images, words, etc. (not like a JPEG image is stored in a computer). (402)

THE BRAIN IS THE PERSON: THE PERSON IS THE BRAIN

We have rooms in ourselves. Most of them we have not visited yet. Forgotten rooms. From time to time we can find the passage. We find strange things … old phonographs, pictures, books … they belong to us, but it is the first time we have found them.

—Haruki Murakami

In two medical novels I co-authored, *Body Trade* and *Unexpected*, the concepts and ramifications of brain injury and brain transplantation are explored and emphasized, stressing the point that the brain is the person (socially, emotionally, intellectually, occupationally, etc.), with the remainder of the body providing the vital and necessary functions to support the brain. (250, 251) To put into context the impact on a person's function after suffering an injury to the brain, let us consider the impact of the injury on other body parts and organs, and for a moment, give thought as to what actually constitutes a person. If an individual suffers an injury to their hand, they are the same person, but they have an injured hand. If they fracture a leg, they are the same person with a fractured leg. However, if they injure the brain, they may be, in essence, a mildly or dramatically different person, because the thoughts, language, memory, perception, awareness, concentration, ambition, attention, emotions, skills, dreams, intelligence, aptitude, hopes, and interpersonal interactions, which for the most part reside within the brain, are the actual person. When these functions are altered through injury, the brain is no longer the same and, therefore, the person is no longer the same. In addition, since the brain controls functioning of the remainder of the body, the remainder of somatic functions may also be impaired and changed.

CONSCIOUSNESS, ARISTOTLE, FLATLANDS, BRANES, AND QUANTUM MECHANICS

The only way of discovering the limits of the possible is to venture a little way past them into the impossible.

—Arthur C. Clarke

The mind-brain dualism relationship has fascinated mankind for two-and-a-half millennia, since the time of ancient Greece. (429) Bridging neuroscience with a quantitative description of inner subjective feelings through the incorporation of advancements in physics, chemistry, and biology may help with this human scientific inquiry. (430) Although the brain remembers images and sounds, there are no photographs or recordings within the brain and no memory storage unit that is similar to a computer made by man. Instead, there are neurons, cell walls, axons, chemicals, neurotransmitters, oligodendrocytes, astrocytes, blood vessels, and CSF. To understand this is to understand a network of unfathomable complexity. (529)

Eric Kandel, who won the Nobel Prize in Physiology or Medicine in 2000 for his research on the basis of memory in neurons, reflected upon the understanding of consciousness in his autobiography, *In Search of Memory*. Kandel stated that "understanding consciousness is by far the most challenging task confronting science." Reflecting on the work of Francis Crick, whom he considered possibly the most influential biologist of the second-half of the 20th century, he mentioned that when Crick first entered biology, he felt that "two great questions were thought to be beyond the capacities of science to answer: What distinguishes the living from the nonliving world? And what is the biological nature of consciousness? Crick turned first to the easier problem, distinguishing animate from inanimate matter, and explored the nature of the gene." Crick teamed with James Watson to crack the genetic code, discovering how DNA makes RNA and RNA makes protein. (520)

Koch notes "consciousness is everything you experience. It is the tune stuck in your head, the sweetness of the chocolate mousse, the throbbing pain of a toothache, the fierce love for your child." (389)

When reflecting upon the concept of consciousness and higher brain functions, a logical question utilizing Occam's razor is to ask where cognitive function in the brain begins. Before analyzing consciousness, let's start with a task seemingly less intricate: the flexion of a biceps muscle. For this relay to occur, a Betz cell (neuron in the gray matter of the primary motor cortex) or other motor neuron must fire an action potential through the corticospinal tract, synapse onto an anterior horn cell in the spinal cord, which then activates a muscle fiber through the neuromuscular junction/ motor end plate. (384, 386) Conceptually and anatomically, this sounds straightforward. The question naturally arises as to where free will at the conscious level originates to initiate this action. It appears that the free will of consciousness did not originate in the motor neuron itself, but required an antecedent action to occur, causing it to fire an action potential. While there may be several thousand synapses from other neurons sending signals to the motor neuron and causing it to subsequently fire, the same question may then be asked as to what caused each of those other neurons to fire. (385) At some level, this higher plane of understanding supersedes the more comprehensible subjects of anatomy, physiology, biochemistry, and physics, and invokes philosophy, spirituality, religion, and other levels of understanding. Aristotle had described the entelechy of vitalism. There may be a point at which the chemistry and physics of the body end, and a higher driving force, the entelechy, begins. (387) As most of this is beyond the scope of this text, I will restrict thoughts to just a few concepts. The analysis of the motor cell firing to move a muscle fiber is anatomically difficult to visualize but easy to conceive of. Asking whether this cell firing is the result of the net summation of thousands of other predictable neurons firing and synapsing upon it leads to the next logical question as to where this theoretically predictable and analyzable sequence of events begins. In other words, the neuron fired as a result of thousands of inputs afferent onto it, but similarly, what caused those neurons to fire. This Gordian knot analysis causes a great conundrum as to where does free will and consciousness start. Seemingly, for that volitional act of flexing a bicep muscle to originate, a motor neuron (or a neuron afferent upon it) would have to fire without another action causing it to fire. This would defy the laws of classical physics and would be equivalent to a billiard ball moving without another ball hitting it. Nevertheless, we are naturally accustomed to thinking that we have this free will of consciousness to move the biceps muscle.

If we don't allow ourselves to be restricted to an analysis based upon classical physics, but instead invoke quantum mechanics, doors are opened up to the concept of the wave-particle duality theory. (383) Heisenberg's uncertainty principle changed the fundamental thought process of Newtonian physics, which was initially introduced by Sir Isaac Newton in his 1687 work entitled *Philosophiae Naturalis Principia Mathematica*. (390) Heisenberg in 1927 stated that it is not possible to simultaneously know the position and momentum of an object. Perhaps this uncertainty may have a role in consciousness and free will, removing the theoretically predictable effects of synaptic summation on neuronal function. Can a person's mind affect the activities of their brain within quantum theory? Henry Stapp noted that Wolfgang Pauli (Nobel Prize in Physics, 1945), Eugene Wigner (Nobel Prize in Physics, 1963), and John von Neumann recognized that quantum theory was about the mind-brain connection. (427) Barry Ward stated "an understanding of consciousness will most likely require a similar paradigm shift found in the disciplines of philosophy, physics and neuroscience when confronted by Newton's gravity, Einstein's relativity and De-Broglie's 'matter-wave' hypothesis." (428)

Koch has studied the neural basis of consciousness. He describes an experiment carried out by Benjamin Libet (neuropsychologist at the University of California at San Francisco) on volunteers in the 1980s in which he wanted to determine the exact moment at which a mental act occurred, related to the urge to raise a hand, before the actual raising of the hand occurred. The experiment involved a green oscilloscope and EEG electrodes on the head. The conclusion was that the beginning of a readiness potential precedes the conscious decision to move by at least half a second. Koch states,

> "the brain acts before the mind decides. ... somewhere in the catacombs of the brain, possibly in the basal ganglia, a few calcium ions cluster close to the presynaptic membrane, a single synaptic vesicle is released, a threshold is crossed, and an action potential is born. This lone pulse cascades into a torrent of spikes that invades the premotor cortex, which is primed, ready to swing into action. After receiving this go-ahead signal, the premotor cortex notifies the motor cortex, whose pyramidal cells send their detailed instructions down to the spinal cord and muscles."

After this occurs precognitively, a cortical structure produces the conscious notion that it just decided to move. The actual decision to move occurred before awareness. (529)

It may be that high resolution maps of the brain are not sufficient, and new technologies in neuroscience should work in harmony with psychoneural concepts to understand how the mind is implemented in the brain. In a specific type of brain injury that involves a lesion in the parietal lobe, patients may experience a visuo-spatial syndrome of extinction. Shown an object on one or the other side of the body, a patient can identify it, but if shown both objects simultaneously, the patient claims not to see one of the objects despite possibly having activation in the relevant face area of the brain. The patient has had an experience of seeing an object, without knowing about it. It appears that the patient has a problem with activation of the neural basis of cognitive access in the frontal and parietal lobes, suggesting that the actual seeing of an object requires the neural basis of cognitive access to seeing an object, as well as the neural basis of the conscious experience of seeing the object. (401)

Steven Pinker states "our minds evolved by natural selection to solve problems that were life-and-death matters to our ancestors, not to commune with correctness or to answer any question we are capable of asking. We cannot hold ten thousand words in short term memory. We cannot see in ultraviolet light. We cannot mentally rotate an object in the fourth dimension. And perhaps we cannot solve conundrums like free will and sentience." (522) Before leaving this construct of a higher understanding of consciousness and free will, above the neuroanatomical constructs, I would like to consider another possibility as an explanation. Just as Newtonian mechanics prevailed for centuries until quantum mechanics was conceptualized, it is quite likely that the truth we seek for ultimate understanding is much deeper than that. In 1884, Edwin Abbott published *Flatland*, a satirical novella in which a 2-D world existed with people represented as geometric shapes. When a sphere from a 3-D world visits the 2-D world, only a circle is seen, and they are not able to see the third dimension. A sphere passing through the 2-D world would be seen as a circle, which first enlarges, and then shrinks. If a Flatlander were asked to look up, to see the third dimension, they would not be able to, as it would not be accessible to them. (391)

Lisa Randall, a theoretical physicist specializing in particle physics and cosmology and involved with testing at the Large Hadron Collider, has described branes (membrane-like objects) as important components of rich higher-dimensional landscapes, and described brane worlds as hypothesized universes in which we live on a brane. Perhaps the answers we are searching for are in other branes. String theory also considers extra dimensions of existence. (399)

Even though we believe that we understand the three dimensions of space, and one of time, in which we live, it is almost impossible for us to understand even these. It is difficult to think of time as always having been there, going backward infinitely, with no beginning. Similarly, it is difficult for us to imagine space as being infinite, with no ending. Perhaps the answers to these questions and some of the questions of the nervous system are available only in other dimensions of thinking, whether they be conceptualized by branes, string theory, or other.

SYMPTOM PROGRESSION, COMORBIDITIES, FAMILY IMPACT, AND AWARENESS OF TBI

Inability to recognize or measure functional changes does not equate to the conclusion that those changes have not occurred. Some damage may also be progressive and worsen with time (as with CTE), before it becomes "noticeable." While an individual's damage may not be outwardly observable at times, based upon their current behavior or objective testing, there may come a time at which it will be. Reasons for this delay may include the following: (1) the decline may be progressive, either from natural progression or from further insults to the brain, causing it to exceed the "tipping point" at which symptoms are apparent; (2) the environmental factors and stresses that may not have elicited symptoms initially may have changed, placing new stresses or requirements upon an individual that were not previously existent, again crossing the threshold of a "tipping point" for symptoms to appear; and (3) our behavioral and cognitive testing abilities (including neuropsychological, neurological, psychiatric, vocational, and social assessments) and technological testing (imaging modalities of the brain, serum, and CSF biomarkers, etc.) will likely continue to improve in the future. It is important to recognize that just because we have not recognized or measured a deficit, does not mean that the deficit does not exist, but rather that our measurement and assessment tools may not have been thorough enough, advanced enough, or detailed enough, or that not enough time has elapsed for the possible progression of symptoms to become apparent.

The study of the brain is ever-evolving and advancing. As we learn more, new tools result in new discoveries that will be retrospectively applied to past clinical data and findings. As this occurs, previous classification methods and scales may become obsolete because they fail to consider new understandings of the intricate workings of the brain. While this may make comparison to historical studies and data difficult, it is inevitable as the field advances. As we answer new questions about the brain, many more questions are created. One would expect nothing less when trying to study the world's most sophisticated and complicated "machine," the human brain.

SUBTLE BUT IMPORTANT CONSEQUENCES OF TBI

TBI is a major cause of morbidity and mortality in the United States. Many individuals suffering a TBI may not seek medical attention, and many may have suffered cognitive and functional impairments without recognizing it. The moderate and severe cases of TBI are easily detected, as these patients usually arrive at an emergency department of a hospital in a severe condition. Many of these patients may suffer lifelong disabilities, requiring various levels of assistive care. Some may never achieve independent living. Some may not be able to walk, comprehend written or verbal language, eat, or talk, and some may require breathing and nutritional support. The devastation to a patient who was previously functioning well, and who is consciously awake enough to recognize that the life they knew has been taken from them, will be devastating, and have with it its own associated psychological, neurological, and psychiatric sequelae.

The cases of mild TBI, which represent 75–90% (depending on the study) of all cases of TBI, may be difficult to understand and detect. Imaging studies of the brain are frequently normal, although advances in imaging are now often able to detect abnormalities. Neuropsychological evaluation may detect abnormalities. While imaging and testing may appear to be quite normal, the real test for these patients is determined by how their subsequent functioning in life is affected, and how well they integrate into the family, work, and social roles in which they were previously engaged. Are they independent in daily living or has that been affected, even in a subtle way? What has happened to their job? Are they able to perform the same skills they used to perform? If they are an accountant, can they process information as proficiently, accurately, and rapidly as they used to? Can they still work with four spreadsheets on a computer simultaneously? If they are a carpenter, is their spatial perception altered, resulting in difficulty visualizing where shelves, cabinets, and doorways will be built? Is their depth perception or ability to see in stereo altered, affecting a pilot's ability to land a plane? Is their hearing or voice altered, affecting a musician's ability to play an instrument or sing, or recognize music properly? Is their comprehension of verbal or written language impaired, affecting their ability to learn new tasks? If they are a student, is their ability to learn affected? In patients who have suffered injury to the frontal lobes of the brain, has their drive, ambition, and mood been altered? Are social relationships with family and friends changed? Are they angry, depressed, or anxious? Do they have difficulty sleeping or experience nightmares? Were there any preexisting cognitive or psychological impairments that might have been aggravated or worsened by the TBI? Are there new physical and emotional stressors in life, which have occurred as a result of the TBI, such as relationship, financial, job, and other, that might interact with each other to worsen any underlying or newly caused TBI-related functioning neuropsychological pathology?

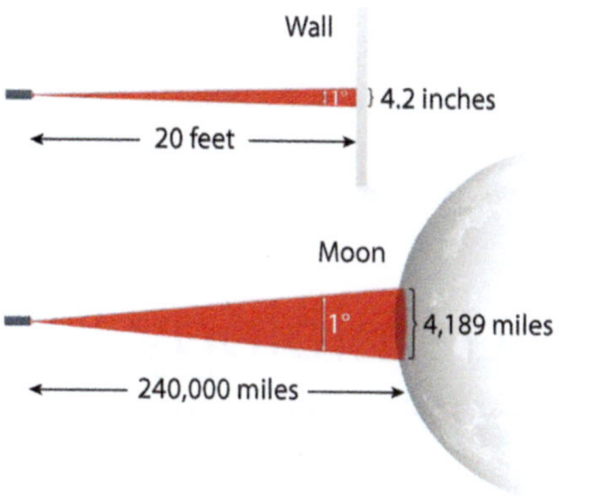

Figure 1.3 Distance is a great amplifier of small changes. A one-degree angulation of a laser beam will move the dot on the wall (which is 20 feet away) only 4.2 inches, while the same one degree angulation will move the location of the dot on the moon (240,000 miles away) by 4,189 miles. In a similar manner, time is also a great amplifier.

TIME AND DISTANCE: THE GREAT AMPLIFIERS

Even small and subtle changes that might affect an individual's cognitive, psychological, and neurological function, are amplified over time. As an example, consider a laser beam that is shown at a wall 20 feet away, and mark the spot on the wall. Next, if the laser is angled one degree, the laser will light a spot on the wall that is 4.2 inches from the original spot. Now, let us shine the laser beam at the moon, which is 240,000 miles away, and mark the spot on the surface of the moon. Again, move the laser one degree, and now the new location where the laser hits the moon's surface will be 4,189 miles away from the initial spot. This tremendous amplification of distance from the original to the new spot, is a result of the 240,000-mile distance to the moon, versus the 20-foot distance to the wall (**Figure 1.3**).

In a similar manner, any subtle changes that a patient who has suffered a TBI experiences will be amplified over time. Small errors in judgment or decision-making, changes in intellect, recognition, perception, and other aspects of functioning may not be immediately noticeable, but over time, there may be profound effects. Future family, social and business opportunities may be missed or no longer available to an individual who has suffered a TBI. Projected years out, even "small" and "subtle" changes to the essence of a person may tremendously impact their future, altering family, relationships, job performance, and many other factors. This is well recognized with repetitive head trauma and CTE. Just as distance is a great amplifier in which small initial changes may have significant eventual consequences, the same is true for time, resulting in greatly magnified future consequences arising from seemingly small changes in the present. Importantly, seemingly small perturbations to brain function at present may have significant ramifications to an individual and those around them in the future.

2

Epidemiology

Before discussing classifications of TBI, we should understand that clinical outcome is not necessarily represented by the nomenclature of traumatic brain injury (TBI). When the term "mild" is used to describe traumatic brain injury, it should not be assumed that the effects on the brain are mild. There may be patients that suffered from large epidural hematomas who leave the hospital soon after an emergency surgery and resume a relatively unaffected life. On the other hand, there may be a patient who has suffered a "mild" TBI, with a negative CT scan of the brain, who may suffer from lifelong sequelae of the brain injury. When it comes to brain injury, the term "mild" is misleading, as the impact which this injury has on the patient and those around them may be severe. The term "brain damage" rather than "traumatic brain injury" or "head injury" may be more appropriate because when axons are sheared and torn, the brain is damaged. With that said, we can move on to the standard nomenclature used throughout the world to describe TBI.

In a paper discussing the symptomatology and functional outcome in mild TBI, McMahon eloquently stated, "what is becoming clear though, is that 'mild' is indeed a misnomer for this disease, because many patients experience significant and persistent symptoms. For these patients, mTBI (mild TBI) is anything but mild." (324)

TBI is a global problem that transcends all geographic, social, and economic barriers, and is one of the most common, disabling, and costly medical problems facing the world. The Centers for Disease Control and Prevention defines TBI as "a disruption in the normal function of the brain that can be caused by a bump, blow, or jolt to the head or a penetrating head injury." (6)

TBI is generally broken down into categories of mild, moderate, and severe. The classification criteria for mild TBI, moderate TBI, severe TBI, and penetrating TBI are given in the chapter on TBI classification, scales, and definitions. The phrases "mild TBI" and "concussion" are implied to have the same meaning, although it may be considered that a concussion is a type of mild TBI, and that a subconcussive injury is one in which there are no acute appreciable clinical symptoms. The major causes of TBI are falls, motor vehicle collisions, and gunshot wounds. Other causes include explosive blasts, sports injuries, and interpersonal violence. Incidence and prevalence of TBI may vary between different studies, due to differences in population samples, geography (country and region within the country), age groups, and methods in which hospitals assess and classify brain injury. In addition, some patients with mild symptoms may not seek medical attention or may under-report them, and those who do seek medical attention may have their symptoms of TBI left unrecognized and undiagnosed by the medical providers examining them. There are estimated to be approximately 42–74 million annual cases of mild TBI worldwide; mild TBI occurs with a 10-fold higher frequency than moderate and severe injury and may represent 70–80% of TBI cases, depending upon the study. (5, 8, 140, 255) According to the World Health Organization, the mortality rate of mild TBI is below 1%, while it is 20–50% for severe TBI, and 2–5% for moderate TBI. (581)

DOI: 10.1201/9781003354154-2

CIVILIAN TBI

In the United States, it is estimated that on a yearly basis, TBI is responsible for 1.1–2.9 million emergency department treatments of which roughly 224,000–285,000 people are hospitalized and 50,000–61,000 die. In one review, of the roughly 230,000 who are hospitalized and survive, approximately 80,000–90,000 people suffer long-term disability. (257) Children less than 18 accounted for about 8% of all TBI hospitalizations in 2017, and about 4.5% of all TBI-related deaths. Motor vehicle collisions were responsible for about 25% of all TBI hospitalizations, while unintentional falls were the cause of about 49% of admissions. The incidence ratio of hospitalizations to deaths per 100,000 people in the general population, were about 67:20 (hospitalizations:deaths) for adults aged 55–64, 103:24 (hospitalizations:deaths) for those aged 65–74, and 321:77 (hospitalizations:deaths) for those over 75 years of age. According to the CDC Surveillance Report, in 2017, males had a significantly higher age adjusted rate than females with respect to TBI resulting from unintentional and intentional mechanisms including the following: "unintentional falls (35.6 versus 23.9); motor vehicle crashes (22.5 versus 10.8; two-fold higher); unintentionally being struck by or against an object (2.3 versus 0.9; more than two-fold higher); intentional self-harm (0.8 versus 0.3; more than two-fold higher); and assault (7.5 versus 1.7; more than four-fold." Similarly, males had a significantly higher age adjusted rate of mechanisms of injury in these categories which contributed to a TBI-related death. (12, 256, 257)

Almost one-third of all injury-related deaths in the United States have been related to TBI. Due to stability and strength issues, younger and older individuals account for a disproportionately higher amount of fall-related TBI. (15) In individuals 75 years of age and older, the rate of hospitalization and death increases, with falls causing 51% of cases of TBI, and motor vehicle crashes causing 9%. It is possible that increased use of aspirin and anticoagulants in older adults may place them at risk for greater incidence of TBI consequences. (16)

In the entire world population, there are an estimated 73 cases per 100,000 people who suffer a severe TBI annually, or approximately 5.5 million people in total. TBI is the main cause of death in one-third to one-half of all deaths related to trauma. (258)

The majority of TBI falls into the mild TBI category. In a review of 20 years of European studies, 235 out of every 100,000 people were hospitalized or died annually from TBI, with a mortality of 15 per 100,000 population. For every severe case of TBI, there were 1.5 moderate cases, and 22.1 mild cases. The authors point out difficulties in longitudinal studies due to diverse outcome measurements, loss to follow-up, and other factors that affect the quality and consistency of findings. In a study of mild brain injuries in San Diego in 1981, 80% of patients hospitalized for an acute brain injury had suffered a mild uncomplicated (no finding on computed tomography [CT] scan of the brain) TBI. (14, 130)

In Germany, where there was an incidence of 332 cases of TBI per 100,000 people per year, it was seen that of 6,783 patients admitted to an emergency department due to TBI, and of 56% who received a GCS/neurological exam, 90% were considered mild, 4% as moderate, and 5% as severe. Of those that were severe, 76% required intubation and 1% died. Even though 90% of patients had a mild TBI, 45% of all patients were still in medical treatment one year after the accident and of those patients who had complaints one year post-injury, 50% had initially been classified as having a mild TBI. In a follow-up survey of subjective complaints one year after injury, 78.7% reported doing as well as pre-injury at their job or school, but 50% of all patients stated they still required treatment. Fifty-two percent of the TBIs were caused by falls and 26% by road accidents. The time lapse between the injury and the initial hospital examination was less than one hour in 63% of all cases. In cases of severe TBI, the time between admission to the hospital and the first CT scan of the brain was less than one hour in 70% of cases. (23)

On a worldwide scale, pediatric TBI has been seen in 47–280 cases per 100,000 children annually, depending upon the country, with the majority of injuries resulting from motor vehicle collisions and falls. Of those, greater than 80% suffer a mild TBI and negative imaging is seen in as high as 90% of the injured. Most children will have a good clinical outcome and neurosurgical intervention is rarely needed. (13)

SPORTS-RELATED TBI

In a study of 3.42 million emergency department visits for a sports- and recreation-related TBI in the United States from 2001 to 2012, about 70%

were for patients aged 0–19 years. These occurred most in males as a result of injuries during bicycling, football, and basketball, whereas for females, the most common activities were bicycling, playground activities, and horseback riding. About 90% of patients were treated and released from the emergency department. Hospitalizations were often associated with bicycle use. (261)

In an assessment of 1,532 high school varsity football players, only 47.3% of those who had suffered a concussion had reported it, mostly for the following reasons: lack of recognition of the seriousness of an injury; concern about being removed from play; and lack of education as to concussion symptoms. (263)

MILITARY-RELATED TBI (INCLUDING BLAST TBI)

The prevailing causes of TBI are different in a military population, when compared to a civilian population. Blast injuries have different mechanisms by which they impact the body and the blast overpressure wave may have a profound effect upon the internal organs of the body. (33)

A review by Meaney found, in comparing the civilian and military population, that TBI in civilians has been found to be the result of falls in 35% of cases, motor vehicle injuries in 17%, being struck by or against an object in 17%, assaults in 10%, and unknown in 21%. In the military population, causes of TBI were explosions in 63% of cases, blunt trauma in 19%, penetrating injury in 11%, and 7% for other causes. In the military population compared to the civilian population, a higher portion of TBIs were moderate or severe and a lower portion were mild. (9) Ten to twenty percent of the soldiers returning from the wars in Iraq and Afghanistan have suffered a TBI, with blast-related injury being the most common cause. (34) The United States Department of Defense reports 468,424 cases of TBI from the year 2000 to the third quarter of 2022. These may have resulted from military training or deployment as well as day-to-day recreational activities and sports. Of these, mild TBI represented roughly 82%, moderate TBI represented roughly 11%, severe TBI represented 1%, and penetrating brain injuries represented 1.2%. Most military personnel who suffered a mild TBI return to full duty within 10–14 days through a progressive approach. (33, 36, 44)

3

Can significant brain damage go unrecognized?

When you divide the brain surgically by midline section of the cerebral commissures the mind is also correspondingly divided. Each of the disconnected hemispheres continues to function at a high level, but most conscious experience generated within one hemisphere becomes inaccessible to the conscious awareness of the other.

—Roger Sperry

Try it. And don't read the literature until after you have made your observations. Otherwise you can be blinded by pre-existing dogma.

—Roger Sperry as remembered by Michael Gazzaniga

In an individual who has suffered a traumatic brain injury, is it possible there is unrecognized significant brain damage despite the best clinical and imaging evaluations? If significant brain injury can go unrecognized by a traditional neurological or neuropsychological evaluation, then it is logical to conclude that a mild brain injury may be more easily unrecognized. As discussed in Chapter 1, brain injury may occur as a result of external trauma, or as the result of surgery of the brain. In this chapter, we will address the intentionally induced trauma to the brain which is caused by splitting of the corpus callosum, a separation of the two hemispheres of the brain, with the intention of helping patients suffering from intractable seizures. The question which arises is whether significant brain damage can go unrecognized.

To address this question, let us first consider Roger Sperry's seminal work *Consciousness, Personal Identity, and the Divided Brain.* (356) Sperry was awarded the 1981 Nobel Prize in Physiology or Medicine for his discoveries on split brains. (543) Sperry studied the effects of the neurosurgical splitting of the corpus callosum in patients, essentially an intentionally and iatrogenically induced brain trauma designed to help patients with intractable seizures. This is still a severe trauma to the brain, resulting in significant intended damage with the hope of significant benefit as well. This procedure may be done for patients who suffer intractable seizures which are not responsive to antiseizure mecidations, and who may experience drop attacks when their seizure crosses from one cerebral hemisphere to the other through the corpus callosum.

Division of the corpus callosum (a major white matter tract connecting the two cerebral hemispheres), known as a corpus callosotomy, has been performed in patients suffering from uncontrolled seizures despite use of antiseizure medications to lessen their seizures. Division of the corpus callosum prevents the seizure spreading from one

DOI: 10.1201/9781003354154-3

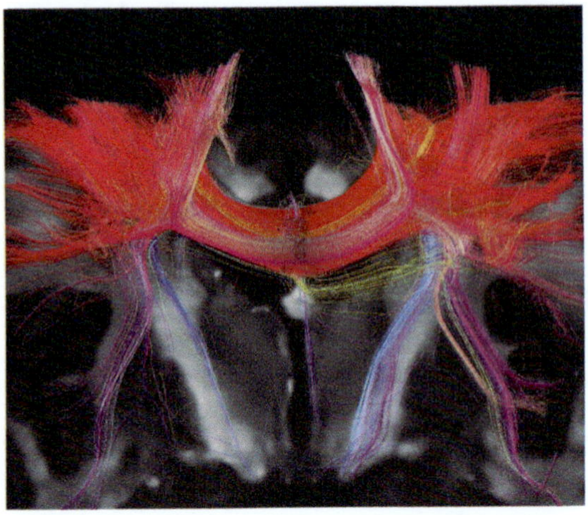

Figure 3.1 Coronal view of corpus callosum with tractography showing nerve pathways (red) that connect the two cerebral hemispheres. (From Sherbrooke Connectivity Imaging Lab / Science Source.)

hemisphere to the other. The procedure involves severing all or a portion of the corpus callosum (the largest white matter fiber system in the brain, containing more than 200 million nerve fibers). **Figure 3.1** shows the corpus callosum with tractography, which connects the two cerebral hemispheres. In doing so, the following are affected: 1) fibers which interconnect the left and right halves of the cortical field for vision (restricting visual perception in each hemisphere to half the normal field of view), 2) fibers which interconnect primary sensory projections and skilled motor control for the right and left hands and feet, and 3) connections to the right hemisphere from the speech and language centers in the left hemisphere (in 95% of the population).

After undergoing such a major operation, Sperry noted "these patients following surgery appear in ordinary, everyday behavior to be very typical, single-minded, normally unified individuals." Sperry noted that his studies were prompted by reviewing a "series of published reports supporting the conclusion that no definite symptoms are detected after surgery, even with extensive neurological and psychological testing." Sperry points out that although a year is required to recover from this extensive brain trauma, two years after the surgery, a typical patient "could easily go through a complete routine medical examination without revealing to an uninformed practitioner that anything is abnormal." In addition, Sperry stated "nor is there any marked change in the verbal scores on the standard IQ test." Importantly, Sperry noted "despite the outward seeming normality, however, and the apparent unity and coherence of the behavior and personality of these individuals, controlled lateralized testing for the function of each hemisphere independently indicates that in reality these people live with two largely separate left and right domains of inner conscious awareness." As result of this, "each hemisphere can be shown to experience its own private sensations, percepts, thoughts, and memories, which are inaccessible to awareness in the other hemisphere." Each surgically disconnected hemisphere essentially has a mind of its own, "cut off from, and oblivious of, conscious events in the partner hemisphere."

To provide an example of a subtle but important deficit following this surgery, patients may be unable to recognize by sight an object they have looked at in one visual half-field if it is subsequently shown in the opposite half-field of view. Objects identified solely by touch with one hand will not be recognized by the other hand. Certain tasks, which an individual claims verbally that they have no knowledge of, are able to be performed manually by pointing, hand signals, and gestures. It appears that although both hemispheres retain mental function at a high level, they are not aware of the mental functions of their partner hemisphere. (356)

It is likely that the processes within the brain, whether connected within one hemisphere or between the two hemispheres, can be viewed as an integrated unit that is different from and greater than the sum of the activities within each hemisphere or the combined hemispheres, thus, leading to the two hemispheres perceiving, thinking, emoting, and learning as a unit. Even while the left dominant hemisphere is involved in processing speech, the right hemisphere is not idling quietly, but rather aiding in the speech by adding tone and expression, inhibiting unrelated activity, and otherwise focusing to help with cerebral processing. (356)

As a result of research on split brains, important questions arise as to the existence of one or two conscious agents in a split brain. (358) As noted by Gazzaniga in 2014, "knowledge about the kinds of mental processes that could be integrated across the great divide created by the surgery, such as emotional and attentional processes, added to the foundations of how to think about the underlying biology of conscious experience ... overall, the dozens upon dozens of studies revealed the parallel and distributed organization of the human brain even though the sense of psychological unity remained intact." (359) There remain questions as to whether dividing the brain divides consciousness and the possibility of whether there are one or two conscious agents in a split brain, or rather some intermediate level of consciousness. (358) In a case study of a patient who had undergone a complete splitting to treat intractable epilepsy, it was reported that each hemisphere independently retained the ability for self-recognition, but only the right hemisphere could recognize others. (541)

4

Traumatic brain injury classification, scales, and definitions

Make everything as simple as possible, but not simpler.

—Albert Einstein

Universal classification scales are important, as they provide a mechanism to standardize assessments and outcome research. By creating and implementing broadly accepted scales for the assessment of brain injury and outcomes, a standardization is applied, which is necessary for consistent guidelines, recommendations, and evaluation of existing literature studies with incorporation of past information into new studies in a consistent manner. The severity of traumatic brain injury (TBI) is generally categorized as mild, moderate, or severe, depending upon the clinical presentation. In some patients, the neurological signs and symptoms may resolve, but in others, there can be severe and permanent disabilities, resulting in "chronic traumatic brain injury disease." The CDC broadly defined chronic conditions as "conditions that last 1 year or more and require ongoing medical attention or limit activities of daily living or both." (53)

It is important to recognize that TBI is not an "event" that is simply treated with rehabilitation and resolves, but is rather a chronic disease process. After a TBI, a number of disorders may ensue over time, including neurological disorders, psychological and psychiatric disorders, sleep disorders, neurodegenerative diseases, Alzheimer's disease, chronic traumatic encephalopathy, Parkinson's disease, neuroendocrine disorders, psychiatric disease, sexual dysfunction, incontinence, musculoskeletal disorders, metabolic dysfunction, and others.

Gleaning conclusive information from the TBI literature is, at times, difficult because of variations in definitions used in different studies, especially with respect to mild TBI. This may in part be attributed to a lack of consistency in timing when the most commonly used Glasgow Coma Scale (GCS) scores were assessed, and study design flaws, including frequent lack of control groups and the grouping of patients with GCS scores of 13, 14, and 15 into one category known as mild TBI. (47, 179)

An interagency initiative involving the National Institute of Neurological Disorders and Stroke (NINDS), the National Institute on Disability and Rehabilitation Research (NIDRR), the Department of Veteran Affairs (VA), the Defense and Veterans Brain Injury Center, and the Defense Centers of Excellence have jointly defined TBI in a position statement from their experts, who made up the Demographics and Clinical Assessment Working Group, as "an alteration in brain function, or

DOI: 10.1201/9781003354154-4

other evidence of brain pathology, caused by an external force." They further define "alteration of brain function" as one of the following clinical signs: "any period of loss of or a decreased level of consciousness; any loss of memory for events immediately before (retrograde amnesia) or after the injury (posttraumatic amnesia); neurological deficits (weakness, loss of balance, change in vision, dyspraxia paresis/plegia (paralysis), sensory loss, aphasia, etc.); any alteration in mental state at the time of the injury (confusion, disorientation, slowed thinking, etc.)." Confounding factors that might complicate this diagnosis include posttraumatic amnesia (PTA) versus loss of consciousness (LOC), delayed LOC, posttraumatic stress disorder (PTSD) causing partial amnesia for the injury, medications whether administered after the injury or substances such as alcohol or drugs consumed by the patient before the injury, and stress, anxiety, and depression. (48)

GLASGOW COMA SCALE (GCS)

There are a number of scales that can be used to assess TBI, both in the acute early phase as well as in the treatment and recovery phase. Different aspects of the patient's neurological exam are assessed with different scales and, therefore, there is a lack of standardization. In assessing clinical severity of brain injuries, the GCS is a widely accepted standard in measuring the level of consciousness. Regarding the use of a scale as opposed to a full neurological evaluation, Teasdale and Jennett in 1974 wrote in their seminal paper titled "Assessment of Coma and Impaired Consciousness: A Practical Scale" published in *The Lancet*, that there are "good reasons for restricting routine observations to the minimum, and for choosing those which can be reliably recorded and understood by a range of different staff."

The GCS (Table 4.1) has gained wide acceptance in the evaluation of patients with impaired consciousness and head injury. The scale has three components, with scores for ocular, verbal, and motor function, and ranges from 3–15. A person who is alert, with normal eye and motor function, would score 15. The GCS score can be affected by variables such as alcohol and drug intoxication, as well as medical sedation. (54, 264)

While GCS measurements for patients with severe TBI have been found to be helpful in predicting morbidity and mortality, this and other traditional methods for evaluation have limited use when it comes to evaluating mild TBI, which creates difficulty in standardizing epidemiologic research of mild TBI. (24)

Table 4.1 Glasgow coma scale

Domain	Response	Score (points)
Eye Opening Response	Spontaneous, open with blinking at baseline	4
	To verbal stimuli, command, speech	3
	To pain only (not applied to face)	2
	No response	1
Verbal Response	Oriented	5
	Confused conversation, but able to answer questions	4
	Inappropriate words	3
	Incomprehensible speech	2
	No response	1
Motor Response	Obeys commands for movements	6
	Purposeful movement to painful stimulus	5
	Withdraws in response to pain	4
	Flexion in response to pain (decorticate posturing)	3
	Extension response to pain (decerebrate posturing)	2
	No response	1

TBI CLASSIFICATIONS: MILD, MODERATE, SEVERE

The Centers for Disease Control and Prevention (CDC) in their "Report to Congress on Traumatic Brain Injury in the United States: Epidemiology and Rehabilitation," referenced Brasure et al., 2012, for their criteria to classify TBI severity as follows:

- *Mild TBI:* Brain imaging is normal; loss of consciousness (LOC) <30 minutes; PTA 0–1 day; GCS score 13–15.
- *Moderate TBI:* Brain imaging normal or abnormal; LOC 30 minutes–24 hours; PTA more than one day and less than seven days; GCS score 9–12.
- *Severe TBI:* Brain imaging normal or abnormal; LOC >24 hours; PTA more than seven days; GCS score 3–8. (6)

The United States Department of Defense (DOD), in their report of 468,424 cases of TBI from the year 2000 to third quarter of 2022, utilized the following classification scale to rate the severity of TBI:

- *Concussion/mild TBI:* "confused or disoriented state that lasts less than 24 hours; or loss of consciousness for up to 30 minutes; or memory loss lasting less than 24 hours. Excludes penetrating TBI. A computed tomography (CT) scan is not indicated for most patients with a mild TBI. If obtained it is normal."
- *Moderate TBI:* "confused or disoriented state that lasts more than 24 hours; or loss of consciousness for more than 30 minutes, but less than 24 hours; or memory loss lasting greater than 24 hours but less than seven days; or meets criteria for mild TBI except an abnormal CT scan is present. Excludes penetrating TBI. A structural brain imaging study may be normal or abnormal."
- *Severe TBI:* "confused or disoriented state that lasts more than 24 hours; or a loss of consciousness for more than 24 hours; or memory loss for more than seven days. Excludes penetrating TBI. A structural brain imaging study may be normal but usually is abnormal."
- *Penetrating TBI, or open head injury:* "a head injury in which the scalp, skull, and dura mater are penetrated. Penetrating injuries can be caused by high velocity missiles or objects of lower velocity such as knives or bone fragments from a skull fracture that are driven into the brain." (44, 714, 715)

(Note: Regarding the above DOD scale, a patient must meet any of the criteria of a single level [mild, moderate, severe], to be classified in that category of severity. If a patient meets more than one category, the higher level of severity is assigned.)

The ACRM definition in 1993 for mild TBI in a person, according to the Mild Traumatic Brain Injury Committee of the Head Injury Interdisciplinary Special Interest Group of the American Congress of Rehabilitation Medicine (ACRM), is a person who has suffered a traumatically induced disruption of brain function with at least one of the following:

- "Any period of loss of consciousness.
- Any loss of memory for events immediately before or after the accident.
- Any alteration in mental state at the time of the accident (e.g. feeling dazed, disoriented, or confused).
- Focal neurological deficit(s) that may or may not be transient.

but where the severity of the injury does not exceed the following:

- Loss of consciousness of approximately 30 minutes or less;
- After 30 minutes, an initial Glasgow Coma Scale (GCS) of 13–15;
- Posttraumatic amnesia (PTA) not greater than 24 hours;

This definition includes:

- The head being struck.
- The head striking an object.
- The brain undergoing an acceleration/deceleration movement (i.e., whiplash) without direct external trauma to the head."

Imaging studies of the brain such as CT, magnetic resonance imaging (MRI), electroencephalogram, and neurological examination may be normal. Some patients might not have a medical evaluation done acutely, but may describe these symptoms at a later medical visit. (319)

According to the CDC, symptoms of a mild TBI and concussion may appear immediately after an injury or may occur hours or days later. They generally improve over time, and most people feel better within a couple of weeks.

The CDC describes symptoms of mild TBI which may involve physical complaints, trouble with thinking and remembering, changes of emotion or social interaction, and changes in sleep patterns.

- Physical complaints may include: disturbance from light or noise, dizziness or balance problems, feeling tired with no energy, headaches, nausea and vomiting, and visual problems.
- Thinking and memory difficulties may include difficulty with attention or concentration, feeling slowed down, feeling groggy or foggy, difficulty with memory (short or long term), and difficulty thinking clearly.
- Emotional or social problems include anxiety and nervousness, irritability and ability to be angered easily, feeling more emotional, and sadness.
- Sleep changes include sleeping less or more than usual and difficulty falling asleep. (320)

Mild TBI, most frequently caused by blunt trauma, has often been diagnosed mainly based upon symptoms, a history of a loss of consciousness for less than 30 minutes, less than 24 hours of PTA, an initial GCS score of 13–15, and patients may have a CT scan of the brain which is normal in about 90% of cases. As mild TBI is generally considered to not show positive findings on CT scans of the brain, those cases of mild TBI in which the CT scans show pathology have been considered to be complicated mild TBI cases. More subtle injuries, such as a small contusion, may be better seen on MRI. (50)

OUTCOME SCALES

To assess the impact of TBI on the outcome of a patient as well as measure the effect that the natural history of the injury and the impact of treatments and rehabilitation have on the patient, standardized tests and outcome scales are needed.

For assessing disability due to physical and cognitive impairment, the following functional measurement scales are frequently used in assessing TBI patients:

- Glasgow Outcome Scale (GOS) with or without extended scores (GOSE).
- Disability Rating Scale (DRS).
- Rancho Los Amigos Scale (RLAS) (8 level scale).
- Rancho Los Amigos Revised Scale (RLAS-R) (10 level scale).
- Functional Independence Measure (FIM).
- Functional Assessment Measure (FAM).
- Community Integration Questionnaire (CIQ).
- Functional Status Examination (FSE).
- Supervision Rating Scale (SRS).
- Sensory Modality Assessment and Rehabilitation Technique (SMART).
- Sensory Stimulation Assessment Measure (SSAM).
- Western Neuro Sensory Stimulation Profile (WNSSP).

The GOSE at six months post-injury is the most reliable and commonly used functional outcome measurement in randomized controlled trials studying TBI. (281–283)

Those patients who have had a good physical recovery may need a neuropsychological and cognitive outcome assessment, possibly including:

- Controlled Oral Word Association for verbal fluency.
- Rey Complex Figure for visuoconstruction and memory.
- Grooved pegboard for fine motor dexterity.
- Symbol Digit Modalities (verbal) for sustained attention. (282)

Health-related quality of life (HRQoL) questions reflect the patients' subjective view of their disease, treatments they receive, and the effect they feel this is having on their life, or in other words, how bothered they are by the problems they are experiencing. The range-of-life functions covered include physical, social, psychological, and daily life activities. The most commonly used HRQoL tests used to assess generic quality of life measures include:

- SF-36 (short form 36 health questionnaire), which contains 36 questions.
- SF-12 (a shorter version).
- WHOQOL.
- SIP.
- EQ-5D.

HRQoL tests specific to TBI include:

- EBIQ
- Quality of Life in Brain Injury (QUOLIBRI)
- Neurobehavioral Symptom Inventory (NSI) (281, 282)

The GOS, published in 1975 by Jennett and Bond, looks at outcomes after TBI and has the following five categories: death, persistent vegetative state, severe disability, moderate disability, and good recovery. It was designed to assess the impact of head injury on functioning in daily life. Jennett and Bond stated in 1975, "it is hoped that the scale proposed will enable outcome after brain damage to be more readily assessed." Jennett later expanded the GOS from five outcome categories to eight, and the expanded scale is known as the Glasgow Outcome Scale Extended (GOSE). The categories in this scale are: death (score of 1), vegetative state (score of 2), lower severe disability (score of 3), upper severe disability (score of 4), lower moderate disability (score of 5), upper moderate disability (score of 6), lower good recovery (score of 7), and upper good recovery (score of 8). The Food and Drug Administration has in the past recommended the use of the GOSE for trials assessing the treatment and rehabilitation of TBI. (56, 57, 266)

For patients who have suffered severe head trauma, the DRS has been found to be more sensitive than the GOS in measuring clinical changes. The DRS consists of eight items divided into four categories: (1) arousal and awareness; (2) cognitive ability to handle self-care functions; (3) physical dependence upon others; and (4) psychosocial adaptability for work, housework, or school. (268)

The RLAS is often used in conjunction with the GCS initially in the acute assessment of brain injury and can be used subsequently during treatment and recovery. The RLAS takes into account the patient's level of consciousness as well as cognitive and physical levels of functioning in addition to degrees of assistance they require. While the original scale ranged from levels 1 (lowest level of function) to 8 (highest level of function), the revised scale is known as the Rancho Los Amigos Revised Scale (RLAS-R) and ranges from I to X. (58)

The NSI is a 22-item self-report questionnaire first published in 1995 that provides the ability to track symptomatic changes in patients with TBI. The NSI has been used in the evaluation of TBI by the DOD and the VA. (265) The SMART may be used for vegetative state and minimally conscious patients (it has excellent reliability between different testers and with repeat testing). (59) The SSAM may be implemented for early evaluation of severe brain injury (a valid and reliable test of overall responsiveness). (624) The WNSSP can assess head-injured patients who are slow to recover. (267)

5

Neurobiology of TBI: Mechanical injury and blast injury

Everything is theoretically impossible, until it is done.

—Robert A. Heinlein

Historically, traumatic brain injury (TBI) has been diagnosed primarily based on clinical criteria. With the advent of modern neuroimaging techniques, including advanced magnetic resonance imaging (MRI) and diffusion tensor imaging (DTI), and with the ability to perform statistical analysis and correlations with TBI clinical outcome studies, biomarkers are providing additional insight into the prediction of outcome severity. Ongoing research will help to further classify and stratify TBI based on imaging and blood biomarkers.

MECHANICALLY INDUCED TBI

The brain is housed within the skull and is essentially floating in cerebrospinal fluid (CSF). There are dural membranes, such as the tentorium and falx cerebri, which separate and support different portions of the brain. The floor of the frontal and temporal fossa of the skull, which sits under the frontal and temporal lobes, respectively, has ridges and is frequently involved in causing commonly seen frontal and temporal lobe brain injuries after an impact to the head. While the immediate result of the primary injury occurs at the time of impact, secondary injury may ensue later as a result of physiologic and biomolecular changes. During a head injury, the brain may sustain translational and rotational vectors of forces, forces of acceleration and deceleration, forces of compression and tension, shearing forces, blast-induced forces, coup (trauma to the brain under the location of impact on the skull) and contra coup (trauma to the brain in a location remote to or on the opposite side of the head from the region of impact to the skull) injuries. These may result in cortical contusions, intracerebral hematomas, subdural hematomas, epidural hematomas, intraventricular hemorrhage, subarachnoid hemorrhage, as well as diffuse axonal injury (DAI) or traumatic axonal injury (TAI). By striking the falx, the cingulate gyrus may experience deformation of the surface gray matter and disruption of long-coursing white matter cingulate bundle fibers, resulting in altered cingulate functions. (64, 448) The corpus callosum may be sensitive

DOI: 10.1201/9781003354154-5

to injury from impacts which result in coronal and horizontal rotations, as they may drive lateral motion of the falx, which is a relatively stiff membrane, in the direction of commissural fibers below. (625)

Anatomy of brain injury

Since the skull is a fixed container, if the brain starts to swell as a result of trauma, intracranial pressure (ICP) increases and herniation of the brain may occur, in which portions of the brain that are suffering from increased swelling are forced into compartments of the brain that have less swelling. When the swelling causes one hemisphere of the brain to push under the falx toward the opposite side of the skull, subfalcine or cingulate herniations occur (**Figure 5.1**). When the brain above the tentorium experiences increased pressure, the medial portion of the temporal lobe is forced in an inferior direction, resulting in uncal herniation. When this occurs, the oculomotor nerve (cranial nerve III) is frequently compressed, leading to dilatation of the ipsilateral pupil. When herniation occurs, forcing the brain across a firm dural membrane (falx, tentorium) that separates compartments within the brain, the cerebral arteries may become compressed and occluded, resulting in ischemia and infarction of brain tissue, which results in further swelling and the downward cascade of events continues. When the supratentorial contents migrate toward the infratentorial compartment, or when there is swelling or hemorrhage arising in the infratentorial compartment, the cerebellum and brainstem can herniate downward through the foramen magnum, leading to cerebellar tonsillar herniation. When this occurs, the brainstem may suffer linear hemorrhages known as Duret hemorrhages, leading to further neurological demise and ultimately death. (64) Increases in water content in the brain causing cerebral edema, may cause an increase in ICP locally in the brain. This may complicate and exacerbate the process that created the edema in the first place, leading to additional edema and to a cyclical worsening of events.

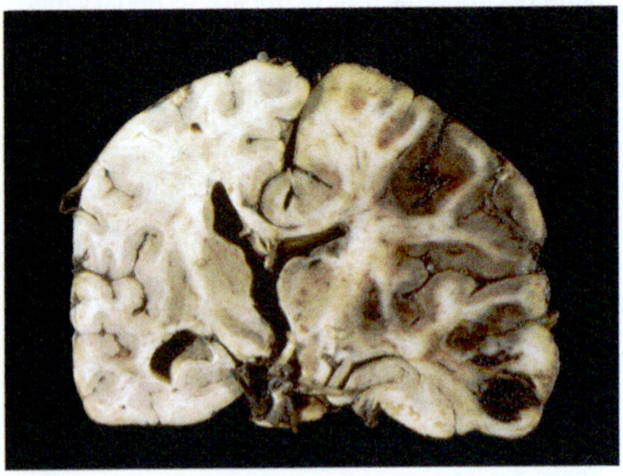

Figure 5.1 Gross specimen showing a coronal section through a brain that has suffered blunt head trauma. The right hemisphere shows extensive hemorrhage (brown and dark brown areas). Bleeding and edema have caused the compression of ventricles, as well as herniation of the cingulate gyrus. (From CNRI / Science Source.)

Brain edema has been thought to occur due to three mechanisms: vasogenic, cytotoxic (water within the cells increases), and osmotic (related to chemical or osmotic differences in the chemical makeup of blood and tissue). Cytotoxic edema, which is characterized by intracellular accumulation of water in neurons and astrocytes, has been found to play a primary role in brain edema. Substances released following TBI and that appear to have a role in vasogenic and cytotoxic brain edema include lactate, glutamate, potassium, calcium, arachidonic acid, free oxygen radicals, and others. The post-TBI pro-inflammatory environment that develops in the brain promotes oligodendrocyte loss and demyelination, a disruption of axonal transport; the glial responses are mediators of neuronal death. (70, 75)

Cerebral edema

The pathophysiology of mild TBI may have a transient cellular manifestation of axonal injury, but axonal function deficits may be present over a longer period postinjury and there may be alterations in dopaminergic signaling that may differ than that in more severe cases of TBI. (55) Mild TBI injuries are typically characterized by a neurometabolic cascade in which injured cells typically recover, although some may degenerate and die. The injuries may involve ionic shifts in the brain, reduced blood flow, and altered neurotransmission. (143) While primary injury to the brain occurs at the time of impact to the brain, a cascade of events may cause a secondary injury to occur over the ensuing hours to weeks. Some of these secondary causes include cerebral edema, increased ICP, cerebral ischemia, vasospasm, meningitis, biochemical changes, neurotransmitter-mediated excitotoxicity, and seizures and may lead to neuronal cell death. (70, 75)

In a study on rats, it was found that TBI-related brain edema was caused by a disruption of the blood brain barrier (BBB) (lasting four days) associated with a decrease in anchoring tight junction proteins as well as cytotoxic and vasogenic components. Cellular edema may be the main cause of brain swelling during the first one to two weeks post injury, which followed an initial brief period (as little as approximately 45 minutes) of vasogenic edema due to BBB compromise. (76, 77) In another study on rats, it was found that TAI did not produce a generalized effect on all axons, but rather different axon subpopulations have different levels of vulnerability and potential for functional recovery. (66)

One of the challenges in studying and understanding TBI, is the difficulty in measuring it in a quantitative manner. The severe TBI cases are easy to identify, as there may be significant findings on physical examination of the patient, as well as on CT and MRI scans of the brain. The mild TBI injuries pose more of a difficulty to evaluate and diagnose. While the traditional imaging studies such as CT and MRI scans may not show positive findings in cases of mild TBI, advanced MRI studies such as DTI and susceptibility weighted imaging (SWI) may show white matter injury and functional MRI may show brain activity changes related to cognitive function, such as memory and concentration. Both structure and function of the brain can be objectively examined with advanced imaging techniques. (50)

It is important to remember that while the resolution of CT and MRI scans of the brain may get down to the millimeter level, the functioning of neurons in the brain is at the micron (1/1,000th of a millimeter) and nanometer (1/1,000th of a micron) level. Damage to neurons at this level, while it may result in neurological changes, may escape detection by imaging studies. The most common visible findings on MRI are hemosiderin deposits within the brain, white matter signal abnormalities, and focal encephalomalacia. (65)

Mechanisms of brain injury and location of damage

When an object collides with the head of a patient, the first impact is to the scalp, then skull, dura, and brain. Skull fractures may be open (exposed through a laceration in the scalp) or closed (non-exposed), linear or comminuted (multiple fragments), depressed (pushing into the brain) or non-depressed, and may occur over the vault of the head or at the skull base (possibly resulting in CSF leaks from the nose known as rhinorrhea). The dura mater, which is a tough covering of the brain, surrounds and helps to compartmentalize the brain.

A blood accumulation between the skull and the dura mater is known as an epidural hematoma, and is often associated with a skull fracture that lacerates the middle meningeal artery. The patient may initially be lucid, but may deteriorate neurologically within minutes to hours if a large epidural hematoma develops, leading to uncal herniation and death. Rapid neurosurgical evacuation of the hematoma is necessary to save the patient's life. (64)

Acute subdural hematomas are blood collections between the dura mater and the brain and can result from the tearing or rupture of bridging veins or superficial cortical arteries. Neurosurgical evacuation is frequently performed. The morbidity and mortality of subdural hematomas can be substantial.

Concussions are temporary alterations in consciousness suffered after experiencing blunt trauma to the head. While traditional brain imaging studies such as CT and conventional MRI scans may not show positive findings, DTI scans and other advanced imaging techniques may detect abnormalities.

Contusions are areas of hemorrhagic necrosis in the crests of cerebral gyri and may occur as a result of the brain striking the adjacent dura-covered skull, especially in the frontal and temporal lobes. Of note, the floor of the anterior and middle cranial fossae (upon which the frontal and temporal lobes, respectively, rest) contains irregular boney contours which during trauma to the head are prone to inflict injury upon the adjacent surface of the frontal and temporal lobes of the brain. For this reason, contusions are frequently seen on the sub-frontal and anterior temporal cortical surfaces. Coup contusions occur deep to the site of impact, while contra-coup contusions occur on the opposite side of the brain. Contusions may evolve and expand over hours to days after an injury. (64)

Penetrating brain injuries, from bullets, shrapnel, screwdrivers, knives, lawn darts, and other objects occur once the object has broken through the skull and has subsequently lacerated the brain.

While the tract of the missile will experience significant injury and bleeding, areas of the brain that are remote from this trajectory may also experience significant injuries of axonal shearing and other damage due to the significant deformation of the brain and blood vessels as a result of energy delivered by the missile. (64)

When shearing forces of trauma to the brain cause damage to axons, this results in DAI, which has also been labeled TAI. This pathology has been found in mild, moderate, and severe TBI. When axoplasmic transport is impaired as a result of TAI, the axon swells and, eventually, the proximal and distal ends of the axon become disconnected; over hours to days, axonal retraction bulbs may form, resulting in Wallerian degeneration over weeks to months, of the distal segment of the axon. When this process occurs diffusely throughout the brain, it is known as multi-focal traumatic axonal injury. (64)

In a study in which rat neurons were plated on a deformable silicone membrane within a culture well and subjected to rapid tensile elongation, periodic breaks of individual microtubules were observed along the axons that corresponded with undulations in the axon's morphology and, subsequently, evolved into periodic swellings within hours. As these axonal undulations and varicosities were found postmortem in human brains following severe TBI, this suggests that in the area of broken microtubules, transport within an axon may be halted, but it may proceed through other regions with intact microtubules. (380)

Following TBI, traumatic intracerebral hematomas may occur due to the rupture of blood vessels within the brain. While they may occur immediately after impact, they can also occur in a delayed manner (hours or days after the injury) and evolve over time in regions of the brain that appeared normal on the initial brain CT scan. Bleeding within the ventricles is known as intraventricular hemorrhage. (64)

Repetitive brain injury has been seen to result in chronic traumatic encephalopathy (CTE), which has been known as dementia pugilistica resulting from repetitive boxing injuries and which itself replaced the term "punch drunk." Clinical findings include slurring dysarthria, memory deficits, ataxia, and changes in personality. Pathological associations may include concussion-related hemorrhages, Alzheimer's disease pathology, amyloid β plaques, neurofibrillary pathology, and tauopathy. (67)

Chronic traumatic encephalopathy (CTE)

CTE, a progressive neurodegenerative pathology, is associated with repetitive concussion, subconcussion injuries, and blast injuries to the brain. As the lesions progress, they may become large and confluent, likely due to continuing tau deposition, without necessarily any continued trauma. To obtain a conclusive diagnosis of CTE, brain tissue must be evaluated histologically and typically shows features of accumulation of hyperphosphorylated tau (P-tau) in neurofibrillary tangles, neurites, and astrocytes surrounding small blood vessels. The definitive lesion of CTE is a neuronal lesion consisting of neurofibrillary tangles and neurites. (10, 68)

In 2005, Omalu presented the results of an autopsy of a retired professional football player, revealing CTE with many diffused amyloid plaques, sparse neurofibrillary tangles, and tau-positive neuritic threads in neocortical areas. This brought attention to "potential long-term neurodegenerative outcomes in retired professional National Football League players subjected to repeated mild traumatic brain injury." (626) In 2014, Omalu noted that CTE "is a progressive neurodegenerative syndrome, which is caused by a single, episodic, or repetitive blunt force impacts to the head and transfer of acceleration-deceleration forces to the brain." Furthermore, although microscopic examination of the brain of a CTE sufferer may show microscopic evidence of primary proteinopathy (tauopathy) and secondary proteinopathy (including amyloidopathy and TDP [TAR (transactive response) DNA-binding protein 43]), the brain may appear grossly unremarkable. (627)

When the brains of deceased former National Football League players were examined, CTE was found in 110 of the 111 football veterans, with findings of "extensive brain atrophy, astrogliosis, myelinated axonopathy, microvascular injury, perivascular neuroinflammation, and phosphorylated tau protein pathology." It is possible that a toxic compound cis P-tau (an abnormal isomer of the normal trans P-tau) is produced by neurons as a result of TBI, as seen in mouse models. CTE appears to be a tauopathy with a perivascular accumulation of hyperphosphorylated tau in neurons and astrocytes within cerebral sulci. (69)

BLAST-INDUCED TBI

Blast overpressure (BOP) or high-energy impulse noise are seen in the military as well as occupational and civilian settings. As a result of an explosive detonation or firing of weapons, there is a significant instantaneous rise in atmospheric pressure. While the injury primarily damages hollow organs such as the ears; lungs and the gastrointestinal tract; solid organs such as the brain, heart, and spleen may be affected; and air emboli, hypoxia, and shock may occur. These injuries frequently subject the patient to additional exposure to toxic gases, smoke, and high heat. Brain injury from the primary blast may result from pathological changes in the outer-layer cortical region and diffuse white matter damage. Consistent brain neuropathological findings after a blast injury include multifocal axonal and neuronal injuries, astroglial alterations, inflammation, BBB abnormalities, and hemorrhages within the brain. Seizures may be more prevalent following a blast injury, due to consistent neuropathological brain changes. (33, 37, 41)

The primary injury is initially caused by the BOP wave, which in animal studies causes changes in the brain similar to DAI. Secondary injuries may result from fragmentation injuries and penetrating trauma from airborne debris. Tertiary injuries may result from transposition of the entire body due to blast wind or structural collapse. Quaternary injuries include all other causes, such as burns, exposure to toxic inhalants, and asphyxia. Mild TBI and posttraumatic stress disorder are often seen together and occur in a substantial portion of military service members who have suffered blast and non-blast mild TBI. The distinction between post-concussive syndrome and PTSD may be difficult as symptoms may overlap. Complaints of fatigue, irritability, impaired attention, altered memory and concentration, and sleeping difficulties may be common to both. The difference between the two disorders will be based on the major symptoms and a postconcussive syndrome may have organic symptoms such as headache, dizziness, hearing loss, visual complaints, cognitive disturbance, and balance issues. PTSD symptoms, on the other hand, may have symptoms of nightmares, avoidance, reexperiencing phenomena, and hyperarousal. It is easier to recognize the neurological and cognitive changes in cases of moderate to severe TBI, but more difficult with a mild TBI. Although PTSD symptoms may occur in both blast and non-blast mild TBI, they may be more pronounced in patients with blast injuries. (34–36)

A study of 163 combat veterans with a history of blast exposure revealed significantly lower bilateral hippocampal volume. (458) In a study in which rats were exposed to repeated BOP of 17 pounds per square inch (psi), chronic glial pathological changes of astrocyte pathology (glial fibrillary acidic protein [GFAP]) and dendritic alterations were seen in the hippocampus and motor cortex regions and the rats also suffered behaviors suggestive of anxiety. The authors felt it is possible that pathologic changes in the hippocampus or motor cortex have a role in psychiatric impairment following blast injuries, but further studies are needed. (71)

BIOMARKERS OF TBI

Biomarkers are objective markers which can be used to identify TBI. As science and the study of medicine evolves through research and collaboration, the sensitivity and specificity of biomarkers will advance. Not only will this allow for more accurate diagnoses, but it will also help to monitor progress of treatment regimens, ultimately leading to better outcomes for patients.

Chemical biomarkers

Biomarkers can help to quantify the assessment of TBI. Biomarkers may be chemical, which can be evaluated in a laboratory, or they may be radiological and seen on imaging studies. This section will focus on chemical biomarkers with imaging covered in another chapter.

As a result of TBI, the BBB may be broken down due to mechanical forces as well as inflammatory and neurometabolic cascades. Neurons and glial cells may release proteins, nuclei acids, and metabolites from their intracellular to the extracellular space and, from there, these biomarkers may enter the bloodstream through the damaged BBB. (74)

To evaluate TBI in an analytical method and stratify its outcomes, biomarkers in the blood serum, CSF through a ventriculostomy or spinal tap, brain extracellular fluid, and brain tissue may be examined. Biomarkers are evaluated in clinical research, but generally not in the daily clinical practice of medicine. As summarized by Khellaf et al.

regarding works of Depreitere and Donnelly, "noteworthy biomarkers in TBI include glia-related biomarkers (GFAP, S100B), neuron/axon-related biomarkers (neuron-specific enolase [NSE], neurofilament light polypeptide [NFL], ubiquitin carboxy-terminal hydrolase [UCH-L1], tau, amyloid β, αII-Spectrin breakdown products among others) and other inflammation-related biomarkers (high mobility group box protein 1 [HMGB1], various cytokines and autoantibodies)." (73) Tau protein is associated with microtubules within axons, and NSE is a glycolytic protein mostly found in the cytoplasm of neurons. (477)

GFAP and S100B are found in astrocytes and ependymal cells of the brain, but S100B is less astrocyte-specific than GFAP and may be released from the death not only of astrocytes, but also of O2A glial progenitor cells, oligodendrocytes, ependymal and plexus epithelial cells, and neurons. (79)

A study of blood biomarkers was performed in 18 college athletes who suffered concussions and had positive findings for neurotoxicity biomarkers and decreased IMPACT cognitive testing scores. The authors suggest that biomarkers of neurotoxicity may assist in the assessment of transient changes in the brain in addition to a neurocognitive assessment and advanced neuroimaging. (477) **Figure 5.2** shows relative elevations and timing (which may vary) of blood biomarkers after a mild TBI of N-acetyl aspartate (NAA), glutamate receptors (GluRs; a family of approximately 25 proteins comprising channel-activated ionotropic and G-protein regulated metabotropic receptors), GFAP, S100B, UCH-L1, C-tau, αII-Spectrin, and myelin basic protein (MBP). As Dambinove cited Nag, injury to the brain causes the parenchymal cells and endothelia to suffer mechanical damage and energy failure, which compromises the BBB within hours to days after the impact. This leads to the acute (within hours after injury) and subacute (up to several weeks after injury) release of proteins into the bloodstream and biological fluids.

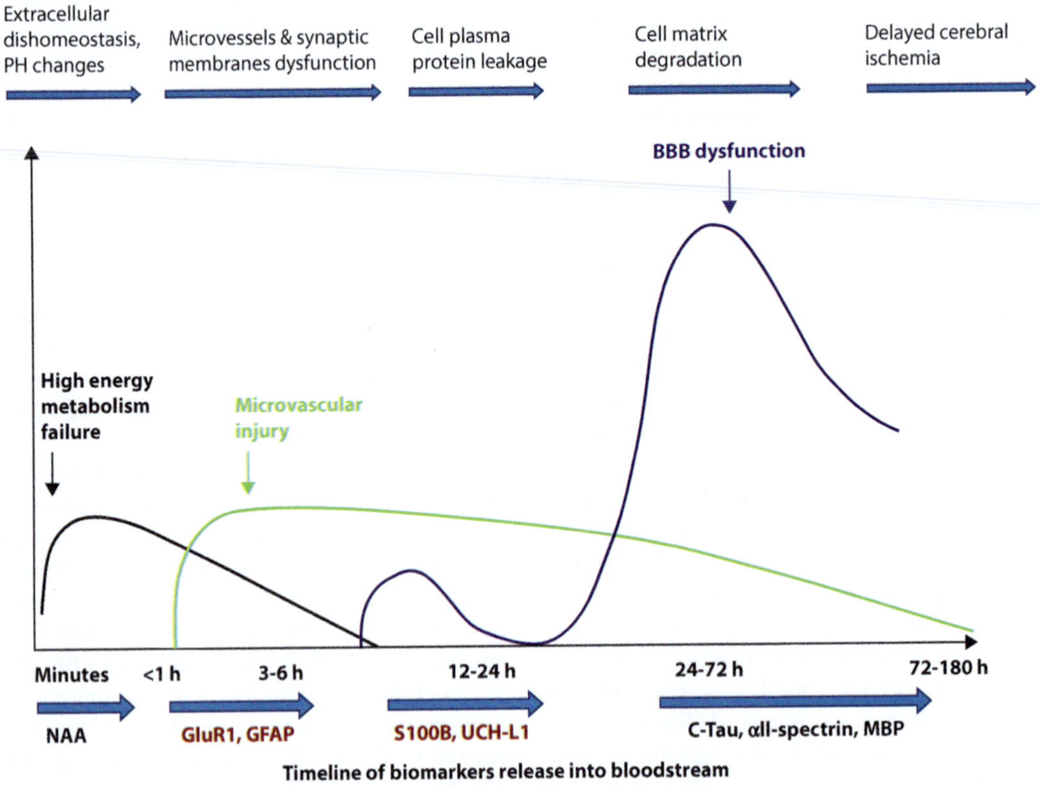

Figure 5.2 Mechanisms involved in development of subtle brain injury after mild TBI and relative timely release of corresponding biomarkers (relative timing is approximate and may vary). (Adapted from [477].) https://creativecommons.org/licenses/by/4.0/legalcode

A positive GFAP, ubiquitin carboxyl terminal hydrolase L1 (UCH-L1) or an S100B blood test within six hours of TBI may be helpful in stratifying degrees of TBI in the emergency department, but they cannot exclude a diagnosis of concussion. (72) A study of blood samples in patients who suffered a mild to moderate TBI were evaluated for levels of GFAP and UCH-L1. GFAP was more accurate in detecting TBI, CT lesions, and predicting neurosurgical intervention than was UCH-L1. (82) Evidence suggests that when used within the initial six hours after a TBI, S100B may be a candidate as a screening tool for traumatic intracranial lesions. GFAP may also be an option, given its stability over time and allowing sampling up to 24 hours post-injury. (84) The blood S100B protein biomarker appears to have an excellent negative predictive value and, therefore, has at times been considered an alternative to a brain CT scan when managing patients with mild TBI. Other biomarkers (GFAP, UCH-L1) when used in conjunction or alone, may improve specificity. (83) In a study of 566 patients with mild TBI who had S100B blood levels drawn prehospital and in the hospital, of 32 patients who were found to have a traumatic intracranial lesion, the sensitivity of an elevated S100B level being detected was 100%. With low levels of S100B, traumatic intracranial lesions were ruled out with a sensitivity of 100%. Specificities were lower. (85)

The neuronal and axonal injury markers neurofilament light protein and total tau and the astroglial injury marker GFAP were measured in the CSF of boxers after a fight and three months later. After the fight, neurofilament light protein and GFAP, but not total tau, were elevated, but three months later, only neurofilament light protein remained elevated when compared to nonathletic controls. The initial increase was significantly higher with more hits or higher impact of hits. It was felt that boxing impairs axonal and astroglial integrity. (80)

NSE is another biomarker that has been found to be elevated in CSF following a severe TBI and it was thought that its increased levels were a better predictor of deterioration to brain death than were CSF levels of S100B. (60)

Tau protein normally plays a role in axonal microtubule disassembly and assembly. Abnormal hyperphosphorylated tau protein (P-tau) forms paired helical filaments and aggregates to form the predominant component of neurofibrillary tangles, which are seen postmortem in human brains after repetitive mild TBI's. In a study of plasma in 217 patients with TBI, it was found that total-tau (T-tau) and abnormal hyperphosphorylated tau protein (P-tau) were elevated in mild, moderate, and severe TBI. It was also found that the acute P-tau levels and the P-tau-to-T-tau ratio were better than T-tau levels alone in correlating with severity of TBI and eventual outcomes. The authors note that even in the chronic phase of TBI, plasma P-tau and the P-tau-to-T-tau ratio may be elevated. Based on these findings, P-tau levels and the P-tau-to-T-tau ratio may be good biomarkers for stratifying brain CT findings and outcomes. (81)

Imaging biomarkers

As imaging has become more advanced, it may serve as a biomarker for TBI. This will be discussed in depth in the Imaging chapter (Chapter 8) of this book.

6

Cognitive function and neuroanatomy of the brain

The history of modern neuroscience is still being written.

—Mark Bear, Barry Connors, Michael Paradiso

NEUROSCIENCE PROGRESS: ONE CENTURY VERSUS FIVE MILLENNIA

Brain research is traditionally conducted on several levels of analysis: 1) molecular neuroscience, 2) cellular neuroscience, 3) systems neuroscience, 4) behavioral neuroscience, and 5) cognitive neuroscience. (483) With the exponentially increasing facilitation of growth and dissemination of knowledge through technology, it is clear that advancement in knowledge of the nervous system is likewise accelerating. While it appears that the sum of human knowledge related to the brain has soared over the last century as compared to the past five millennia, this knowledge gain would not have been possible without the foundation provided from those millennia. The first written reference to the brain appears to be provided by the ancient Egyptians, likely written in 1700 BC, but probably a copy of an older manual for military surgeons from around 3000 BC. The writings of Hippocrates, who lived circa 460–370 BC, were collected by scholars after his death and are contained in the work *Corpus Hippocraticum*, which contains many references to the brain and also deals with epilepsy. Plato, who lived 424–347 BC, felt that the brain is the sole organ of reasoning, a spiritual force unique to humans, providing them

DOI: 10.1201/9781003354154-6

with thought and intelligence. Aristotle, who lived 384–322 BC, felt that the psyche cannot exist as a purely spiritual entity without the body, but the psyche retains a spiritual-like property that can be regarded as a form of vitalism. (424)

During his dissections, Claudius Galen (129–200 AD) had developed instructions on how to remove the brain from the skull by using iron knives and other tools. He described the meninges, dura mater, and pia mater and explained how to cut the brain, exposing the corpus callosum. Galen described many other regions of the brain. Galen has been acknowledged as the earliest neuroscientist. Leonardo da Vinci (1472–1519), recognized as a genius who excelled in art, engineering, mathematics, and mechanics, felt that the brain provided the essential vital energy for life. Others who have advanced neuroscience were René Descartes (1596–1650) (first account of the reflex), Thomas Willis (father of modern neurology), Du Bois-Reymond (discovery of the action potential), Hermann von Helmholz (measured speed of nerve impulse), Gabriel Valentin (first detailed description of an individual brain cell, likely a Purkinje cell), Camillo Golgi (silver impregnation stain for nerve cells), and Santiago Ramón y Cajal (1852–1934) (founder of modern neuroscience, established neuron doctrine of individual cells and synaptic organization of the nervous system). Golgi and Cajal, both great pioneers of neuroanatomy, shared the 1906 Nobel Prize in recognition of their work on the nervous system. (424)

Although shown to not have any plausible physiological basis, phrenology, which was originated by Franz Joseph Gall (1758–1828), asserted to be able to identify psychological and personality traits based on palpation of protrusions or bumps on a person's skull. (349, 530) In 1865, Paul Broca, the father of localization theory, localized the inability to produce speech (motor aphasia) to the third left frontal convolution. (354) As noted by Nieuwenhuys, Carl Wernicke (1848–1905) subsequently reported on a language disorder involving the inability to comprehend speech with speech production relatively unaffected and attributed this sensory aphasia to the region of the left cerebral hemisphere where the occipital, parietal, and temporal regions meet. Alois Alzheimer (1864–1915) discovered neurofibrillary tangles and plaques in a demented patient, and the disease was named after him.

Appreciation of the function of the previously-felt-to-be-silent frontal lobes was gained from a work-related injury. The case of Phineas Gage has been considered one that greatly contributed to and influenced 19th century neuropsychiatric discussion of the mind-brain relationship and regions of the brain that affect personality. In 1848, Gage, a 25-year-old man was injured while working on railroad construction. During a rock-splitting job, Gage put gunpowder in a hole, pressed a long rod into it, and an unintentional explosion resulted, propelling the bar to enter his left cheek, damaging his left eye and piercing the left frontal region of the brain to exit the skull (**Figure 6.1**). Despite a few seizures, Gage awoke and walked. After several weeks of treatment (wound infection, anemia, transient coma), Gage was walking around the city within two months of the injury with intact strength, cognition, and memory, but with significant changes in personality. While once considered to have a gentle personality, he became rude, disrespectful, irritable, and profane with disregard

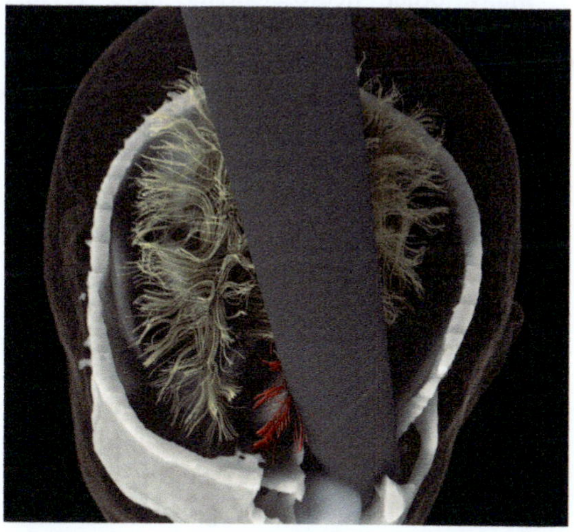

Figure 6.1 Estimation of possible trajectory of the tamping iron that caused penetrating injury to left frontal lobe of Phineas Gage (seen from above the frontal region of head) with potential interruption of fiber pathways in brain. (From the USC Mark and Mary Stevens, Neuroimaging and Informatics Institute [www.ini.usc.edu]; Dr. Arthur W. Toga, Director; Sidney Taiko Sheehan, Communications Manager; Jim Stanis, Medical Illustrator.)

for the future and for consequences of his actions. Due to these changes, Gage lost his friends. Gage's case was one of the first to provide scientific medical evidence that the frontal lobes are significantly involved with controlling personality, social interaction, and emotions. (424, 426, 523)

Wilder Graves Penfield, a neurosurgeon who specialized in the surgical treatment of epilepsy, developed a surgical technique in which he stimulated the brain of a conscious patient to map motor, sensory, and language regions of the brain. This allowed him to surgically resect regions of the brain in a safer manner to treat epilepsy. In 1931, when Penfield was stimulating the left temporal lobe of a woman who suffered from epilepsy, she stated that she saw herself re-enacting giving birth to a baby girl, even though this had really occurred many years earlier. Another time, a similar temporal lobe stimulation caused a 14-year-old girl to report experiencing herself walking through a meadow while being followed by a man holding a snake, which the patient's mother verified to be a genuine memory, and a memory that, at times, warned the mother of her daughter's impending seizure. (424)

Many other neuroscientists have further advanced the understanding of the brain. Subsequent studies revealed that specific centers within the brain were responsible for certain mental functions. Comprehensive maps of the brain based upon regional differences in cytoarchitecture of the human cerebral cortex were described by Korbinian Brodmann, Alfred Campbell, and others. Although Brodmann acknowledged that the various regions of the brain do not operate in isolation from each other, he excluded the interconnecting fiber architecture from his work. As cited by Sporns, Campbell was among the first neuroanatomists who, in 1905, recognized the connecting cortical fiber bundles. Sporns also noted that Karl Lashley in 1929 recognized the distributed nature of brain function, rather than viewing the brain as having specialized regions with localization of function. (349) As cited by Sporns, in 1965, Geschwind reported on "disconnection syndromes" involving damage to association pathways either within or between the cerebral hemispheres, as causing numerous cognitive deficits, including word-blindness without agraphia, word-deafness, etc. These represented a type of "conduction aphasia."

David Hubel and Torsten Wiesel, who shared the 1981 Nobel Prize in Physiology or Medicine, were recognized for their break-through research into the ability of the brain to interpret the code of impulses from the eyes. Their research showed that the visual cortex is divisible into discrete columns, and within each column the receptive-field axis orientation is the same. They found that the ability of the visual cortex to interpret messages from the retina is developed shortly after birth and that deprivation of this information from an eye for only a few days after birth will result in permanent functional changes in the visual cortex, which will not correct to its normal function despite later exposure to light stimulation. (397, 398)

Currently, as imaging techniques, cytoarchitectonic studies, and tract tracing of the brain improve, connectivity-based parcellation along with probabilistic maps of cellular microanatomy will likely improve correlations between brain structure and function at the microscopic level. (349) Software has been used to fully automate parcellation, based upon identifying sulco-gyral structures. This type of probabilistic sulco-gyral atlas, one of which produces a detailed parcellation of the cortex into 74 different structures per hemisphere, was felt to be reproducible and practical for large data sets and is less time consuming than manual labeling of the cortex. (524) In 2005, Sporns, Tononi, and Kötter proposed the use of the word "connectome" to describe the network of elements and connections forming the human brain. (527) They noted that non-invasive magnetic resonance imaging (MRI) image mapping of the connectomes of the brain using diffusion tensor imaging (DTI), high angular resolution diffusion imaging (HARDI), q-ball, and diffusion spectrum imaging (DSI) have been accomplished using deterministic approaches (finding optimal streamlines of fiber tracts within the tensor field) and probabilistic approaches (using statistical estimates to map the fiber pathways). Sporns noted that when applying clustering methods to structural and functional brain networks, the brain may be seen as "a set of interconnected communities of structurally and functionally related elements, arranged on multiple scales from cells to systems." (349) Cortical connectivity may consist of the existence of a structural core composed of regions that are densely interconnected. (528) To understand the function of the brain requires embracing the concepts of neuroscience, neuroanatomy, and the science of complex networks. More specifically, knowledge is required regarding the components of the network (anatomical structures of the brain and nervous system) as well as the way in which these components interact and the properties of their interactions through their intricate web of connectivity. While no single nerve can carry out an individual's complex behaviors and emotions, shape their thoughts, allow for speech and comprehension, form and retrieve memories, or be responsible for consciousness and awareness, when a multitude of nerves are linked together in networks and organized in a nervous system, these irreducible thought patterns become possible. According to Sporns, "we cannot fully understand brain function unless we approach the brain on multiple scales, by identifying the networks that bind cells into coherent populations, organize cell groups into functional brain regions, integrate regions into systems, and link brain and body in a complete organism." Three types of brain connectivity are structural (anatomical connections that are relatively static and not time dependent), functional (highly time dependent and modulated by external task demands, sensory stimulation, and internal state of the organism), and effective (describes network of causal effects between neural elements) connectivity. (349)

NEUROANATOMY AND FUNCTION

Historically, different regions of the brain were felt to be responsible for certain functions. With better understanding of the connectome and with functional imaging studies, it appears that that complex behaviors require the input of various brain regions and that interruption of these can lead to symptoms. Injury along the connecting pathways of different cortical regions can cause symptoms that appear to be related to a cortical region, despite the cortical region being intact. (553)

This portion of the chapter will be broken down into discussing neuroanatomy and function. The two cannot be separated, as they are intertwined in nature. Human knowledge has increased over time and the understanding of and responsibilities and function ascribed to various regions of the brain continues to morph. Our discussion of neuroanatomy will review different structural regions of the brain and will be followed by a review of function of the brain. Since the multitude of regions of the brain are inextricably connected on both a macroscopic and microscopic level, understanding their connections becomes crucial. These connections will be reviewed on a broad level grouped together by region and on an individual level, tract by tract, to the extent that they are currently understood, and it is within the scope of this book to do so. Pathology resulting from any of these levels may cause a variety of symptoms, which will be studied and discussed whether they arise from pathology of a specific region of the brain or from a connecting bundle of white matter tracts, which may involve several regions of the brain.

Knowledge from the study of anatomy and function of the brain could fill many tomes. The goal of this chapter is to present basic concepts and ideas on this topic, which can be used as a foundation for understanding the effects of traumatic brain injury (TBI).

NEUROANATOMY

Traditionally, knowledge of the neuroanatomy of the brain has been essential to understanding which regions of the brain are related to various aspects of brain function. Despite additional concepts regarding neural networks, which may help us to understand cerebral and cognitive processing, this knowledge is a prerequisite to evaluating compromise of function in an injured brain and how the changes in anatomy of the brain relate to changes in function. In putting together the complexities of TBI evaluation and how it affects an individual, it is essential to have an understanding of: 1) anatomy of the normal brain; 2) functioning of the normal brain; 3) correlations between normal anatomy and normal functioning; 4) changes in anatomy of the injured brain when compared with the normal brain; 5) changes in functioning of the injured brain compared to the normal brain; and 6) correlations between anatomy and functioning of the injured brain. To gain an understanding of brain anatomy in a patient, we can use the best imaging technology available. To gain an understanding of functioning of the brain, we use clinical input from physicians (neurosurgeons, neurologists, psychiatrists), neuropsychologists, nurses, therapists (physical therapists, occupational therapists, vocational rehabilitation specialists), social workers, and other medical personnel, as well as functional imaging.

Classically, different regions of the brain were thought to correspond with specific functions. Understanding the anatomy and function of the brain is significantly improving with the advent of advanced imaging capabilities.

In 1909, Korbinian Brodmann, a pioneer in the field of brain mapping through his studies of the cytoarchitectonic parcellation of the human cerebral cortex, published a seminal textbook *Brodmann's Localisation in the Cerebral Cortex* (textbook translated by Laurence Garey) that described "a topographic analysis of the human cerebral cortex based on its cellular structure … the emphasis would be not only on gross divisions of the brain, such as lobes and gyral complexes, but also on the smallest gyri and parts of gyri … to describe topographical parcellation and localisation in the cortex that would also be of value for clinicians." (341). Brodmann established 52 regions of the brain. More than a century later, this classic work remains important in advancement of the field and has been cited more than 170,000 times (as of July 2018). (342)

As neuroimaging studies have advanced, so has the understanding that traditional neuroanatomical maps do not provide the precision to match some aspects of functional segregation. (343) Brain atlases often present brain organization from a single perspective. (392)

To understand what symptoms and neurological examination findings may be encountered following a TBI, in it important to understand the anatomy and function of the brain. Next is a basic overview of anatomy and function of the brain. An excellent detailed description is provided in *DeJong's the Neurologic Examination*, 7th edition. (264, 269–272)

The brain, which is enclosed within the skull, is surrounded by the pia mater, the arachnoid, and the dura mater. The dura mater forms the falx cerebri (separates the two hemispheres of the brain) and the tentorium cerebelli (separates the cerebral hemispheres from the cerebellum). Blood is supplied to the brain by the carotid arteries and the vertebral arteries. The brain is bathed in cerebrospinal fluid (CSF), which cushions the brain. Within the brain are the ventricles, which also contain CSF. The left and right hemispheres of the brain are connected by the corpus callosum and contain gyri and sulci. (269, 478) White matter makes up about 50% of the human brain and myelination indices of the various white matter tracts vary according to age, fiber tract, and hemisphere. (479)

The "dominant hemisphere" is the one to which a function is lateralized, and in humans, this is true for language, interpretation of sensory stimuli (gnosis), and complex motor function (praxis). The majority of people are left hemisphere dominant. Broca's area, located in the inferior frontal gyrus, functions for speech production in the dominant hemisphere. The superior temporal gyrus contains Wernicke's area, which is responsible for the ability to understand spoken and written words. (270, 478)

The majority of the population (approximately 90–95%) is right-handed, with the left cerebral hemisphere being dominant for language in 99% of right-handed individuals, and for 60–70% of those who are left handed. Of the remaining individuals who are left-handed, about half are right-hemisphere dominant, and half have a mix of dominance in both cerebral hemispheres. (629)

A general overview of brain anatomy is seen in **Figure 6.2** which shows a type of 3-D rendering of the brain as seen from a sagittal view.

Frontal lobes

The frontal lobes, on their lateral aspect, comprise roughly the anterior one-third of the cerebral cortex, lie in the anterior fossa of the skull, and are easily injured during trauma to the head. Although myelination in the central nervous system continues until the age of roughly three years, myelination of the frontal lobes may continue into the early 20s. The posterior-most gyrus, the precentral gurus, contains the premotor area and lies just posterior to the precentral sulcus and anterior to the central sulcus. The motor strip is located in the precentral gyrus. The frontal lobe also contains the supplementary motor and premotor regions, and the dominant hemisphere contains the motor speech area (Broca's area) in the inferior frontal gyrus. (269, 270, 478, 482, 486)

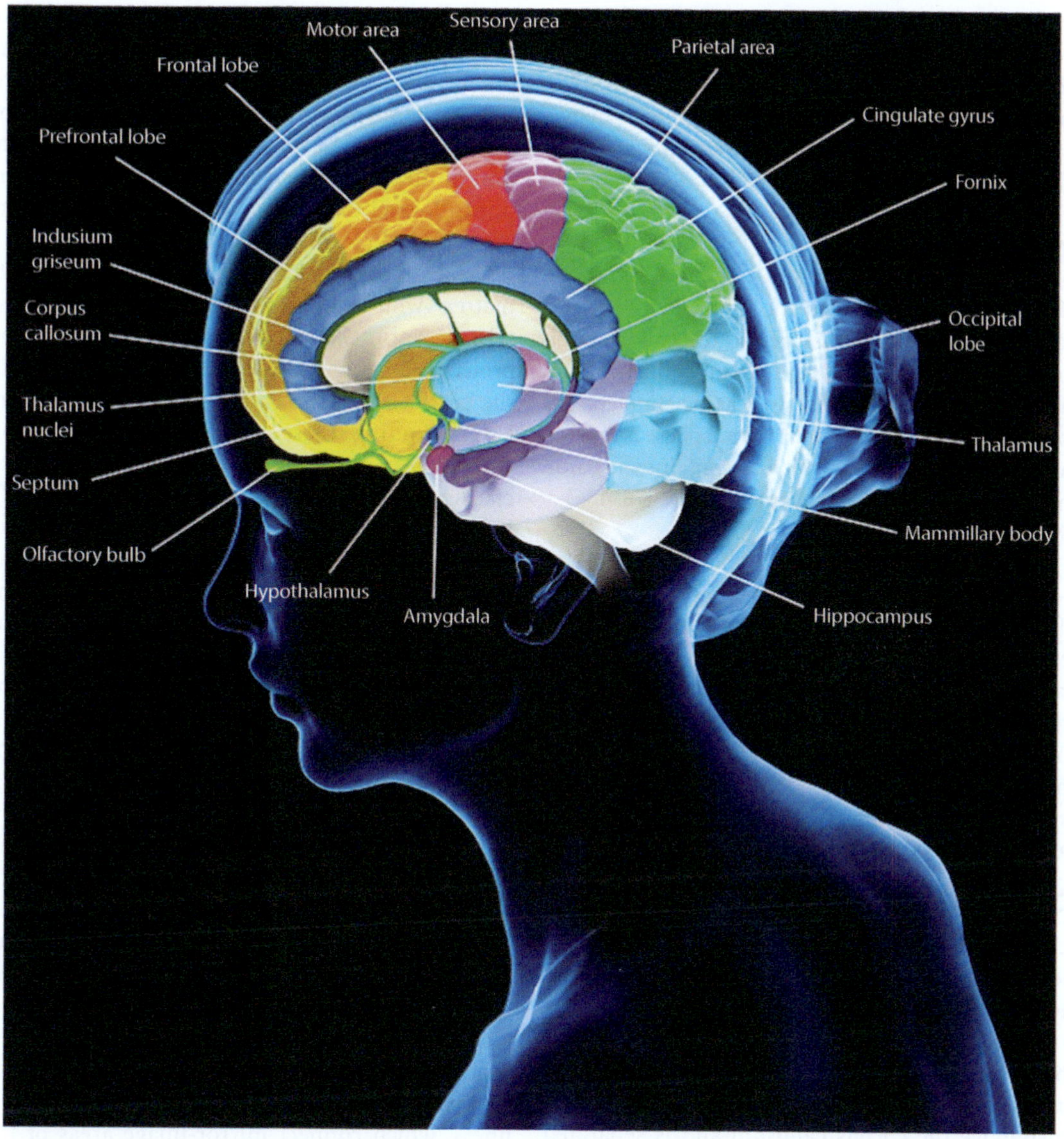

Figure 6.2 Illustration of a 3-D section through the human brain showing the various areas and structures. (From Fernando Da Cunha / Science Source.)

Parietal lobes

The parietal lobe is located between the frontal and occipital lobes and lies above the temporal lobe. It is posterior to the central sulcus, anterior to the occipital lobe, and superior to the temporal lobe. The primary sensory cortex is located in the post-central gyrus. Also located in the parietal lobe is the somatosensory association area and association cortex for somatosensory, visual, and auditory functions. (269, 478, 482, 486)

Occipital lobes

The occipital lobe, at the posterior aspect of the cerebral hemisphere, extends from the occipital pole to the parieto-occipital sulcus. The cortical tissue on each bank of the fissure forms the primary visual cortex and is known as the striate cortex (calcarine cortex). Destructive lesions in this region result in defects in the visual field. The visual association cortex is comprises the parastriate and peristriate regions, as well as other extrastriate visual areas. This association cortex projects pathways to the angular gyrus, temporal gyri, frontal lobe, and limbic system, as well through the splenium of the corpus callosum to the opposite hemisphere. Disruption of these pathways may result in disconnection syndromes. (269, 270, 478)

Temporal lobes

The temporal lobe lies in the middle fossa of the skull below the sylvian fissure and rests on the floor of the middle cranial fossa. It contains the primary auditory cortex and the auditory association cortex, part of which in the dominant hemisphere is known as Wernicke's speech area. It also contains the parahippocampal gyrus and the uncus. (269, 478, 486)

Limbic lobe

The limbic lobe, which because of its function rather than anatomy may be considered a separate lobe of the brain, contains the hippocampus, the fornix, mammillary bodies, anterior nucleus of the thalamus, cingulate gyrus, and the parahippocampal gyrus and resembles a "C"-shaped structure. Beginning in the paraterminal gyrus and subcallosal area beneath the rostrum of the corpus callosum, the full connection of the components of the limbic lobe are known as the Papez circuit. The classical Papez circuit is the neural loop which goes from the hippocampal formation to the mamillary body, to the anterior nucleus of the thalamus, to the cingulate gyrus/part of parahippocampal gyrus, and then back to the hippocampal formation. (655) The cingulate gyrus lies just above the corpus callosum and is separated by the callosal sulcus. The rhinencephalon (nose brain) is the basal portion of the forebrain contains olfactory bulbs and tracts, olfactory trigone, and part of the amygdala and is involved with olfaction and emotion. (269, 478)

Cerebral cortex, deep structures and white matter fibers

The cerebral cortex, which in the adult human measures about 1,100 cm^2, is an ultracomplex six-layered structure with about one-third of its contents on the surface of the brain and the remainder within the fissures and sulci. Its thickness ranges from 1.3 to 4.5 mm. The cortical mantle gray matter, which generally has six layers and may contain about 15–30 billion neurons, sends and receives input from other parts of the brain through fibers. The two hemispheres are incompletely separated by the longitudinal cerebral fissure (which is the location of the falx cerebri) and at its floor is the corpus callosum, the large myelinated fiber tract that connects both hemispheres. (269, 270, 478, 530)

Beneath the cortical gray matter lies the white matter, which contains glial cells, blood vessels, and also the association, commissural, and projection axons that connect the neurons in the cortical mantle to other regions of the brain. Understanding these connections, as we will explore later in this book, is important for appreciating the mapping of tractography using DTI imaging and applying this to the normal and injured state of the brain. While the association fibers connect cortical regions within the same hemisphere, commissural fibers connect to the opposite hemisphere and projection fibers connect to lower portions of the brain and, eventually, the spinal cord. An example of a projection fiber is the corticospinal tract. Association fibers may be very short, connecting close regions of the cortex, or may be long and may gather in bundles, gaining and losing axons along their path. Significant long-association bundles include the superior and inferior longitudinal fasciculi, superior and inferior occipitofrontal fasciculi, and many other association fiber tracts. Connecting the parietal, temporal, and occipital lobes is the accurate fasciculus, which provides communication between the receptive speech center (Wernicke's) and the motor speech center (Broca's). Commissural fibers, which connect mirror-image areas of the two opposite hemispheres, consist of the major connections known as the corpus callosum, the anterior commissure, the hippocampal commissure, and many smaller ones. The corpus callosum is the largest commissural system, and connects portions of the frontal lobes (including speech areas), parietal, temporal, and occipital lobes. (269, 478, 486, 530)

Efferent projection fibers descend from the cortex to caudal structures, including the basal ganglia, thalamus, brainstem motor nuclei, reticular formation, and spinal cord. There are also afferent projection fibers that ascend from the striatum and thalamus and deeper structures to the cortex. (269)

The internal capsule comprises the convergence of the efferent and afferent fibers that connect to the cortex in a fan-shaped corona radiata. Many of the fibers are thalamic radiations, but the remainder travel to lower structures. Below the internal capsule, fibers travel inferiorly to become the cerebral peduncle in the midbrain. There are many other intricate connections, which are beyond the scope of this discussion. (269)

The thalamus functions as a relay station that integrates, coordinates, and modulates communication between numerous systems and is involved with motor, sensory, arousal, cognitive, limbic, memory, and behavioral functions. The thalamus receives all ascending sensory tracts (with the exception of olfaction) and then projects them to the cortex. There are many other intricate functions of the thalamus, which are beyond the scope of this discussion. (269, 478)

Association areas of the brain can be broken down into modality-specific (unimodal) and high-order (heteromodal). Each primary sensory area is combined with a modality-specific sensory association area. The somatosensory unimodal association cortex is located in the parietal lobe directly posterior to the primary somatosensory areas. The visual unimodal association cortex surrounds the primary visual striate cortex. The auditory unimodal association cortex flanks the primary auditory cortex. The high-order heteromodal association areas (polymodal or supramodal) receive afferent from other unimodal areas, other heteromodal areas, and paralimbic areas. It may be that most of the human neocortex is occupied by association areas and their boundaries are different than those cytoarchitectonic fields described by Brodmann and others. (530)

Brainstem and cerebellum

The brainstem is situated above the spinal cord and below the cerebral hemispheres, passes motor and sensory fibers between the two, and is responsible for consciousness, involuntary life sustaining functions (breathing, regulation of the heart), and other functions. The brainstem contains the midbrain, pons, and medulla. The reticular activating system is responsible for arousal. Long tracts ascending and descending through the brainstem include the spinothalamic tact, corticospinal tract, and others. The majority of the cranial nerves have their nuclei in the brainstem and they enable sensory and motor function of the head and neck. Roughly 90% (about 20 million) of the axons that pass through the midbrain synapse on neurons in the pons, and relay information to the cerebellum through this "switchboard" (pons derives from the Latin word for "bridge"), which is responsible for the ventral bulge of the pons. (269, 478)

The cerebellum rests in the posterior fossa and is connected to the brainstem by the cerebellar peduncles. There are four layers in the adult cerebellar cortex, which from superficial to deep are: 1) the molecular layer, 2) the Purkinje cell layer, 3) the granular layer, and 4) the white matter. There are both inhibitory neurons (Purkinje, Golgi, stellate, and basket cells) and excitatory neurons (granule and unipolar brush cells). Granule cells project their axons to the molecular layer to form parallel fibers that synapse with inhibitory neurons of the molecular layer. Mossy (from the brainstem and spinal cord) and climbing fibers are excitatory. (622) Purkinje cells carry inhibitory signals to the cerebellar nuclei. The anatomy is shown in **Figure 6.3**. A fluorescent light micrograph also shows the Purkinje cells and surrounding architecture in **Figure 6.4**.

The cerebellum helps with the coordination of movement, by choreographing the simultaneous movement of opposing muscle groups (agonist muscles, antagonist muscles, synergist muscles and fixating muscles) to deliver smooth movement in the body. Injury to the cerebellum may cause uncoordinated and disorganized movement of the body, tremor, slowed movement, impaired rapid alternating movements, hypotonia, dysarthria, and nystagmus. (272, 478)

Anatomy of vision and balance

The central nervous system connections which control and monitor vision and balance are extremely important. These networks span the brain from the brainstem to the cerebral hemispheres, and are readily evaluated with a neurological evaluation in the office, as well as by additional testing. In the event of abnormalities, a neuro-ophthalmologist and a neuro-otologist may be consulted to add significant insight.

The anatomy of vision and the anatomy of balance are discussed in Chapter 11, "Long-term prognosis and outcome" of TBI.

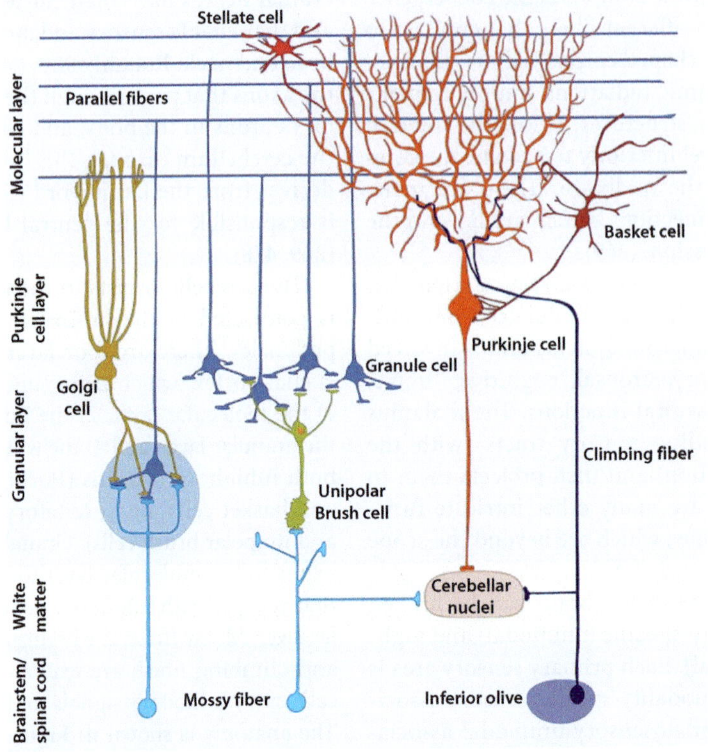

Figure 6.3 A schematic cytoarchitecture of cerebellum, showing four layers (molecular, Purkinje cell, granular, and white matter). Both inhibitory neurons (Purkinje, Golgi, stellate, and basket cells) and excitatory neurons (granule and unipolar brush cells) are present. Purkinje cell axons send inhibitory signals to cerebellar nuclei, while mossy and climbing fiber collaterals send excitatory afferents to the cerebellar nuclei. Source (622) https://creativecommons.org/licenses/by/4.0/legalcode

White matter tract connections

While cortical regions and their associated function are very important, it is the white matter fibers that allow for complex interactions by working together in a symphony of information exchange and processing that is almost incomprehensible. Disruption of white matter connections may result in disconnection syndromes. Studying the detailed connections between neurons and the connectome is extremely difficult because synapses can be precisely identified only by using electron microscopy, requiring very thin 50 nm sections of tissue (478)

Most of the white matter of the cerebral hemispheres is composed of connection fibers. The white matter connections within the brain are responsible for many higher functions and damage to them may result in various disconnection syndromes. (352, 355) In 1956, Ludwig and Klingler created an excellent atlas entitled *Atlas Cerebri Humani* in which brains from cadavers were prepared using the Klingler method. Using a Swiss watchmaker's forceps and a spatula of soft and elastic linden wood, under visual Loupe magnification, meticulous white matter tract dissections were performed and photographed. (560)

DTI is an excellent advanced magnetic resonance imaging tool that evaluates the white matter structure of the brain. The brain has white matter tracts, many of which can be seen on DTI images (depending on the hardware and software) using tractography tools. They can be classified into three main groups (projection, association, and commissural fibers) with additional tracts as discussed depending upon which regions of the brain they connect:

- *Projection fibers:* Connect the cortex with the brainstem, cerebellum, and spinal cord and can be seen on DTI (corticospinal, corticobulbar, and corticopontine fibers; thalamic radiations, geniculocalcarine fibers [optic radiations]).

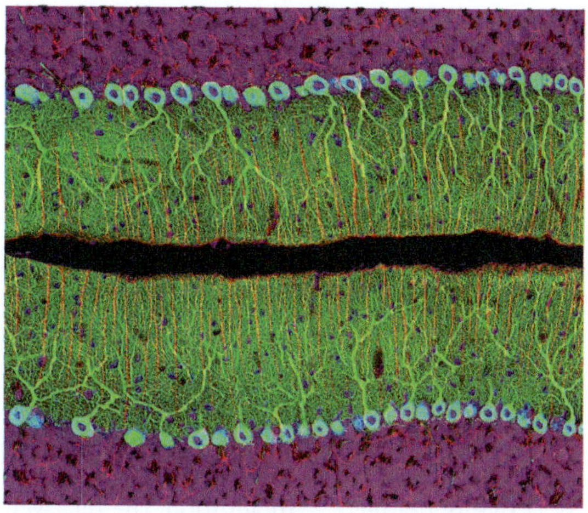

Figure 6.4 A fluorescent light micrograph of Purkinje cells (green) in the cerebellum of the brain. Purkinje nerve cells have a flask-like body from which numerous highly branched dendrites extend. They are found in the gray matter (cortex) of the cerebellum, at the boundary between the granular layer (purple/red) and the molecular layer (diffuse green). The dendrites relay signals to the cell body, which passes them on through its single axon in the granular layer. The cerebellum is a structure at the base of the brain that plays an important role in motor control, sensory perception, and learning. Magnification: 200 × when printed 10 cm wide. (From Thomas Deerinck, NCMIR / Science Source.)

- *Association fibers:* Connect cortical regions within the same hemisphere and most are reciprocal (cingulum, superior occipitofrontal fasciculus, inferior occipitofrontal fasciculus (inferior fronto-occipital fasciculus), uncinate fasciculus, superior longitudinal fasciculus, arcuate fasciculus, inferior longitudinal fasciculus).
- *Commissural fibers:* Connect analogous cortical regions (homotopic) or non-corresponding areas (heterotopic) of the two hemispheres (corpus callosum, anterior commissure, posterior commissure).
- *Additional tracts:* Fornix, cerebellar peduncles (inferior, middle, superior), stria terminalis, frontal aslant tract, central tegmental tract, decussation of the superior cerebellar peduncle, medial lemniscus. (321–323, 530)

Radwan has produced a comprehensive description of white matter anatomy using advanced magnetic resonance imaging and probabilistic constrained-spherical deconvolution. The arcuate fasciculus (AF) (**Figure 6.5a**), frontal aslant tracts (FAT) (**Figure 6.5b**), and inferior fronto-occipital fasciculus (IFOF) (**Figure 6.5c**) are shown. (336)

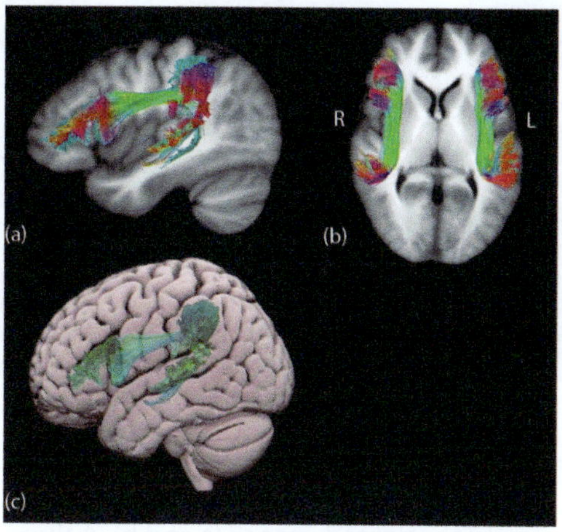

Figure 6.5a Arcuate fasciculi (AF) are overlaid in directional color coding on magnetic resonance imaging sagittal and axial slices of T1-weighted images (a and b). A three-dimensional lateral projection of the left arcuate fasciculus in green is superimposed on a semitransparent MNI pial surface (c). L = left, R = right, MNI = Montreal Neurological Institute. Adapted from (336) https://creativecommons.org/licenses/by/4.0/legalcode.

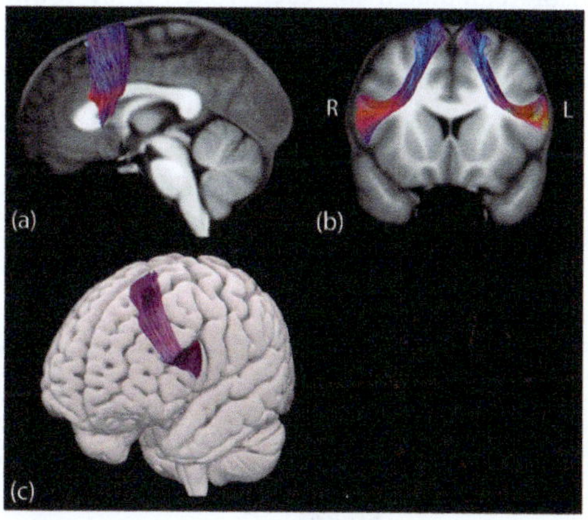

Figure 6.5b Frontal aslant tracts (FAT) are overlaid in directional color coding on magnetic resonance imaging sagittal and coronal slices of the T1-weighted images (a and b). A three-dimensional oblique anterior projection of the left FAT in purple is superimposed on a semitransparent MNI pial surface (c). L = left, R = right, MNI = Montreal Neurological Institute. Adapted from (336) https://creativecommons.org/licenses/by/4.0/legalcode.

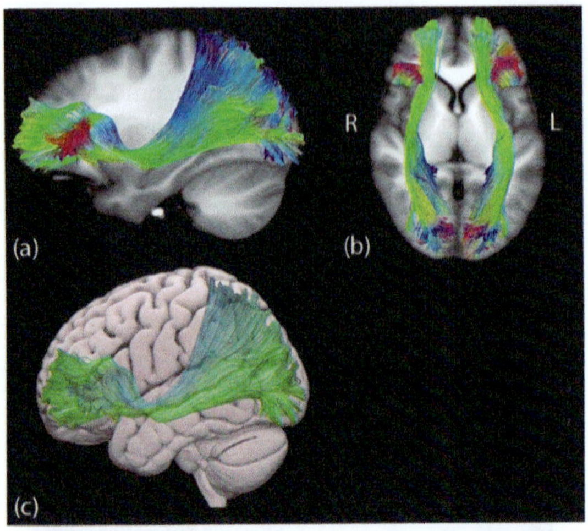

Figure 6.5c Inferior fronto-occipital fasciculi (IFOF) are overlaid in directional color coding on magnetic resonance imaging sagittal and axial slices of T1-weighted images (a and b). A three-dimensional lateral projection of the left IFOF in green is superimposed on a semitransparent MNI pial surface (c). L = left, R = right, MNI = Montreal Neurological Institute. Adapted from (336) https://creativecommons.org/licenses/by/4.0/legalcode.

In a study of the developing brain, 59 pediatric subjects underwent diffusion kurtosis imaging (DKI) imaging with diffusion and kurtosis tensors calculated for each voxel. They found a progressive increase in fractional anisotropy (FA) and mean kurtosis (MK) values for seven white-matter regions (genu/splenium of corpus callosum, frontal white matter, parietal white matter, anterior/posterior limbs of internal capsule (IC), external capsule(EC)) and two gray matter regions (thalamus, putamen), from ages birth to four years seven months **(Figure 6.6a and b)**. The corpus callosum showed higher FA and MK values than other white-matter regions. This increase in anisotropy in white matter occurs as myelination progresses and it is most notable in the first two years when, as Paydar cites Lebel, Mukherjee, Cheung, and Provenzale in stating, "myelination is the dominant contributor to the increase in the microstructural complexity of WM (white matter) .... In addition, the relatively higher FA in the corpus callosum throughout all ages may be attributed to its more tightly packed and anisotropic architecture." DKI can detect MK values, and since MK (like FA) increases in white matter regions, DKI has shown increases in anisotropy related to age, in the developing brain. This increase is likely due to an increase in myelination, as seen in DKI tractography images at birth, 6 months, 11 months, and 2 years and 1 month (Figure 6.7). The changes seen during growth are likely a function of progressing myelination. (438) Other studies also conclude that the brain microstructure develops rapidly in infancy and early childhood, mainly due to increased myelination. Into adulthood, the development of the brain microstructure continues, but may mainly due to axonal packing. (587)

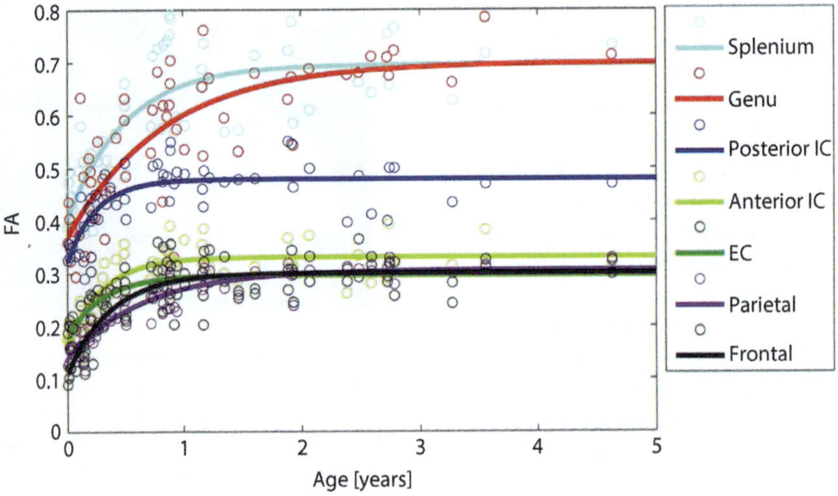

Figure 6.6a FA curves demonstrate a change in FA value as a function of age in seven white-matter regions. Reproduced with permission from American Society of Neuroradiology. (438)

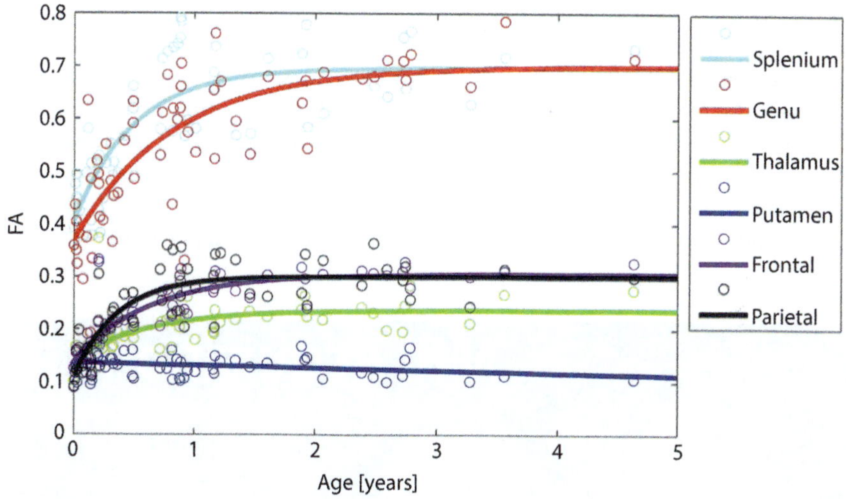

Figure 6.6b FA curves demonstrate a change in FA values as a function of age in two gray-matter regions (thalamus and putamen); FA curves for four white-matter regions from Figure 6.6a are also included in this graph for comparison. Reproduced with permission from American Society of Neuroradiology. (438)

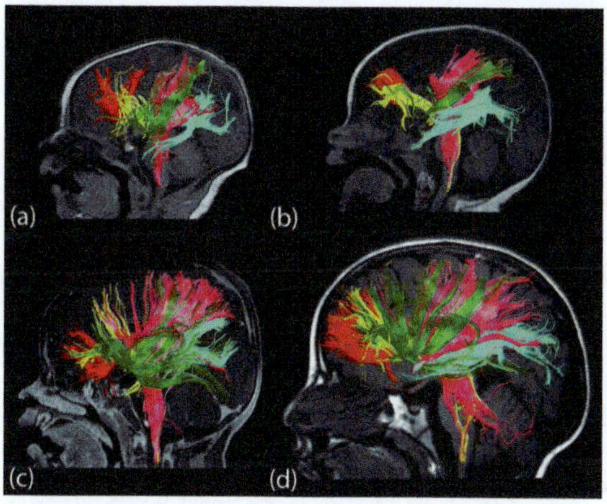

Figure 6.7 DKI tractography at various stages of development, including birth (a), 6 months (b), 11 months (c), and 2 years 1 month (d). Fiber tracking is displayed for the genu (red), splenium (cyan), anterior internal capsule (yellow), posterior internal capsule (pink), and external capsule (dark green). Reproduced with permission from American Society of Neuroradiology. (438)

The human connectome

On a yearly basis, more than 30,000 neuroscientists gather to share information, and yet there is still a tremendous amount that needs to be learned about how the brain works. While there is a good amount of knowledge about individual neurons and molecules as well as the gross organization of the brain, there is much knowledge missing about what happens in-between. The wiring diagram (connectome) is advancing with technology and research. (393)

Two approaches can be used to determine single-cell connectivity, with one being based on physiology and the other on electron microscopy. To map the entire circuit with single-neuron precision, a technique of barcoding individual neuronal connections can be used so that the analysis can be performed with high-throughput DNA sequencing. (394, 395) Brodmann in 1909 identified 52 regions of the brain. (341) Using multi-modal magnetic resonance images from the Human Connectome Project (HCP), 180 areas per hemisphere were delineated with the use of an objective semi-automated neuroanatomical approach (localizing sharp and reproducible parcellated brain images), of which 97 areas are new and 83 areas were previously reported using post-mortem microscopy. (340) Data from the HCP was utilized by the Brainnetome Project to create the *Brainnetome Atlas*, which contains 210 cortical regions and 36 subcortical regions with anatomical and functional connections. Multimodal MRI data used consisted of structural MRI, resting state functional MRI (fMRI), and diffusion MRI (dMRI). Major fiber bundles connecting subregions with the rest of the brain were identified using probabilistic fiber tractography. A connectivity matrix was created showing structural connectivity between all identified subregions for intrahemispheric and interhemispheric connections. (392)

Hagmann used DSI to map pathways within and across cortical hemispheres in human participants. They performed network analysis for 998 regions (average size of 1.5 cm^2), including the entire cortices of both hemispheres, but excluding subcortical nodes and connections. They used network measure metrics including degree, strength, betweenness, centrality, and efficiency. This work resulted in extraction of a whole brain structural connectivity network (**Figure 6.8**; 528).

Functional anatomy is not necessarily constrained by anatomic distinctions and even within one sulcus, the upper bank may be functionally

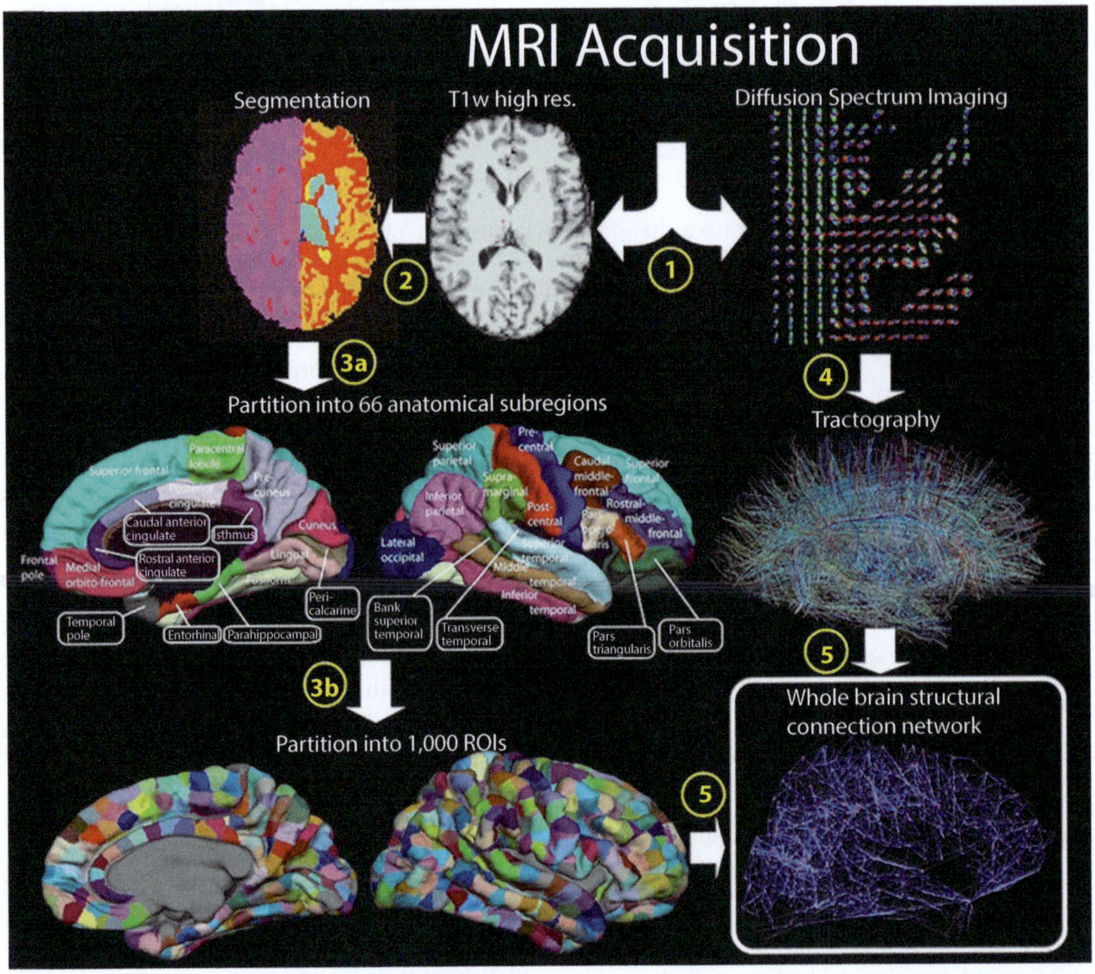

Figure 6.8 Extraction of a whole brain structural connectivity network. High-resolution T1-weighted and DSI is acquired. DSI is represented with a zoom on the axial slice of the reconstructed diffusion map, showing an orientation distribution function at each position represented by a deformed sphere whose radius codes for diffusion intensity. Blue codes for the superior-inferior, red for left-right, and green for anterior-posterior orientations (1). White and gray matter segmentation is performed from the T1-weighted image (2). Sixty-six cortical regions with clear anatomical landmarks are created (3a) and then individually subdivided into small regions of interest (ROIs) resulting in 998 ROIs (3b). Whole brain tractography is performed providing an estimate of axonal trajectories across the entire white matter (4). ROIs identified in step (3b) are combined with result of step (4) to compute the connection weight between each pair of ROIs (5). The result is a weighted network of structural connectivity across the entire brain. From (528) https://creativecommons.org/licenses/by/4.0/legalcode

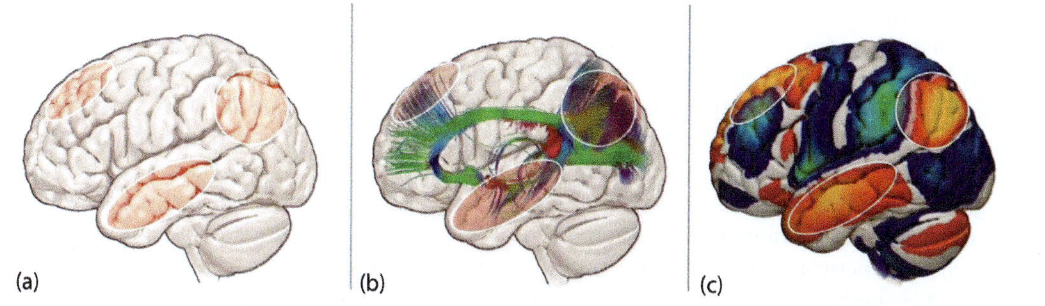

Figure 6.9 Lesions in different brain locations may cause the same symptoms (a) and can be overlaid on a map of anatomical connectivity (b) or functional connectivity (c). From (553) copyright 2018 Massachusetts Medical Society. Reprinted with permission from Massachusetts Medical Society.

distinct from the opposite side. (337) Transcranial magnetic stimulation has also been used for diagnosis and treatment, and has been used to perform functional mapping of the motor cortex as well. (347)

Insights into the human connectome may have importance in the attempt to preserve neurological function in a patient undergoing supratentorial surgery on the brain, as connectomics have contributed to the understanding of human language and other brain functions. (339) Knowledge of the human connectome and the connectivity of functional regions of the brain (**Figure 6.9**; 553) is also helping to gain insight into lesion network mapping, where lesions that cause the same symptom may be located in different brain locations. Improvements in maps of the human connectome may serve as a valuable resource for mapping complex neurologic and neuropsychiatric symptoms. (553) It is possible that all areas of the brain have a significant role, but injury to some regions may be more noticeable in day-to-day life than it is to other regions of the brain. As an example, disorders of emotional regulation have been seen commonly after injury to the right prefrontal cortex. (338)

Instead of thinking of regions of the brain as silent, these areas may instead be portions that are redundant in function. If so, this changes the concept of eloquent versus non-eloquent areas of the brain and, rather, suggests these are areas of the brain that, if injured through trauma, may have obvious or more subtle changes in the functioning of a patient. (337)

Another way of asking this important question is to ponder whether it is likely that a portion of the brain can be damaged and remain silent to the functioning of an individual or whether it is more likely that we do not yet have the proper tools or are not correctly using the tools which we have to assess the damage? Much of the brain's higher executive function may not be easily recognized if there is a small amount of damage, but does our inability to recognize the effect of brain injury mean that the brain is functioning normally?

The brain, especially in the young, has significant powers of recuperation and, despite the loss of an essential node, the brain's capacity to re-route and re-express itself may enable the individual to slowly regain lost function. (529)

By appreciating how exquisite and delicate the brain is on both a macroscopic and microscopic level, it is easy to recognize how trauma to the brain, with compressive, translational, rotational and shearing forces, can tear vital connections to and within the brain, and can result in neurological, cognitive, functional, and neuropsychological changes ranging from subtle to dramatic.

Large-scale brain networks

A number of large-scale networks within the brain are involved with higher executive processing. These networks are highly complex, functionally and anatomically connected, involve interaction of different regions of the brain, and are interconnected to enable higher executive functioning. These networks include the default mode network, salience network, central executive network, dorsal and ventral attention networks, sensorimotor system, language system, limbic system, and visual system.

The largest of the multiple networks of functionally correlated brain areas is the default-mode network (DMN). (564) This network has been evaluated with tractography and fMRI, participates in internal modes of cognition, and may have a higher level of activity when an individual is not focused on the external environment. Multiple cortical areas of the brain may be involved including the medial temporal lobes, medial prefrontal regions, cingulate cortex, and lateral parietal lobes, as well as the thalamus and basal forebrain. (563–565) This network may comprise multiple dissociated components, which become active depending upon the mental task one is undertaking. (566) This network may have relevance for understanding mental disorders including autism, schizophrenia, and Alzheimer's disease. (565)

The salience network, the essential function of which remains uncertain, refers to brain regions whose cortical hubs are the anterior cingulate and ventral anterior insular cortices (includes the amygdala, hypothalamus, ventral striatum, thalamus and specific brainstem nuclei). (631) The network, with its integral hub located within the insula, functions to segregate the most relevant of internal and extrapersonal stimuli, in order to guide behavior, and generate appropriate behavioral responses to salient stimuli. (632) Seeley cites Goodkind and Sha in noting that clinical examples of dysfunction of or alterations in the connectivity of the salience network are disorders of social-emotional function, including behavioral variant frontotemporal dementia, schizophrenia, bipolar disorder, major depression, attention-deficit/hyperactivity, anxiety states, autism, spectrum, and substance abuse disorders. (631)

The insula, which plays a role in the salience network, may also have a role in facilitating the central executive network and the default mode network. The executive network includes the dorsolateral prefrontal cortex (DLPFC) and the anterior cingulate cortex (ACC). Heinonen cites Geary, Ellamil, Beaty, and Raichle in noting that the executive network and the default mode network appear to have an important role in creative thought. Heinonen found that the central executive network, default mode network, and the salience network support focused and goal-oriented creative processes. (633)

The dorsal attention network and the ventral attention network interact dynamically with each other to provide flexible attention control. Both systems are specialized for attentional subprocesses such as controlled attentional selection and the detection of unexpected but relevant stimuli. (634) In a study of patients who suffered a moderate to severe TBI, studies using fMRI and DTI revealed that successful memory encoding was associated with activation of the dorsal attention network, the ventral visual stream, and medial temporal lobes, with decreased activation in the DMN. Those who had impaired memory, had decreased left anterior prefrontal activity, and white matter microstructure of the encoding networks was significantly reduced. (635)

Unilateral spatial neglect is common after a patient experiences an injury to the right cerebral hemisphere. An alternative to attributing the neglect to structural damage of specific brain regions, it may possibly be explained by dysfunction of distributed cortical networks. Deficits may involve coding of saliency, control of spatial attention, as well as deficits of reorienting, target detection, and arousal/vigilance. Reduced arousal and vigilance may be important components of neglect, and Corbetta notes that patients with right hemisphere injuries suffer from lower arousal than those with left hemisphere injuries. (636)

Other important networks include the sensorimotor system, language system, visual system, and limbic system.

A retrospective study was performed on 100 consecutive patients who underwent surgery for intra-axial brain tumor resection. Using the Quicktome platform (Omniscient Neurotechnology) to analyze preoperative brain MRI studies with T1-weighted and DTI sequences, evaluation was performed on the peroperative integrity of nine large-scale brain networks: language, sensorimotor, visual, ventral attention, central executive, default mode, dorsal attention, salience, and limbic. Those patients who experienced noticeable neurologic deficits had a higher number of altered networks (average of 3.42 networks) when compared to those who did not (average of 2.19 networks). Eighty-seven percent of patients had at least one large-scale network affected peroperatively. The highest incidence of affected networks in descending order were as follows: central executive network, default mode network, dorsal attention network, language network, ventral attention network, and visual network (the least affected). The authors point out that a preoperative neuropschological assessment was not performed, which they indicate created some limitation of the neurological examination. (630)

Lesion network mapping

Through use of the connectome, it is possible to study and link lesions in different locations of the brain that may cause the same symptom (**Figure 6.10**; 553). The disconnection of connecting pathways may lead to disconnection syndromes. This lesion network mapping has been utilized to study psychiatric symptoms as well as pain, coma, and cognitive or social dysfunction. Traditionally, different regions of the brain have been thought to subserve specific functions, but it has been seen that lesions that disrupt certain functions are often located remotely from the location typically attributed to that function. Despite being remote from the extrastriate visual cortex, lesions in the brainstem can cause visual hallucinations. (437, 553) Fox cites Catani, Fornito, Carrera, Von Monakow, and Geschwind

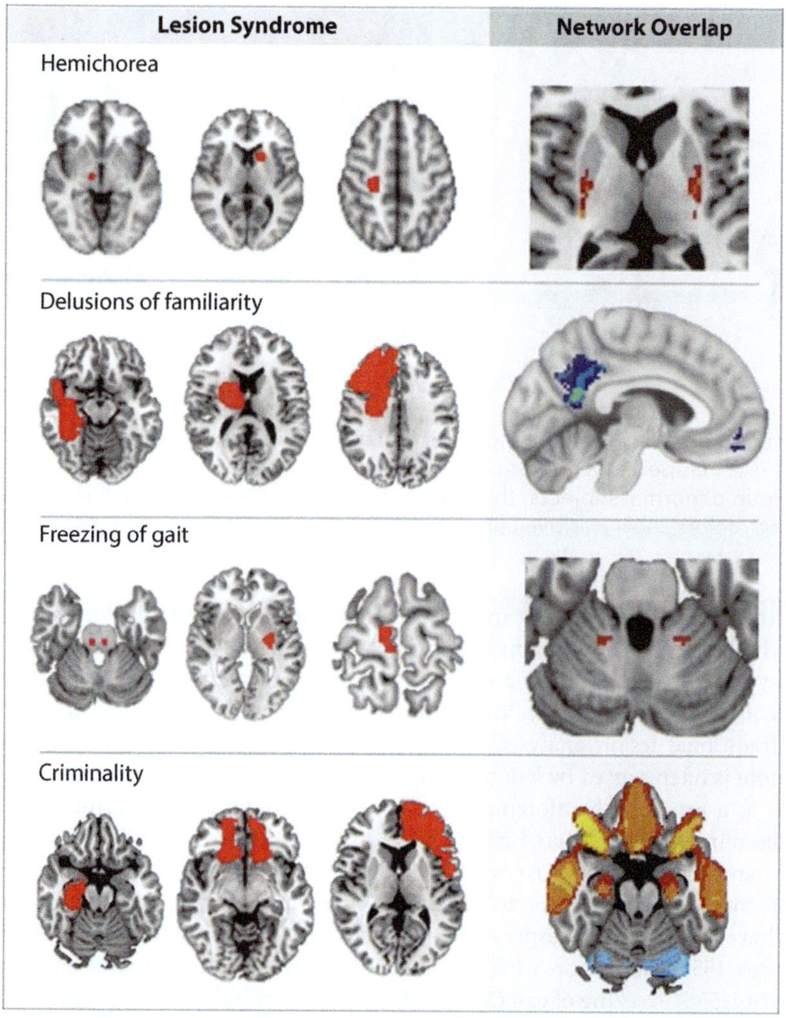

Figure 6.10 Lesion network mapping of neuropsychiatric symptoms with unknown localization. Many symptoms are caused by lesions in different locations (three examples for each symptom are shown in red). More than 90% of lesion locations that cause the same symptom are functionally connected to the same brain regions (right column). Lesion locations that cause hemichorea are connected to the posterolateral putamen, a region implicated in motor control. Lesion locations that cause delusions of familiarity are connected to the retrosplenial cortex, a region activated by familiar stimuli. Lesion locations that cause freezing of gait are connected to the dorsal medial cerebellum, a region activated by locomotion tasks. Lesion locations that are associated with criminality are connected to the orbitofrontal cortex, a region activated by moral decision making. From (553) copyright 2018 Massachusetts Medical Society. Reprinted with permission from Massachusetts Medical Society.

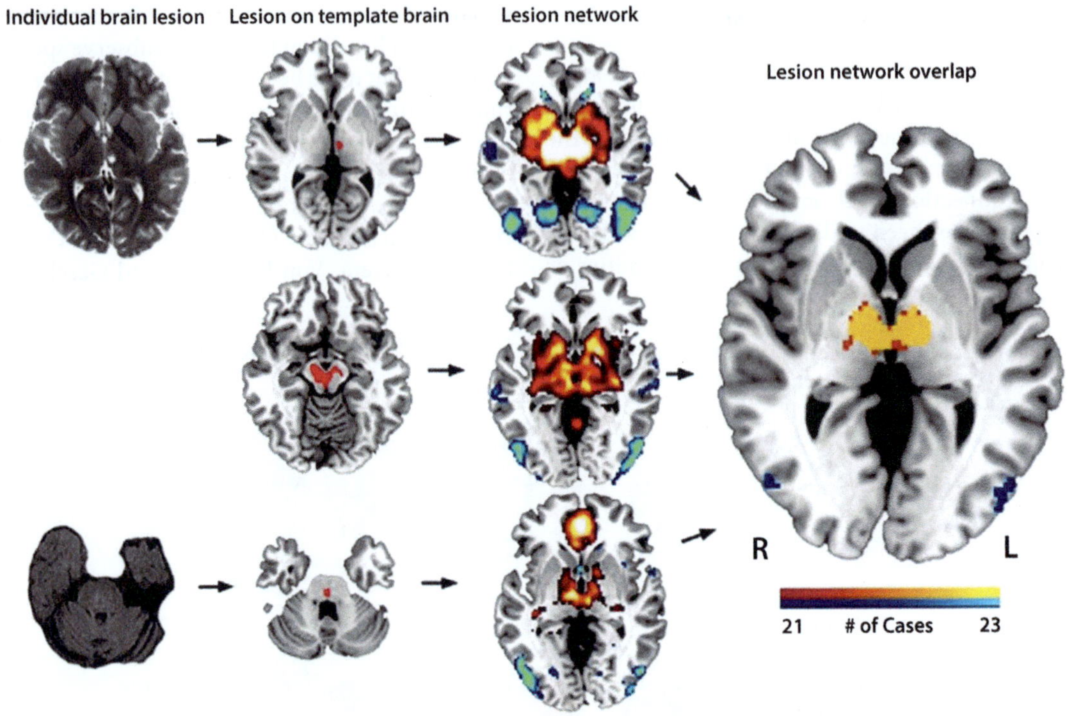

Figure 6.11 Twenty-three lesions resulting in peduncular hallucinosis were identified, three of which are illustrated here, mapped to a reference brain (column 2). Using resting state functional connectivity from a large group of normal subjects, the brain network associated with each lesion was determined (column 3). "Hot" colors show positive correlations and "cool" colors show negative correlations. (437)

in finding that the human connectome can be used to determine whether lesions at different sites can cause similar symptoms if those sites are within the same brain network. Fox stated, "this is an advance over traditional lesion analysis, because the same symptom is often caused by lesions in different locations as a result of the aforementioned connectivity, disconnection and diaschisis." (553) Hub locations may have significant roles in various aspects of cognition and injury to specific locations may have severe and widespread cognitive consequences. (554) Hemichorea (555), delusions of familiarity (556), freezing of gait (557), and criminality (558) have been studied by Fox and colleagues. Importantly, it was found that lesions that cause the same symptom are part of a single brain network despite possibly being located in different regions of the brain and they are defined by their functional connectivity (**Figure 6.10**; 553).

A study looking at network localization of neurological symptoms from focal brain lesions produced interesting findings. Patients with peduncular hallucinations (visual hallucinations following subcortical lesions) (**Figure 6.11**; 437), central post-stroke pain, auditory hallucinations, and subcortical aphasia were evaluated. Due to overlap in functional connectivity networks, lesions may produce similar neurological deficits even though they were present in different locations, because despite their differing locations, they affect the functional connectivity of the brain. (437)

Diffuse axonal injury may cause neurological impairment by disrupting brain networks. An example of a late complication of this may interact with neuroinflammation and neurodegeneration in the pathogenesis of Alzheimer's disease and chronic traumatic encephalopathy. (713)

FUNCTION

Assessing function of the cortical regions and white-matter tracts is difficult, in part because it is not possible to evaluate anatomy through brain sectioning in a living person. Approaches to evaluating brain function have relied upon 1) neurological, neuropsychological, and psychiatric evaluation of patients with brain injuries; 2) *in-vivo* diagnostic studies which in combination provide information about both structure and function, such as MRI, DTI, fMRI, positron emission tomography (PET), electroencephalography (EEG), magnetoencephalography (MEG), etc.); and 3) post-mortem examination. (355)

With the understanding that function of the brain is not restricted to an isolated area of the brain and that the connectome is important, there are certain regions that are viewed as critical for a large component of function. As brain anatomy and function are entwined in a most intricate, subtle, and interconnected manner, it is not truly possible to ascribe function to one particular locus of the brain, although it is convenient to do so and we must do our best with the tools which we have at present. As David Poeppel has stated "a statement such as 'Broca's area underpins language production' (or 'speech,' or 'syntax' or other broad categories of linguistic experience) is not just grossly underspecified, it is ultimately both misleading and incorrect. Broca's region is not monolithic but instead is comprised of numerous subregions as specified by cytoarchitecture, immunocytochemistry, laminar properties, and so on." Even the domains of language, which we refer to as "syntax," are descriptors of complex underlying representations and computations. (400)

Frontal lobe function

Function of the frontal lobes involves the motor strip, premotor and supplementary motor areas, prefrontal region, frontal eye fields, and motor speech areas. The motor cortex contains the large Betz motor neuron cells and transmits signals through the corticospinal and corticobulbar tracts. Injury can affect movement on the contralateral side of the body. The premotor cortex, which is just anterior to the motor cortex, participates in the planning and execution of movements. The supplementary motor cortex is involved in planning movements from memory and coordinates movements of both hands. Lesions of the supplementary motor area may cause difficulty with movement to command in the contralateral limbs, hemineglect, and apraxia. Injury to the frontal eye fields may cause an ipsilateral gaze, while seizures in this area cause a contralateral gaze. Injury to the motor speech area (Broca's area) may cause aphasia. Frontal lobe lesions are also associated with incontinence and gait disorders. (270)

The prefrontal cortex is important in daily life, as it is involved in the executive control of behavior. When there is damage to this region, a patient's perceptual ability, motor behavior, and intelligence may appear to be normal, but they may be unable to function effectively in everyday life. They may be unable to travel alone, as they may board the first bus that arrives. A job such as serving in a restaurant may become impossible due to the inability to respond to competing demands. (270, 284)

- Frontal lobe disorders:
  - Cognitive (memory, attention, executive problems), neurological symptoms (dizziness, headaches, vertigo, imbalance, movement), neuropsychiatric/emotional impairment (depression, anxiety, irritability, mania, impulsivity, disinhibition); Broca's aphasia (speech) (typically left hemisphere).

    Additional details of symptomatology provided below.

The prefrontal cortex has function related to the planning and execution of tasks and utilizes its ability to benefit from experience. It is involved with abstraction, motivation and cognitive flexibility, oculomotor control, voluntary eye movements and inhibition of reflex saccadic eye movements, perception, anticipation of outcomes, decision-making, sense of time, personality, calculating, and thinking. The DLPFC is involved with organization of self-ordered tasks, and along with the cingulate cortex, is critical for the monitoring of events in the working memory. Injury may interfere with these functions, and due to connections with the limbic system, may cause disinhibition syndromes ranging from inappropriate behavior to mania, emotional lability, poor judgment and insight, distractibility, sexual promiscuity, memory loss for recent events, inability to conduct business affairs or personal finance, inability to deal with new problems, loss of attentiveness, loss of ability to acquire and associate new material, fatigue, emotional lability and mood swings, outbursts of crying or rage or laughter, apathy, indifference, abulia (difficulty initiating and completing movements and decreased display of emotions, speech and social interaction), slowed intellectual processing of problems, difficulty linking the past with the present, confusion, and disorientation. When there are significant bifrontal injuries, akinetic mutism or unresponsiveness may occur. (270, 284, 325, 486, 514)

A summary of the vast array of symptoms and syndromes which can occur with frontal lobe lesions falls into several categories:

- *Impaired initiation:* apathy, abulia, hypobulia, akinetic mutism, athymhormia, anhedonia, affective flattenint, attentional impairment, emotional withdrawal, impaired abstract thinking, incoherence.
- *Disinhibition:* echopraxia, echolalia, social disintegration, loss of judgment, loss of insight, inappropriate social behavior, loss of empathy, irritability, aggression, excessive jocularity, hyperactivity, hypersexuality.
- *Working memory:* difficulty multitasking, dysmemory, decreased ability to make decisions, decreased ability to plan and sequence events, difficulty searching memory and activating past memories.
- *Attention:* impaired alertness, decreased set/sensory/motor readiness, decreased interference control.
- *Monitoring:* perseveration, impersistence, ideational apraxias.
- *Emotional control:* impaired empathy/social behavior impairment (euphoria, depression, inability to control emotions).
- *Language:* Broca's aphasia (usually left hemisphere), expressive aprosodia (usually right hemisphere), aphemia (nonfluent speech, normal comprehension and writing, initial muteness).
- *Motor:* eye movement disorders, alien hand syndrome, contralateral body weakness.
- *Behavioral:* obsessive compulsive disorder, other symptoms described above. (325, 484, 485, 487)

The lesion that Phineas Gage (injured railroad worker discussed previously) suffered was a left prefrontal injury. (270, 284, 325, 486, 514) Using computer models, it has been found that while the left frontal lobe did experience significant damage, there was a large impact on the connectedness between directly affected and other brain areas, likely having a great effect on both acute and long-term behavior (**Figure 6.12a, b**; 523 and **Figure 6.12c**).

Parietal lobe function

Function of the parietal lobes involves the reception, correlation, analysis, integration, and interpretation of sensory signals from the thalamus. Hoffman cited Cavanna in finding that based upon functional imaging, the precuneus (portion of the parietal lobe) has the highest metabolic activity of all brain regions, and this region is involved in the integration of different neural networks responsible for self-consciousness. The primary sensory cortex, the initial reception center for afferent impulses, receives signals for tactile, pressure, and position sensation. Injury may result in loss of sensation from the contralateral side of the body. The sensory association areas synthesize and interpret these inputs, enabling appreciation of similarities and differences, spatial relationships, recognition of changes in form and weight, two dimensional qualities, and localization of sensory input. It integrates somatosensory, visual, and auditory information through connections with the temporal and occipital lobes. Injury to this association cortex area may affect recognition (gnosis) of sensation, with associative functions being impaired while retaining simple primary sensory abilities. Injury to the parietal association cortex may cause deficits of higher-level sensory function, including two-point discrimination, tactile localization, stereognosis, and graphesthesia. When a patient experiences an injury to the non-dominant parietal lobe, they may suffer apraxia, hemineglect, hemi-attention, and anosognosia. (270, 325)

- **Deficits related to right or left parietal lesion syndromes:**
    - *Cortical sensory impairment:* Tactile agnosia; astereognosis (loss of depth perception); impairment of two-point discrimination; agraphesthesia (impairment of palm number tracing); ahylognosia (difficulty recognizing density of material such as liquid, metal, wood); abaragnosia.
    - *Visuospatial disturbances:* Balint's syndrome (Simultagnosia: Inability to perceive more than one object at a time; visual apraxia and ataxia); optokinetic reflex

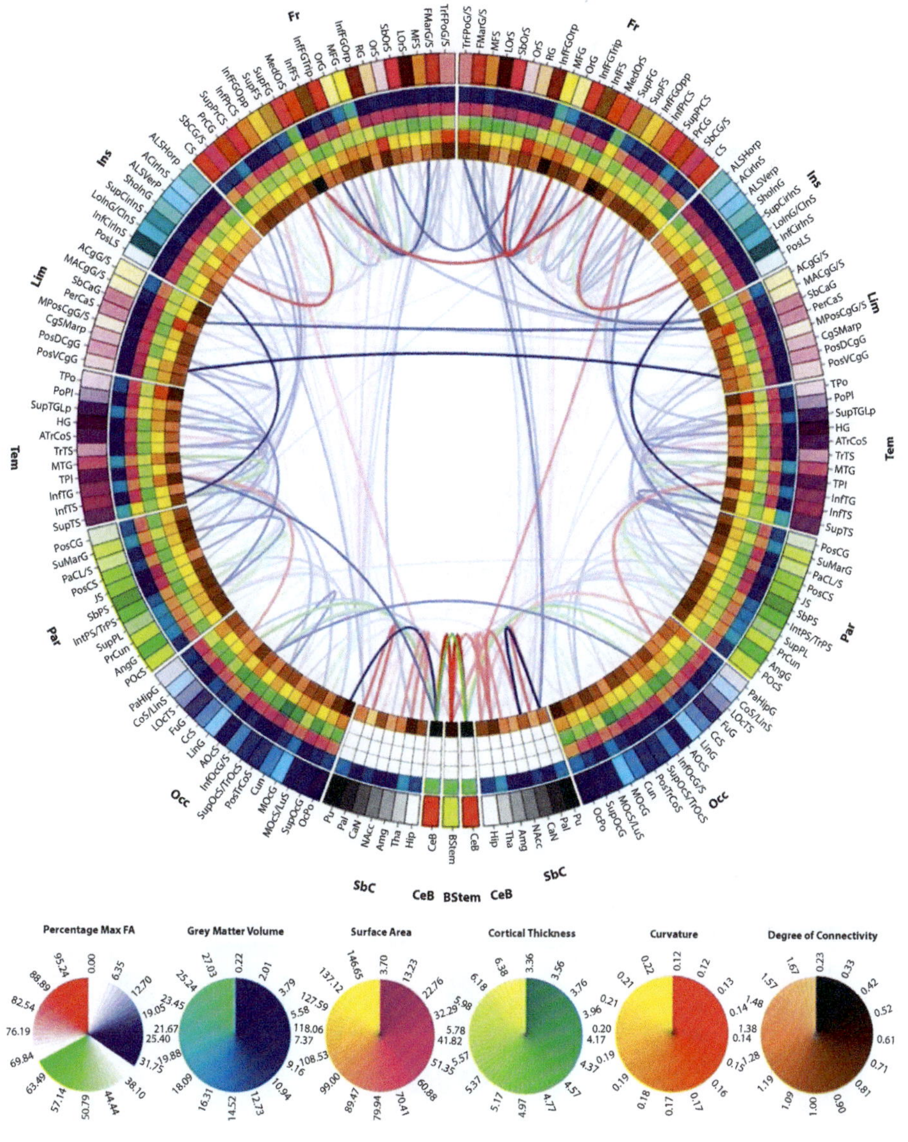

Figure 6.12a A connectogram of normal cortical anatomy and white-matter connectivity, which was obtained from 110 normal right-handed males. The outermost ring shows the various brain regions arranged by lobe. fr = frontal; ins = insula; lim = limbic; tem = temporal; par = parietal; occ = occipital; nc = non-cortical; bs = brainstem; CeB = cerebellum, and further ordered anterior-to-posterior based upon the center-of-mass of these regions in the published (Destrieux atlas [Ref 524]). The left half of the connectogram represents the left hemisphere of the brain and the right half represents the right hemisphere. The five sets of rings (from outside to inside) represent average (1) regional volume, (2) surface area, (3) cortical thickness, (4) cortical curvature of each parcellated region, and (5) the innermost ring shows the relative degree of connectivity of a specific region with respect to white-matter fibers emanating from that region, indicating the degree of connectivity of that region with others. The links show degrees of connectivity with other regions, with blue representing DTI tracts in the lower third of distribution of FA, green in the middle third, and red in the top third. The circular color bars at the bottom describe the numeric scale for each regional geometric measurement and its associated color on that anatomical metric ring of the connectogram. The circular "color bars" at the bottom of the figure describe the numeric scale for each regional geometric measurement and its associated color on that anatomical metric ring of the connectogram. From (523) https://creativecommons.org/licenses/by/4.0/legalcode

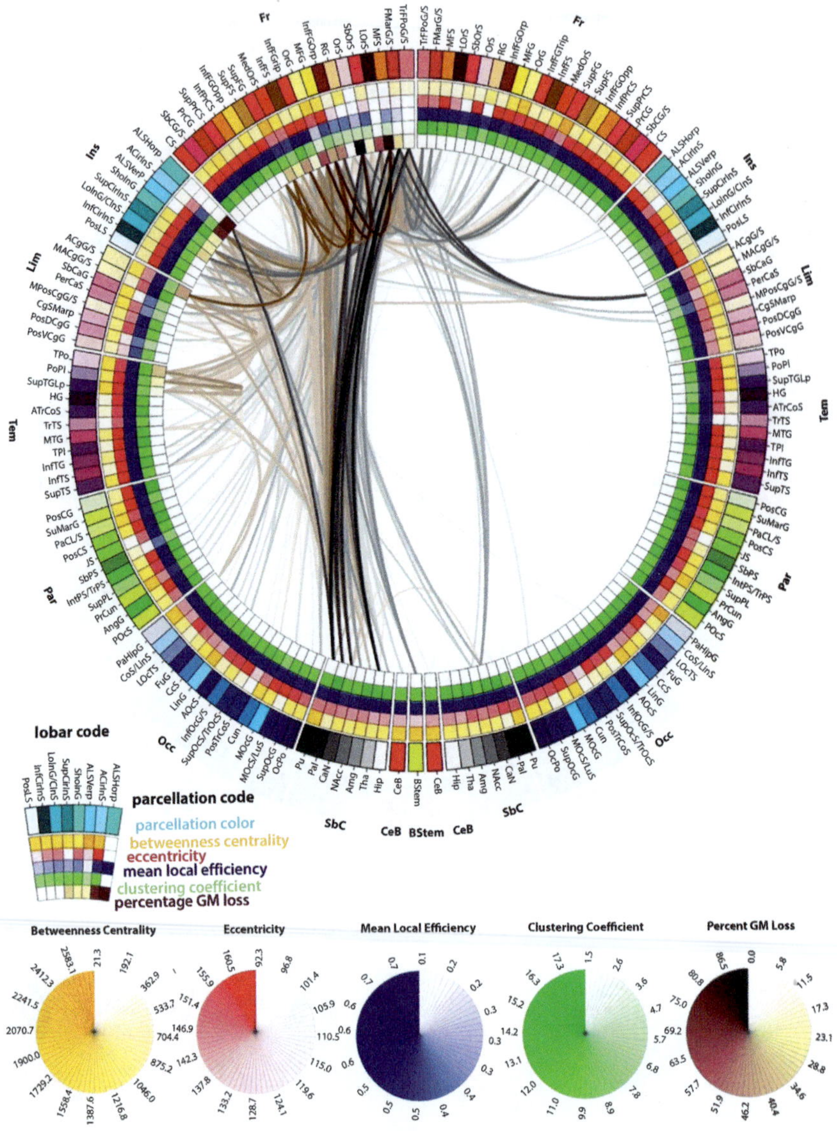

Figure 6.12b A computer-modeled connectogram of Phineas Gage, who suffered a penetrating injury from a tamping iron traversing a portion of the left frontal region. The lines in this represent the connections between brain regions that were lost or damaged by the passage of the tamping iron. Fiber pathway damage extended beyond the left frontal cortex to regions of the left temporal, partial, and occipital cortices as well as to basal ganglia, brain stem, and cerebellum. Inter-hemispheric connections of the frontal and limbic lobes as well as basal ganglia were also affected. Connections in grayscale indicate those pathways that were completely lost in the presence of the tamping iron, while those in shades of tan indicate those partially severed. Pathway transparency indicates the relative density of the affected pathway. The inner four rings of this connectogram indicate (from the outside inward) the regional network metrics of betweenness centrality, regional eccentricity, local efficiency, clustering coefficient, and the percent of GM loss, respectively, in the presence of the tamping iron, in each instance averaged over the N = 110 subjects. (From the USC Mark and Mary Stevens Neuroimaging and Informatics Institute [www.ini.usc.edu]; From (523) Dr. Arthur W. Toga, Director; Sidney Taiko Sheehan, Communications Manager; Jim Stanis, Medical Illustrator.) https://creativecommons.org/licenses/by/4.0/legalcode

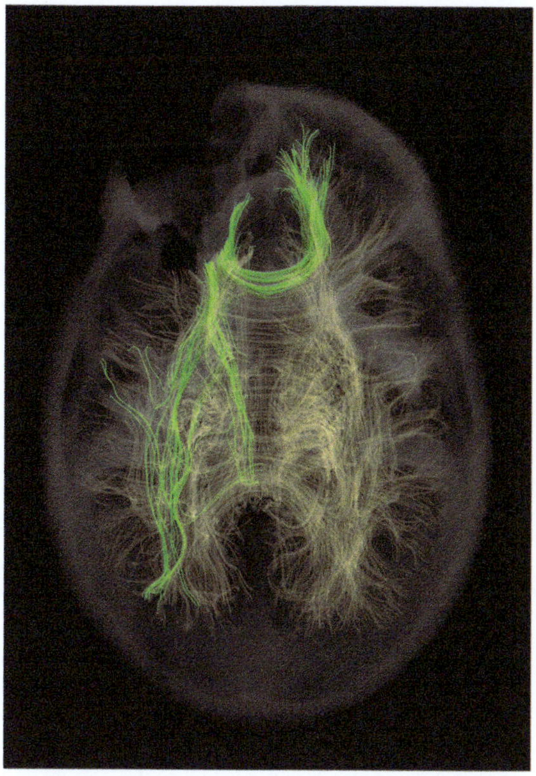

Figure 6.12c Possible extent of left frontal lobe white-matter fiber damage in Phineas Gage's brain due to injury to by tamping iron. (From the USC Mark and Mary Stevens Neuroimaging and Informatics Institute [www.ini.usc.edu]; Dr. Arthur W. Toga, Director; Sidney Taiko Sheehan, Communications Manager; Jim Stanis, Medical Illustrator.)

and nystagmus affected; smooth pursuit/saccadic eye movement disorders.

- *Precuneus and claustrum:* Attention and consciousness hubs, which, if injured, may result in minimally conscious or transcendental states.
- *Temporo-occipito-parietal junction and other cross-modal abnormalities:* Autoscopy (seeing one's double from an out-of-body experience); acquired synesthesia (sensory stimulus in one modality triggers sensations in another modality); Cotard's syndrome (as Hoffman cited Ramirez-Bermudez); autokinesis (impression of movement of objects in the dark).
- Sensory impairment for opposite side of body (hot, cold, numbness, proprioception, pain); deficits with pain processing; phantom limb pain.
- Conversion disorders. (325, 503, 512, 530)

- **Impairment of the left parietal lobe**: Anomias; apraxias; Gerstman's syndrome (acalculia, agraphia, finger anomia, difficulty with right/left orientation), autotopagnosia. (325, 488, 501)
- **Impairment of the right parietal lobe**: Aprosodia (difficulty comprehending or expressing changes in tone of voice); visuoconstructive impairment; neglect syndromes; visuospatial impairment; anosognosia (inability of brain to recognize illness of itself or the individual's own body); geographic disorientation (inability to orient oneself in their surroundings); allesthesia (perception of one receiving a stimulus on the body that is remote to where it was actually applied); impairment of three-dimensional sense appreciation; phonagnosia (inability to recognize familiar voices); dressing apraxia; event timing; perception of sound movements. (325)
- **Left hemisphere disorders**: Apraxia.
- **Right hemisphere disorders** (right hemisphere is important for attention attributes in both hemispheres (left hemisphere is responsible for attention only contralaterally) and emotion: Difficulty with attention, prosody, neglect, anosognosia for hemiparesis, visuospatial function). (325)

As noted by Nieuwenhuys, in right-handed individuals, the left hemisphere is mainly involved with verbal and linguistic functions, mathematical skills, and analytical thinking. The right hemisphere in those persons is primarily involved with spatial relationships, musical and artistic functions, and recognition and expression of emotions. (530) Along with functional differences are also structural differences. Broca's speech region (Brodmann areas 44 and 45) was found to have significantly higher cell densities in area 44 (not in area 45) on the left than the right side of the brain, in five out of five male and three out of five female brains. (361) In situations when a right-handed individual experiences aphasia following damage to the left hemisphere, homologous areas of their right hemisphere have, at times, been able to compensate, but if this does occur, it may need time to develop. (360)

Occipital lobe function

Function of the occipital lobes includes visual, perception of color, size, form, motion, and illumination impressions. The primary visual cortex (striate cortex) receives primary visual impressions, such as color, size, form and motion. While electrical stimulation or seizure activity may produce unformed visual hallucinations (such as light flashes), lesions in this area produce visual field defects. The visual association cortex (parastriate and peristriate regions) is required for the recognition and identification of objects. It projects to the ipsilateral and contralateral (through the splenium of the corpus callosum) hemispheres and interruptions of this may result in disconnection syndromes. The visual association cortex stores visual memories and is involved in visual recognition, perception, visual association, and spatial orientation. Injury to this area may cause deficits in a patient's visual attention, visual memory, stereoscopic vision, localization and discernment of objects, spatial orientation including judgment of distance, ability to discriminate size / shape and color, ability to localize themselves or objects in space, ability to voluntarily direct gaze, as well as ability to clearly see objects without a distorted perception (metamorphosia). Bilateral occipital lobe lesions may result in visual loss such as cortical blindness. If the parietal lobe is also involved, there may be defects of higher cortical function, including color agnosia, prosopagnosia, and simultagnosia. Patients may lack awareness of the deficits and it may be interpreted that a patient confabulates or hallucinates their environment as the patient walks but may stumble over objects. The patient may have awareness, but deny that a deficit exists (Anton's syndrome). Despite having normal visual acuity and visual fields, a patient with damage to the occipital lobe may have difficulty reaching for objects using visual guidance (optic ataxia), and have difficulty with voluntary direction of gaze (optic apraxia). The occipital lobe is also involved in control of eye movements. (270)

Vision-related deficits related to the occipital cortical regions:

- Hemianopsias, scotomas.
- Simple hallucinations, phosphenes, photopsias (perception of light in the absence of light stimulus).
- Visual agnosia (apperceptive and associative).
- Cortical blindness (loss of vision without ophthalmological causes).
- Anton's syndrome (denial of visual loss with confabulation in setting of cortical blindness). (326)
- Astereopsis.
- Riddoch phenomenon / syndrome. (325, 530, 542)

Temporal lobe function

Function of the temporal lobe is related to hearing and language. There are many connections between this lobe and other regions of the brain, including the occipital lobe, hippocampal formation, and limbic system. Injury to one temporal lobe will not cause deafness because this function is served bilaterally by both temporal lobes, but there may be difficulty with sound localization, and a decrease in auditory acuity. Bilateral injury to the temporal lobes may cause deafness, although patients may be unaware that they cannot hear. Seizures involving the temporal lobe may cause auditory, olfactory, and gustatory hallucinations. Injury to the dominant hemisphere temporal lobe may cause Wernicke's aphasia. Patients with injury to the visual and auditory association areas of the temporal lobes may experience perceptual deficits (agnosias). Those with a visual object agnosia may not be able to recognize objects, but can draw them. This contrasts with patients who suffer from a parietal cortex injury, who may be able to recognize objects, but have difficulty drawing them. Temporal lobe lesions may cause auditory distortions and illusions, despite not creating a disturbance in hearing. Difficulty with balance or equilibrium may result from damage to the temporal lobe vestibular area.

Other lesions of the temporal lobe may cause visual field deficits (injury to Meyer's loop) pathways), Klüver-Bucy syndrome (bilateral anterior temporal injury causing visual agnosia, psychic blindness, rage, loss of fear, hypersexuality, bulimia, and memory loss, but the complete syndrome rarely occurs). During complex partial seizures, patients may experience perseveration and visual hallucinations, which may have an auditory component, alteration of consciousness and amnesia for the event, and disorders of recognition in which they feel they have already had an experience (déjà vu). (269–272, 284, 530)

Temporal lobe-related disorders

- Right or left and bilateral temporal lobe
  - Vertigo, disequilibrium, olfactory hallucinations, gustatory (taste) abnormalities.
  - *Neuropsychiatric:* Klüver-Bucy syndrome, anxiety, agitation, paranoia.
  - *Cognitive:* Memory (Korsakoff amnestic state), cortical deafness, auditory agnosia and hallucinations/paracusias, difficulty with time perception, illusions.
- Left temporal lobe disorders
  - Right upper quadrantanopsia.
  - Wernicke's aphasia, verbal amnesia, visual agnosia, lexical amusia (difficulty reading music), synesthesia.
- Right temporal lobe disorders
  - Left upper quadrantanopia.
  - Visuospatial amnesia, prosopagnosia, auditory agnosia, amusia (receptive and expressive), delusional misidentification syndromes, semantic dementia. (325)

White-matter tracts by group and individually

Function of various regions of the brain, and the symptoms which result if damage occurs to these regions, has been discussed previously. Now, we will review potential neurological consequences that may occur if groups of connecting fibers between the various regions become injured as well as discuss the function of individual white-matter tracts. When connecting white-matter fiber tracts are disrupted, disconnection syndromes and disconnection phenomena may result. It is important to remember that this is a ever-changing science. With additional research constantly utilizing improved anatomical and functional imaging, the understanding of white-matter pathways, and insights into normal and injured states of the brain is also advancing.

WHITE MATTER TRACTS BY GROUP

The dorsal and ventral visual streams play a role in integrating visual function with processing of shape, color, depth, and motion occurring downstream in various ventral and dorsal stream cortical regions. (325) While it has been thought that the anatomically distinct ventral (occipitotemporal) and dorsal (occipitoparietal) pathways subserve different functions (object perception and object localization respectively), there may be some overlap of function (329). Described below are the generally ascribed roles of each, and potential deficits related to injury.

Vision-associated deficits related to ventral stream disorders: The three standard ventral tracts are the uncinate fasciculus (UF), IFOF, and temporo-frontal extreme capsule fascicle (ECF). (327, 650). The ventral stream links the primary visual cortex to inferior regions of the occipito-temporal cortex. The ventral stream, utilizing "top-down" information from visual and semantic memory, may provide perceptual representations (which can serve visual thought, recognition, planning and memory). (648)

- Ventral stream disorders may result in achromatopsia (inability to see colors), color anomia, color agnosia, hyperchromatopsia, color hallucinations, prosopagnosia, facial intermetamorphosis, object agnosia/anomia/aphasia, environmental agnosia, micropsia, macropsia, synesthesia (stimulation of one sensory modality causes experiences in another (as in a colored grapheme, in which viewing letters and numbers induces a perception of color), pareidolia, lilliputian hallucinations (325)

Vision-associated deficits related to dorsal stream disorders: The fiber tracts comprising the dorsal stream are the arcuate fasciculus (AF) and the superior longitudinal fasciculus (SLF). (649) The dorsal occipitoparietal pathway has been felt to subserve object localization and visually guided action, although it may have a role in object perception. (329) The dorsal stream links the primary visual cortex to superior regions of the occipito-parietal cortex. The dorsal stream may provide a "bottom-up" visual guidance for movements, and may govern the visual control of movement without intervention from vision awareness. (648)

- Dorsal stream disorders may result in simultagnosia, optic ataxia, oculomotor apraxia, Balint's syndrome, motion hallucination, palinopsia, polyopia, entomopia, visual perseveration, visual fading, visual extinction, visual allesthesia, inverted vision, visual vestibular disorders, heautoscopy, autoscopy, extracampine hallucinations, paroxysmal perceptual alteration. (325)

Injury to Papez' circuit: Papez' circuit (described by Papez in 1937) involves the following structures (mammillothalamic tract, medial mammillary nucleus, anterior nucleus of the thalamus, cingulate gyrus, cingulum, entorhinal cortex, subiculum, hippocampus, fornix) and has been thought to play a significant role in memory. It has been felt that a new conceptualization is needed as a result of recent anatomical and functional findings, which have shown interactions between the anterior thalamic nuclei and the hippocampal formation, along with neocortical interactions, to support episodic memory. (656)

- Injury to Papez' circuit affects consolidation of short- and intermediate-term memory into long-term memory (333)

WHITE-MATTER TRACTS INDIVIDUALLY

White matter tracts in the brain have an important role as they interconnect various regions of the brain, and also allow the brain to send signals via the brainstem to the spinal cord, thus serving the entire body. The white-matter tracts have various inputs, and there is some variability in the specifics as to which cortical and deep regions are connected by different tracts. In addition, additional anatomical and functional data is being studied. Understanding this, the ascribed functions of the tracts may vary depending upon the study and, in some cases, the function of a tract remains unclear at this time. Fibers from different regions of the brain may join and leave the white matter tracts as they go to and from their destinations. The long association fasciculi are bidirectional and, historically, the superior longitudinal fasciculus and the AF were regarded as a single fiber bundle, although they no longer are. (480)

As described above, association fibers connect cortical regions within the same hemisphere, commissural fibers connect to the opposite hemisphere, and projection fibers connect to lower portions of the brain and, eventually, the spinal cord. Described below are some of the major white matter tracts, with some of the neurological functions which are ascribed to them. As this is a continually evolving field, the understanding of the anatomy and function of these tracts is constantly improving, and therefore evolving.

- Association fibers
  - *AF:* Language processing. (531)
  - *Cingulum (CG):* Executive control, emotion, pain (dorsal cingulum), episodic memory (parahippocampal cingulum). (532)
  - *Fornix:* Left fornix = verbal memory; right fornix = visuospatial memory; they also are involved in object recognition and other functions. (Senova citing Cameron and McMackin). (533)
  - *FAT:* Speech initiation, verbal fluency, executive function/inhibitory control (Radwan citing Dick, La Corte, Pascual-Diaz). (336)
  - *IFOF:* Ventral vision and language streams (there is debate in literature): Right IFOF = facial recognition/semantic visual stream; left IFOF = semantic language functions. (Radwan citing Caverzasi, Herbet, Almairac). (336)
  - *Inferior longitudinal fasciculus:* Visual memory, visual emotion. (321)
  - *Middle longitudinal fasciculus:* High-order function related to acoustic information. (534)
  - *Superior longitudinal fasciculus:* Integration of auditory and speech nuclei. (321)
  - *UF:* Auditory verbal and declarative memory. (321)
  - *Vertical occipital fasciculus:* Perception of visual categories (words, faces, etc.). (535)
- Commissural fibers
  - *Anterior commissure:* Involved with neospinothalamic tract for nociception and pain sensation. (321)
  - *Corpus callosum:* Connectivity of sensorimotor and auditory function between the hemispheres; potentially seven regions, including prefrontal, premotor and supplementary motor, motor, sensory, parietal, occipital, and temporal. (336, 321)
- Projection fibers
  - *Medial lemniscus:* Spinothalamic information of proprioception, vibration, fine touch, two-point discrimination. (536)
  - *Optic radiation:* Visual processing. (336)
  - *Optic tract:* Each optic tract carries half of the visual field. (537)
  - *Corticospinal tract:* Carries motor signals from the cerebral cortex to the spinal cord. (321)
  - *Thalamic radiations:* Transmit sensory and motor information to precentral and postcentral cortex. (321)
  - *Cerebellar bundles (dentato-rubro-thalamic tract, inferior cerebellar peduncle, middle cerebellar peduncle):* Balance, posture (via integration of proprioceptive sensory and motor functions), modulation of skilled manual motor function (Radwan cited Lingford-Hughes). (336)

7

Agnosias, aphasias, apraxias, agraphias, etc.

Higher executive processing and functioning of the brain (which may involve connections between primary sensory processing areas of the brain, as well as association portions of the cortex), when injured, may result in a variety of complex, sometimes obvious and sometimes extremely subtle, cognitive and neurological changes. Even very subtle changes may have profound impacts upon a patient's ability to function in their daily life, interpersonal relationships and skills, work skills, judgement, management of their independence, and their finances. This category of cognitive impairments may be undiagnosed or misdiagnosed, which may have significant long-term consequences for patients. Not all of the disorders listed here are necessarily related to traumatic brain injury (TBI). On the other hand, it is possible that because of the subtle nature of some of these conditions, they may go unrecognized in patients who have suffered a TBI. The anatomic basis of some of these disorders may not yet be known, although improving imaging technology and continued post-mortem neuropathological evaluation is likely to lead to greater insight in the future. Many of these may be cortical lesions, or they may be lesions affecting the connecting white matter, with varying degrees of disconnection phenomena and disconnection syndromes occurring.

Self-awareness is multifaceted and requires the coordination of a hierarchy of physiological and psychological body systems, which are represented in the brain. It is the mental representations of oneself that provide a platform for self-awareness and allow an individual to compare a subjective view of themselves with an objective reality. Patients may be unaware of their symptoms and refuse treatment. Disorders that may interfere with self-awareness include the following: phantom limbs (subjective feeling of limb presence despite having undergone an amputation), somatoparaphrenia (individual feeling a body part does not belong to them), anosognosia for hemiplegia (individual denies having hemiplegia despite being paralyzed on one side of the body), facial feature and body size (incongruence between objective features and mental representations of oneself), mirrored self-misidentification (individual looks in the mirror and no longer recognizes themselves), body dysmorphic disorder (excessive preoccupation with a perceived defect in one's appearance), anorexia nervosa (individual restricts food due to unrealistic view of their body size and weight), panic disorder, illness anxiety disorder, somatoform pain disorder, agency (individual feeling that the action of their body is controlled by an external force), and alien limb phenomenon (perceiving a limb as having a mind of its own, and even naming the limb). (521)

This category of deficits can be easily missed on evaluation. Acquired visuoperceptual deficits are rarely reported. Patients may deny their own deficit, which may be due to a focal lesion or to involvement of a complex brain network. (503) Since visual agnosia often presents with deficits of visual field and changes in eyesight and attention, it is easy to go unnoticed. (500) The clinician must also be

DOI: 10.1201/9781003354154-7

cognizant of the fact that any clinical, radiological, or other biomarker findings which may be identified are likely the "tip of the iceberg."

EXAMPLES OF BRAIN DISORDERS AND CONSEQUENCES

Examples of this category of brain disorder include:

- A child with verbal agnosia, who was felt to have hearing loss despite intact hearing function and could respond to music but not words. (504)
- A patient with difficulty recognizing objects and shapes perceived through the left hand, but could appreciate basic sensory features presented tactually to the same hand flawlessly: Left-hand tactile agnosia is due to a disconnection syndrome resulting in this case from a hemorrhage in the posterior corpus callosum. (506)
- A patient with severe impairment in non-auditory comprehension without impairment to speech comprehension: Severe auditory agnosia for non-verbal sounds due to left posterior temporal and parietal damage (Wernicke's area), causing nonverbal auditory agnosia. (507)
- An individual with the sudden onset of bizarre and random fire-setting behavior (arrested for felony arson); neuropsychological tests showed impaired executive function (attention, memory, consistent with frontal lobe) although they were normal two years earlier; current scans showed lesion in anterior internal capsule. (508)
- A patient who developed cortical blindness after cerebral infarct in distribution of both posterior cerebral arteries, who, upon recovery, had color blindness in left visual field but not in right. (509)
- A patient with landmark agnosia, restricted to recognition of newly learned landmarks only (note: Elaborate neuropsychological screening and virtual reality-based tests of navigation ability); deficit can occur in the absence of difficulty in processing route information; possibly related to right temporal lobe and right hippocampus. (510)
- Balint's syndrome (visual disorientation/simultagnosia [inability to see visual field as a whole], ocular apraxia [impaired visual scanning], optic ataxia [deficit in pointing and reaching under visual guidance]): Lack of awareness may cause misdiagnosis of blindness, psychosis, or dementia. (512)
- A patient with verbal auditory agnosia, who suffered a TBI, with subsequent inability to follow oral commands or repeat or dictate words, despite maintaining fluent and comprehensible speech, preserving the ability to read and write words and sentences without motor weakness. Verbal auditory agnosia tends to be easily misdiagnosed as hearing impairment, cognitive dysfunction, and sensory aphasia. (512)
- Somatoparaphrenia in a patient with a right thalamic hematoma, who, despite being alert, had anosognosia (unaware of their left hemiplegia), profound left spatial neglect, but also reported that her sister's hand was in her bed and it was hard and unable to move. Despite being shown her own arm, she stated that it was her sister's arm. (519)
- A patient with visual agnosia, who, when looking for his hat, "reached out his hand and took hold of his wife's head, tried to lift it off, to put it on. He had apparently mistaken his wife for a hat! His wife looked as if she was used to such things." (516)

This category of cognitive disorders discussed in this chapter can have profound effects upon an individual's life. Prosopagnosia (face blindness), which is the inability to recognize faces (even familiar ones), may lead to social isolation and shyness because those affected have difficulty recognizing and naming people with whom they are speaking. Coping strategies may involve focusing on a specific feature, such as a mole, shape of nose, ear, bright shirt, or a voice, but changes in hairstyles and makeup will impede recognition. On the other hand, Capgras delusion is characterized by an individual claiming that their spouse has been replaced by an alien (who acts exactly as their spouse did). The individual recognizes the face of their spouse, but has no autonomic reaction of familiarity. An individual with akinetopsia has motion blindness, and "the individual with this disorder is banished to a world lit only by strobe lights," in which movement is only seen when illuminated by each flash. The motion blind individual can only assume that objects have moved by noting their relative positions in time, but they are unable to see them move. Other aspects of vision remain intact. (388)

LIST OF COGNITIVE DISORDERS (ALPHABETICAL ORDER)

Below is a review, in alphabetical order, of various conditions and syndromes. At times, the region of the brain to which a disorder may be localized is provided. Many times, the condition may involve several regions of the brain, or may involve the white matter connections of the brain. At times, the responsible region may be unknown. As the field of understanding anatomy of the brain as it relates to function is fluid and evolving (especially with some of the subtle deficits), the regions felt to be attributed with certain disorders may change as knowledge and research advance.

- *Abaragnosia:* loss of weight perception. Region: right or left parietal lobe.
- *Abulia:* Apathy, lack of drive or initiative for action, speech and thought. Regions: anterior cingulate cortex, bilateral medial frontal lobes, frontal convexity, focal subcortical lesions (caudate nucleus, anterior thalamus, globus pallidus, internal capsule, midbrain), disconnections of limbic tracts.
- *Acalculia:* Impairment of mathematical calculation abilities.
- *Achromatopsia:* Impairment in color perception and discrimination (not due to eye). Region: Cerebral cortex.
- *Affective prosopagnosia:* Difficulty with recognition of facial expressions.
- *Agnosia:* (gnosis is the Greek noun for knowledge) is the inability to process or difficulty with higher processing of sensory information.
- *Agnostic alexia:* Inability to recognize words.
- *Agrammatism:* Leaving out prefixes, suffixes, function words from speech.
- *Agraphia:* Disorder manifested by inability to write or difficulty with writing.
- *Ahylognosia:* Inability to identify textures and weight (wood, cotton, metal, liquid, etc.).
- *Akinetopsia:* Inability to perceive visual motion. Region: Cortical.
- *Alexia:* Impairment in reading (vision, intelligence, language intact).
- *Alexithymia:* Lack of effect, low emotionality (limits creativity). Region: Characterizes a person with a split brain.
- *Alien hand syndrome:* Phenomena in which one hand is not under control of their mind. Regions: corpus callosum, posterior parietal cortex, supplementary motor area, anterior cingulate cortex.
- *Allesthesia:* Perception of one receiving a stimulus on the body that is remote to where it was actually applied.
- *Amnesia:* Memory disorder, non-specific.
- *Amorphognosia:* Inability to identify object size and shape by touch.
- *Amusia:* Inability to recognize music.
- *Anomia:* Difficulty in coming up with words.
- *Anosmia:* Impairment in odor perception.
- *Anosodiaphoria:* Person who has a brain injury has lack of concern (insouciance) for it.
- *Anosognosia:* Inability to recognize a person's own condition or disease.
- *Anton-Babinski or Anton syndrome:* Visual anosognosia (denial of vision loss), with confabulation, in setting of cortical blindness. Regions: Visual cortices, bilateral lateral geniculate bodies, posterior limbs of internal capsules, optic radiations, corpus callosum.
- *Aphasia:* (phasis is from Greek for utterance) Language disorder, comprehending and/or producing; inability or difficulty with producing or comprehending words. Region: Language area, usually in left hemisphere.
- *Apperceptive visual agnosia:* Abnormality of visual perception and discriminative process, despite absence of elementary visual deficits (unable to recognize objects, draw, copy a figure). Regions: Parietal, occipital cortex.
- *Apraxia:* (praxis is the Greek word for action or doing) Disorder in using extremities, with difficulty or inability to use limbs or express gestures with them in a coordinated manner, despite having the physical ability and the intention to do so. The inability to perform or difficulty with performing a motor task, in the absence of weakness or other deficit involving the affected body part. This disorder does not arise from physical difficulties with the extremities.
- *Apraxia (speech):* Awkward and labored articulation, sound distortions, substitutions (speech organs are intact).
- *Aprosodia:* Inability to express or understand the variations of tone in language. Region: right cerebral hemisphere.
- *Asomatognosia:* Experience that one's body has faded from awareness; may be associated with feeling of loss of ownership or agency over a limb.
- *Associative visual agnosia:* Difficulty understanding meaning of what is seen (can draw and copy, but not know what they have drawn). Regions: Bilateral inferior occipitotemporal cortex.
- *Athymhormia:* Abnormality or deficiency in motivation. Region: Frontal lobes.

- *Attention blink:* After identification of target in rapid sequential stream of stimuli, temporary impairment in identifying a second stimulus shortly after the first.
- *Auditory agnosia:* Inability to recognize sounds (hearing is intact). Region: Right temporal.
- *Auditory paracusias:* Auditory hallucinations, which are sensory perceptions of hearing in the absence of an external stimulus.
- *Autokinesis:* Impression of movement of objects in the dark.
- *Autoscopy:* Seeing one's double from an out-of-body experience.
- *Autotopagnosia:* Inability to localize, identify or recognize one's own body part.
- *Balint's syndrome:* Paralysis of eye fixation with inability to look voluntarily to peripheral visual field, optic ataxia, neglect of peripheral visual field. Regions: Large bilateral parietal lesions.
- *Binding problem:* Difficulty determining which elementary visual features (color, shape, size) belong to same stimulus.
- *Broca's aphasia:* Group of speech disorders (loss of ability to produce articulate speech with intact speech comprehension). Region: Usually left frontal lobe (Broca's area).
- *Capgras delusion:* False belief that an identical person has replaced a person close to them. Region: May be due to disconnection of cerebral pathways, but pathophysiology is unclear due to rare nature of syndrome.
- *Category-specific agnosia:* Deficit in ability to identify members of a specific category.
- *Central dyslexia:* Reading disorder of impaired higher reading function.
- *Cerebral akinetopsia:* Inability to perceive movement. Region: Cortical visual area responsible for processing motion.
- *Circumlocution:* A target word cannot be retrieved (instead produce a multiword response).
- *Color agnosia:* Inability to identify and distinguish colors (despite intact basic vision mechanisms). Region: Left occipitotemporal.
- *Color anomia:* Inability to name a color when shown, but able to point to the name of the color and to match colors.
- *Conceptual apraxia:* Loss of mechanical knowledge, such as about the use of tools like a hammer.
- *Conduction apraxia:* Impaired at imitation on command.
- *Cortical blindness:* Loss of vision without ophthalmological causes (normal pupillary light reflexes). Region: Occipital lobes.
- *Cortical deafness:* Inability to hear, despite no damage to ear anatomy. Regions: Bilateral temporal lobes.
- *Cotard syndrome:* delusional belief that one is dead or non-existent. Region: Right hemisphere (disorder leads to perceptual and somatosensory feelings of unreality).
- *Creativity complex:* Influences on creativity (reflect personality, attitude, affect, cognition).
- *Crossed aphasia:* Aphasic deficits following right hemisphere injury in right-handed individuals.
- *Deep dyslexia:* Characterized by semantic errors.
- *Dissociation apraxia:* Modality-specific apraxia (such as for verbal commands), no difficulty with imitation or use of objects.
- *Divergent thinking:* Ideation and problem-solving move in different directions.
- *Dressing apraxia:* Inability to dress oneself.
- *Dysarthria:* Impairment of motor speech system affecting articulation, rate, resonance, loudness, and voice quality of speech.
- *Dyscalculia:* Impairment of mathematical calculation abilities.
- *Dysgraphia:* Disorder of spelling and writing.
- *Dysmetria:* Impairment of control of force and direction of muscle contraction (disruption of multijoint movements).
- *Dysosmia/Parosmia:* Distortion in smell.
- *Dysphasia:* Impairment in the production of speech.
- *Dysprosody:* Abnormal rhythm, articulation, and melody of speech.
- *Dyskinesia:* Involuntary movements appearing as fragments of normal movements.
- *Echolalia:* Meaningless repetition of another person's spoken words.
- *Echopraxia:* Involuntary imitation of movement of others.
- *Entomopia:* A type of polyopia, in which one sees a grid-like pattern of multiple copies of a single visual image.
- *Environmental agnosia:* Inability to recognize familiar places and surroundings.
- *Extracampine hallucinations:* Feeling of a silent and emotionally neutral human presence, perceived as a vague feeling of somebody being near. These are not perceived as visual hallucinations.

- *Finger agnosia:* Inability to name or differentiate the fingers of themselves or others (part of Gerstmann's syndrome).
- *Gerstmann's syndrome:* Characterized by four symptoms: 1) writing disability (agraphia, dysgraphia), 2) inability to understand rules for calculation of arithmetic (acalculia, dyscalculia), 3) inability to distinguish right from left, 4) inability to identify fingers (finger agnosia). Region: Left angular gyrus with probable cortical extension.
- *Gustatory agnosia:* Inability to identify taste sensations.
- *Heautoscopy:* Pathological experience of visual duplication of one's body with an another body, and a disturbing sensation of owning the illusory body..
- *Hemineglect:* Inattention to one side of space.
- *Hemiparesis:* Weakness on one side of the body.
- *Hemiplegic:* Paralysis on one side of the body.
- *Homonymous hemianopsia:* Cortical blindness in one visual field.
- *Hyperchromatopsia:* Colors appear very vivid and bright; increased activity in color cortex.
- *Hyposmia:* Decreased perception of odors.
- *Ideomotor apraxia:* Severe errors when asked to pantomime transitive acts to verbal command (spatial and temporal movement errors).
- *Ideational apraxia:* Inability to carry out series of acts that lead to a goal.
- *Intermetamorphosis:* Belief that an individual is transformed physically and physiologically into another person.
- *Jargon aphasia:* Speech in which most of nongrammatical elements are neologisms.
- *Klüver-Bucy syndrome:* Group of impairments, including visual agnosia, anger, memory difficulties, behavioral changes, and hypersexuality. Regions: Damage to bilateral mesial temporal lobes.
- *Korsakoff syndrome:* Neuropsychiatric syndrome with symptoms of amnesia and confusion (typically caused by deficiency of thiamine, and commonly seen with alcohol abuse).
- *Lexical amusia:* Impairment in reading music. Region: left temporal lobe.
- *Lilliputian hallucination:* Hallucination of human, animal or fantasy entities of minute size.
- *Limb kinetic apraxia:* Loss of ability to make finely graded and precise movements of individual fingers.
- *Literal (phonemic) paraphasia:* Sound substitutions or additions (result in unintended real-word or nonsense utterance).
- *Macropsia:* Condition in which objects are seen to be larger than they really are.
- *Manual praxis:* Difficulty carrying out movements with hands and arms, not due to weakness or immobility, and despite minimal spatial constraints placed by environment on purposeful actions.
- *Metamorphopsia:* Perception of faces or objects in a distorted manner. Region: visual association cortex.
- *Micropsia:* Condition in which objects are seen visually to be smaller than they really are.
- *Neglect (extinction):* Failure to attend to events on opposite side of a lesioned hemisphere (may have extinction that is transient neglect when events occur on both sides of space simultaneously). Region: Posterior parietal.
- *Neologism:* Meaningless word production.
- *Nonverbal auditory agnosia:* Inability to comprehend nonverbal sounds (sparing of speech).
- *Object agnosia:* Impairment of recognition of common objects.
- *Object anomia:* Inability to name objects.
- *Object aphasia:* Inability to name objects.
- *Oculomotor apraxia:* Inability to perform voluntary eye movements.
- *Olfactory agnosia:* Inability to recognize smells.
- *Ophthalmoplegia:* Impairment, weakness or paralysis of ocular muscles, causing diplopia.
- *Optic aphasia:* Inability to name a visually presented object (can identify through gesture).
- *Optic apraxia:* Deficit in ability to perform voluntary eye movements.
- *Optic ataxia:* Inaccurate reaching for targets presented visually.
- *Orientation-dependent visual agnosia:* Failure to recognize objects from unusual views.
- *Orthographic paralexia:* Paralexia in which response shares at least 50% of its letters with the target word.
- *Osmophobia:* Sensitivity to odors.
- *Palinopsia:* Persistent or repetitive perception of seeing an image after the image is removed from sight.
- *Paragrammatism:* Production of grammatically confused and incorrect speech, with incorrect function of words, prefixes, suffixes.

- *Paralexia:* Incorrect production of a word in oral reading.
- *Paraphasia:* Deficit in which there is production of unintended sounds within a word, or replacing an entire word; selecting an incorrect word results in clear-cut substitution of one word for another (words may be inappropriate).
- *Pareidolia:* Tendency to perceive a meaningful image in a random visual pattern.
- *Paroxysmal perceptual alteration:* Hypersensitivity of perception, psychedelic experience (colors appear brighter, contrast appears sharper, vision is distorted) and somatic schema distortion (feeling that one is floating, or their extremities are being pulled and elongated).
- *Peduncular hallucinations:* Visual hallucinations following subcortical lesions.
- *Peripheral dyslexia:* Interference with processing of visual aspects of a stimulus.
- *Perseveration:* Unintended repetition of idea or verbal utterance.
- *Person identification deficit:* Inability to access biographical information about people, but able to recognize familiar from unfamiliar people.
- *Phantom:* Proprioception, perception, and other sensations from missing or deafferented parts of the body; may be related to missing limbs (phantom limb), absent vision (phantom vision), etc.
- *Phantom movement:* Incorrect impression that one is moving a limb in the presence or absence of a proprioceptive deficit; a patient with hemiplegia may have anosognosia for hemiplegia and misperceive they are moving their paralyzed arm.
- *Phonagnosia:* Inability to recognize familiar voices. Region: Sound association region.
- *Phonemic paraphasia:* Substitution of sounds in speech.
- *Phonologic dyslexia:* Preserved ability to read familiar words, inability to read unfamiliar words.
- *Phonology:* System of contrastive relationships among speech sounds.
- *Phonophobia:* Sensitivity to sound.
- *Photopsia:* Perception of light in the absence of light stimulus.
- *Polyglot aphasia:* Aphasic deficits in one or more languages in individuals who knew two or more languages before brain injury.
- *Polyopia:* Perception of seeing two or more images, after fixation on an image, especially with one eye.
- *Prosody:* Melody, stress, intonation of speech (affected by aprosodia).
- *Prosopagnosia:* Inability to recognize faces (elementary vision is intact). Region: Inferior temporal cortex in the fusiform gyrus (right fusiform face area, left frontal regions).
- *Prosopometamorphopsia:* Visual disorder in which there is an altered perception of faces.
- *Reduplicative paramnesia:* Belief that a familiar place, person, body part, or object has been duplicated.
- *Riddoch phenomenon / syndrome (also known as statokinetic dissociation):* The ability to perceive visual motion consciously in a blind visual field.
- *Semantic dementia:* Language deficit, which involves comprehension or words and their semantic meaning. Produced is empty, garrulous speech with thematic perseverations, semantic paraphasias, and poor category fluency.
- *Semantic paralexia:* A paralexia that consists of a real word that is related in meaning to the target word.
- *Simultagnosia (dorsal):* Inability to recognize objects when they appear together (inability to see more than one object). Regions: Bilateral occipitotemporal cortex.
- *Simultagnosia (ventral):* Inability to recognize objects when they appear together (inability to identify more than one object, although they can see more than one object). Regions: Left inferior occipital area.
- *Somatoparaphrenia:* Delusional belief that the limb contralateral to a brain pathology does not belong to the person. Region: Extensive right-sided lesions, but may also be involved with posterior (parietal-temporal) and insular damage.
- *Somatosensory agnosia:* Agnosia for touch.
- *Statokinetic dissociation (also known as Riddoch phenomenon):* The ability to perceive visual motion consciously in a blind visual field.
- *Surface dyslexia:* Difficulty with whole word recognition and spelling; Impairment characterized by reliance on sounding out strategy with words.
- *Synesthesia:* A “union of the senses” where two or more of the five senses which are normally

experienced, are involuntarily joined together (for example, hearing music but seeing shapes).

- *Tactile agnosia:* Inability to recognize objects by touch (able to name objects by sight).
- *Tactile asymbolia:* Impaired recognition by touch (amorphognosia and ahylognosia not present).
- *Topographical agnosia:* Inability to orient to surroundings (unable to interpret spatial information). Region: Right posterior cingulate.
- *Verbal amnesia:* Deficits of both recall and recognition. Region: Mediodorsal thalamic nucleus, temporal lobes.
- *Verbal auditory agnosia:* Selective inability to recognize verbal sounds.
- *Verbal auditory agnosia/pure word deafness:* Inability to comprehend spoken words, intact reading, writing, speaking.
- *Verbal fluency:* Ability to quickly generate words in a semantic category.
- *Verbal paraphasia:* Substitution of real word for a verbal target.
- *Vestibular agnosia:* Attenuation of vestibular sensation of self-motion, despite intact peripheral and reflex vestibular function; in settings of acute TBI (TBI patients with benign paroxysmal positional vertigo are seven times less likely to be referred for treatment if there was concurrent vestibular agnosia), may reduce clinician's awareness of presence of active balance disorders. Region: Possibly right inferior longitudinal fasciculus.
- *Visual agnosia:* Total or partial loss of ability to visually recognize and identify familiar objects or people.
- *Visual extinction:* A form of visual neglect, in which one half of the visual field is not reported when another stimulus is simultaneously introduced to the other half of the visual field.
- *Visuospatial amnesia:* Difficulty reproducing abstract complex figures from memory.
- *Wernicke's aphasia:* Impaired language comprehension and fluent error-containing speech. Region: Usually posterior portion of left temporal lobe (Wernicke's area).

(270, 325, 326, 374, 409–423, 480, 484, 485, 501, 502, 505, 511, 513, 571–576, 243, 628, 637, 638, 639, 640, 641, 642, 643, 644, 645, 646, 647, 651, 652, 653, 654)

8

Imaging

In the future, recognition, assessment, diagnosis, treatment, and prognostication of traumatic brain injury will certainly involve significant utilization of advanced diagnostic imaging as a vital tool in the armamentarium of medical providers caring for TBI patients.

—Gary E. Kraus

With the sophistication of imaging technology, *in vivo* dissections of regions of the brain and fiber tracts can be essentially performed and evaluated, whereas prior to this evolving technology, only *in vitro* laboratory dissections were possible. In the future, recognition, assessment, diagnosis, treatment, and prognostication of traumatic brain injury (TBI) will certainly involve significant utilization of advanced diagnostic imaging as a vital tool in the armamentarium of medical providers caring for patients. Today, diffusion tensor imaging (DTI), diffusion kurtosis imaging (DKI), and connectomes are at the forefront of knowledge to assess TBI patients, but this is a constantly evolving field as ever-improving technology becomes available.

Imaging of the brain can be generally broken down into three categories: 1) structural, 2) functional, and 3) metabolic. The different categories are useful for evaluating different aspects of structure and function, and using them in conjunction with each other, along with a proper clinical evaluation, helps to obtain an accurate diagnosis, and ultimately prognosis, and may help to evaluate the effectiveness of treatment modalities.

- *Structural:* X-ray; computed tomography (CT); conventional magnetic resonance imaging (MRI); advanced MRI (GRE, SWI, DTI, etc.); imaging post-processing (volumetric analysis using Freesurfer, NeuroQuant, Neuroreader, etc.)
- *Functional:* Functional MRI (fMRI); magnetic resonance spectroscopy (MRS); positron emission tomography (PET); single photon emission computed tomography (SPECT); magnetoencephalography (MEG); arterial spin labeling (ASL)
- *Metabolic:* PET, MRS

DOI: 10.1201/9781003354154-8

Imaging of the brain is commonly performed after a patient has suffered a TBI. In the acute setting, a CT scan of the brain is usually performed, especially if there is a moderate or severe TBI. While the CT scan is often negative in the emergency setting when a patient has suffered a mild TBI, other advanced imaging studies performed in the future may detect abnormalities. A CT scan is important in the emergency setting to evaluate for intracranial hemorrhages, which might require an emergent life-saving neurosurgical operation on the brain. Traditional MRI may be subsequently performed to obtain additional detail of the anatomy of the brain. More advanced imaging studies such as diffusion weighted imaging (DWI), DTI, fluid attenuated inversion recovery (FLAIR), gradient echo imaging (GRE), susceptibility weighted imaging (SWI), quantitative susceptibility mapping (QSM), high angular resolution diffusion imaging (HARDI), diffusion spectrum imaging (DSI), perfusion weighted imaging (PWI), MRS, (118, 138) functional magnetic resonance imaging (fMRI), MEG, (119, 120) PET (121–125, 315, 316), and SPECT, (126) among others, may be incorporated to provide additional information about the brain, its cortical structure and function, and the white matter connecting anatomical pathways.

Segmentation protocols may be incorporated into MRI images to evaluate volumes of various regions of the brain, comparing right and left sides of the brain, as well as making comparisons to normal controls. Volumetric assessments may also be repeated on the same patient over a period of time, with longitudinal studies looking for any changes. (127, 131, 368, 431)

Imaging of the brain following a TBI can be broken into several phases, as different information is beneficial at various stages during treatment of TBI patients. Initially, when a patient who has suffered a TBI arrives at an emergency department, depending upon the level of severity of the head injury, different studies will be performed. In the acute phase of injury, a CT scan of the head takes little time to acquire (a few seconds of scan time with modern machines) once the patient is positioned in the scanner. If the patient is on a ventilator, the machine can be brought into the room. CT scanning is excellent for detecting skull fractures and it also detects hemorrhages in the brain parenchyma (**Figure 8.1**), ventricular, subdural, and epidural spaces well. (86)

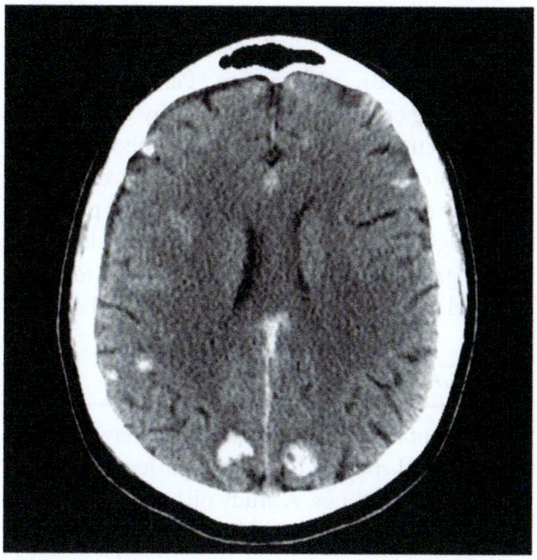

Figure 8.1 Axial slice of CT scan of the brain, showing multiple regions of hemorrhage (white areas within the brain) with edema, which is typical of moderate and severe TBI. (From Living Art Enterprises, LLC / Science Source)

In attempting to quantify TBI and arrive at predictions of prognosis, biomarkers are important to help standardize methods of analysis. As neuroimaging techniques improve, insight into TBI improves, and this creates imaging biomarkers for TBI. Understanding the structure and function of the brain is critical. Multimodal neuroimaging has been important in understanding not only the cortex of the brain, but also critical white-matter pathways, which interconnect various portions of the brain and descend into the spinal cord to reach the body. Traditional CT and MRI of the brain are not sufficient to evaluate the subtleties of many TBI abnormalities and how they pertain to long-term cognitive and behavioral symptoms. Additional and advanced MRI sequences (FLAIR, SWI), diffusion imaging techniques (HARDI, DTI, DSI, among others), and fMRI are very useful. Understanding the structure of the brain and any damage to it, as well as brain connectomics, and comparing this information to normative data and outcome data using statistical analysis will help in the quest for biomarkers, which may help to prognosticate the clinical impact of TBI, and aid in assessment of new treatment regimens. DTI can be used to perform tractography, which gives information about fiber-tract length and connectivity density in the white matter, providing detail about the brain architecture. Personalized profiles can be created to assess atrophy and changes in connectomics (white-matter connections) that may occur over time, as acute injuries evolve to the subacute and chronic phase. This type of personalized longitudinal study may help to provide insight into a patient's clinical course and help to assess their rehabilitation treatment protocols. (127)

CT SCAN

CT scans of the brain in patients who have suffered a minor TBI may be limited to patients with certain clinical findings. A study of 1,429 consecutive patients was broken into two phases and included patients with minor head injury and a normal Glasgow Coma Scale (GCS) score, who underwent a CT scan of the brain. Of the 6.5% of patients (93 patients) who showed positive findings on brain CT scans (contusions and subdural hematomas were most common), all experienced one or more of seven findings: "headache, vomiting, an age over 60 years, drug or alcohol intoxication, deficits in short-term memory, physical evidence of trauma above the clavicles, and seizure." The conclusion was that indications for CT scans of the brain in patients who have suffered minor TBI may be limited to patients with the clinical findings listed here and that these symptoms had a 100% sensitivity for identifying patients with positive CT scans. (109)

TRADITIONAL MRI SEQUENCES

Traditional or conventional MRI imaging has limited value in the assessment of TBI, especially mild and moderate TBI. Although severe TBI is associated with hemorrhagic lesions or contusions, which are readily visible on conventional MRI, the micro-hemorrhages often seen with mild and moderate TBI are often not visible on these studies. While conventional MRI is useful for the evaluation of many pathologies within the brain, when evaluating TBI, it often underestimates the extent of injury, correlates poorly with functional deficits, and lacks the ability to provide quantitative biomarkers that may help to determine prognosis and assess treatment responses. (368)

MRI, DWI, DTI, DSI, GRE, FLAIR, SWI, DKI, CSD, DTT, FBA, AND OTHER ADVANCED MRI SEQUENCES

Advanced imaging plays a significant role in the treatment of TBI. With the advent of advanced imaging such as DTI and other technologies, studying the cerebral cortex and white-matter fiber tracts for traces of injury, which will correlate with neurological function, helps with the understanding, diagnosis, treatment, and prognostication of TBI. The remarkable technologies now available, bring light into an arena in which there was darkness.

MRI imaging techniques helpful for the evaluation of TBI include DTI, SWI, GRE, and FLAIR. Three-dimensional (3-D) T1 MRI helps with volumetric evaluation of different regions of the brain (cortical structures and hippocampi). DTI is an advanced MRI study which looks at the integrity of the white matter fiber tracts in the brain. There are additional techniques that may help to resolve crossing fibers within the brain, including DKI, constrained spherical deconvolution (CSD), super-resolved CSD (super-CSD), and Q-ball imaging (QBI). (442)

DTI, DSI, DWI, DKI, DTT, and others

Imaging of the brain has been improved by utilizing advanced MRI techniques. DWI uses a tissue water diffusion rate to produce images. In a glass of water, the water molecules will move, due to Brownian motion, in all directions in a uniform fashion and travel equal distances in all directions, a type of diffusion pattern known as isotropic diffusion (*iso* comes from the Greek meaning of "equal"; *tropic* comes from the Greek meaning of "pertaining to a turn"). If water molecules encounter obstructions and becomes constrained (such as by obstruction from the wall of a cell located within a white-matter tract) and can no longer move equally in all directions, the diffusion becomes directional and is labeled anisotropic (*an* comes from the Greek meaning of "not or without"). Directionality in the diffusion of water is therefore known as anisotropy. A higher directionality (or constraint in the direction in which it may diffuse) corresponds to a higher anisotropy, while a lower directionality (water has less constraint in the direction in which it may diffuse) corresponds to a lower anisotropy. In other words, the higher the anisotropy, the greater the diffusion directionality which the water experiences. Water diffusion in the brain, when the water is contained within the cerebrospinal fluid (CSF), will occur in all directions, as the water is relatively unconstrained and can travel in any direction. On the other hand, if the water molecules are located within a boundary, such as a cell membrane of an axon, their pathway of diffusion will be partially obstructed in certain directions but permitted in others, and the diffusion signal on an MRI scan will reflect this. In addition, if the boundaries are organized, such as within a white-matter tract, then the signal characteristics of this region will be affected by the orientation of the diffusion gradients. DTI may add to this measure of anisotropy the vector information about which direction the water is diffusing. The addition of vector information to a volume element (voxel) of DWI information can be used to measure water diffusion along an axon in many directions. This directional vector component allows DTI to image the structure (location, orientation, anisotropy) of white matter. Fractional anisotropy (FA), which summarizes the general status of underlying tissue architecture, can reflect the health of an axon and allows quantification of the directionality of diffusivity. Due to the highly uniform collinear structure of normal white-matter tracts within the brain, DTI is well suited to the assessment of traumatic axonal injury (TAI), which can qualitatively and quantitatively demonstrate pathology not detected by other CT and MRI imaging modalities. (128, 317, 318, 382, 567)

Commonly used quantitative parameters of the diffusion tensor, which can be calculated for each voxel, include the apparent diffusion coefficient (ADC) also known as the mean diffusivity (MD) or the "trace," axial diffusivity (AD), radial diffusivity (RD), and FA, which describes the amount of diffusion in a voxel. The diffusion tensor can be described using eigenvalues and eigenvectors, with the axes of the 3-D coordinate system of x-y-z containing eigenvectors, and the "lengths" of their measures called eigenvalues. The AD takes into account the eigenvalue and eigenvector of the diffusion along the axis of the predominant direction of diffusion (such as along the direction of an axon), whereas the RD takes into consideration and is the average of the two eigenvalues and two eigenvectors, which are perpendicular to the main diffusion direction (such as perpendicular to the direction of an axon). The MD takes into consideration all three eigenvalues (therefore the AD and the RD) and is the average of the sum of the three eigenvalues. The FA represents the weighted information about the quantity of directionality and is calculated from a method incorporating the square root of the differences of the squares between several of the eigenvalues. The FA can range from a value of 0 (when there is no constraint to diffusion, and water diffuses in a spherical direction) to 1 (where water would diffuse perfectly in one direction with essentially no axial diffusivity). In an unorganized biologic compartment, diffusion will take on a spherical shape as there are no constraints and, therefore, the ADC is independent from the direction of measurement. AD and RD describe the direction and magnitude of tissue water diffusion (**Figure 8.2**; 481). When the radius of diffusion is constrained (such as when the water molecule is located within a cell and confined by the cell membrane, which may be longer

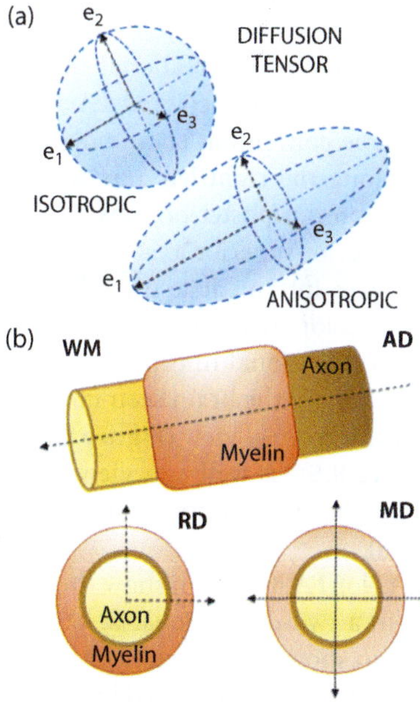

Figure 8.2 Principles of MRI diffusion and diffusion tensor and its association with neural tissue microarchitecture. Isotropic (spherical) and anisotropic (ellipsoid in three dimensions) diffusion tensors are illustrated in (a), showing eigenvalues (e_1, e_2, e_3) with associated eigenvectors. The AD, RD, and MD are seen with respect to white matter (WM), showing a schematic view of an axon in cross section with myelin surrounding it (b). Adapted from (481) https://creativecommons.org/licenses/by/4.0/legalcode.

in one direction and narrower in another), the radius of diffusion may be reduced, compared to the axial diffusion (parallel with the length of the cell membrane, if the cell is not spherical). Analysis including whole brain tractography (showing illustrated fiber tracts from 3-D reconstruction of tensor tracts), region based tractography, graph-based connectivity models, histogram analysis, region of interest analysis, voxel-based analysis, and others may be used to interpret and study the data. (128, 317, 318, 382, 481, 567, 589)

FA ranges from 0 to 1, and does not represent any type of units. (439) Since FA is a measure of the degree of directionality of diffusion, an FA value of 0 indicates that there is no directional dependence on diffusion, while a value of 1 describes diffusion along a single direction. (440)

Unlike qualitative radiological assessments, DTI techniques enable quantitative metrics to be derived from the diffusion tensor to describe information about the complex microstructure of tissue, which can be used to statistically compare patient groups. (128, 317, 318)

When the FA with directional information is shown on MRI slices, a colored FA map may be produced. The convention commonly used is that diffusion along the right/left axis is colored red, along the anterior/posterior axis is green, and along the inferior/superior axis is blue. When diffusion involves intermediate directions, a mixing of the three colors will result. (623) The color FA maps reveal directional information about white-matter anatomy in the brain seen in an axial view (**Figure 8.3**), a coronal view (**Figure 8.4**), a sagittal view (**Figure 8.5**), as well as a view of the region of the fornix/hippocampus/mammillary body (**Figure 8.6**).

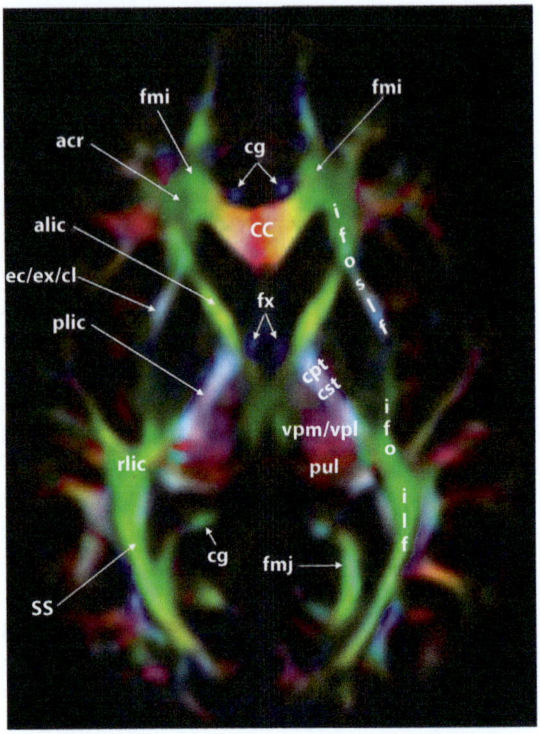

Figure 8.3 Axial color FA map of brain. This axial (cross sectional) color DTI image depicts the major white-matter tracts in the brain. By convention, tracts oriented from anterior to posterior (front to back) are green, tracts oriented from side to side are red, and tracts oriented superior to inferior (head to toe) are blue. Cpt = corticopontine tract, cst = corticospinal tract, ilf = inferior longitudinal fasciculus, cg = cingulum, fx = fornix, ifo = inferior frontal occipital fasciculus, ss = sagittal stratum, cc = corpus callosum, acr = anterior corona radiata, fmi = forceps minor, fmj = forceps major, pul = pulvinar of thalamus, vpm = ventral posterior medial thalamic nucleus, vpl = ventral posterolateral thalamic nucleus, ec = external capsule, ex = extreme capsule, slf = superior longitudinal fasciculus, rlic = retrolenticular internal capsule plic = posterior limb internal capsule, cl=claustrum, alic=anterior limb internal capsule. (From Living Art Enterprises / Science Source)

While color FA maps can show the direction of diffusion in a two-dimensional (2-D) plane, tractography can show white-matter fiber direction in a 3-D view. This can be achieved by using a variety of algorithms, in which data in three dimensions can be used to create a 3-D map of the connecting fibers of the brain.

White-matter fiber tracking using diffusion MRI provides the ability to map brain connections. To create tracks (also known as streamlines) that represent the white-matter tracts within the brain (tractography), several processing steps are taken: (1) the diffusion-weighted images are pre-processed (eddy current, motion, and phase distortion correction); (2) fiber resolving is performed (fiber orientation); (3) fiber tracking is achieved (deterministic or probabilistic method, etc.); and (4) post-tracking processing is performed. (335). TBI connectomics (mapping of neural connections in the nervous system to create a connectome) allows

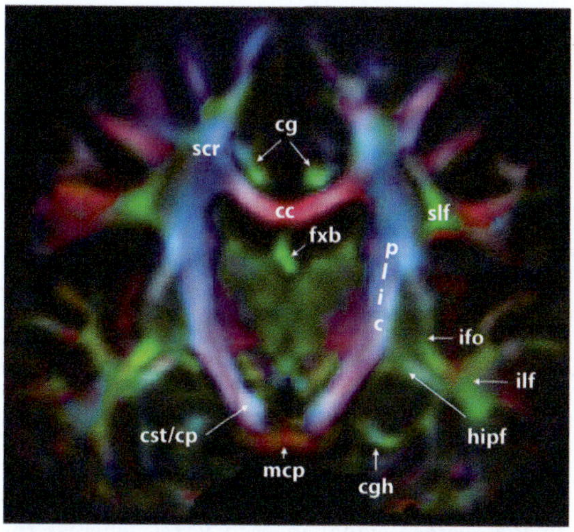

Figure 8.4 Coronal color FA map of brain. This coronal (seen from the front) color DTI image provides information and depiction of the major white-matter tracts in the brain. By convention, tracts oriented from anterior to posterior (front to back) are green, tracts oriented from side to side are red, and tracts oriented superior to inferior (head to toe) are blue. Cp = cerebral peduncle, cst = corticospinal tract, ilf = inferior longitudinal fasciculus, cg = cingulum, ifo = inferior frontal occipital fasciculus, cc = corpus callosum, slf = superior longitudinal fasciculus, fxb = body of fornix, hipf = fimbria of hippocampus, cgh = hippocampus of cingulum, mcp = middle cerebellar peduncle, plic = posterior limb of internal capsule, scr = superior corona radiata. (From Living Art Enterprises / Science Source)

for evaluation of cortical regions and connectivity as a patient's recovery evolves, allows comparison to populations, and may be used to create a personalized atrophy profile for a patient, which may help with personalized rehabilitation treatments by informing the medical team about recovery prospects and guiding evaluation and need for long-term care. (334).

DTI can be used to show fiber tracts of the entire brain (**Figure 8.7**). Individual tracts that can be analyzed using advanced imaging techniques include the following: arcuate fasciculus (AF); cingulum (CG); fornix; frontal aslant tract (FAT); inferior fronto-occipital fasciculus (IFOF); inferior longitudinal fasciculus (ILF); middle longitudinal fasciculus (MdLF); superior longitudinal fasciculus (SLF I, II, and III); uncinate fasciculus (UF);

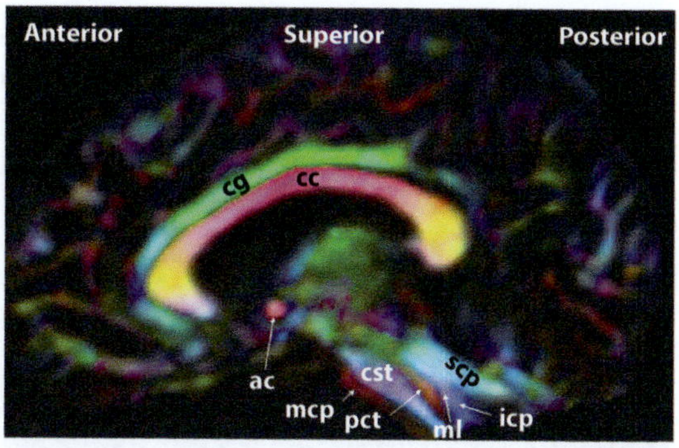

Figure 8.5 Sagittal color FA map of brain. This sagittal (viewed from the left side) color DTI image depicts the major white-matter tracts in the brain. By convention, tracts oriented from anterior to posterior (front to back) are green, tracts oriented from side to side are red, and tracts oriented superior to inferior (head to toe) are blue. Cc = corpus callosum, cg = cingulum, mcp = middle cerebellar peduncle, scp = superior cerebellar peduncle, icp = interior cerebellar peduncle, ml = medial lemniscus, pct = ponto-cerebellar tract, ac = anterior commissure, cst = corticospinal tract. (From Living Art Enterprises / Science Source)

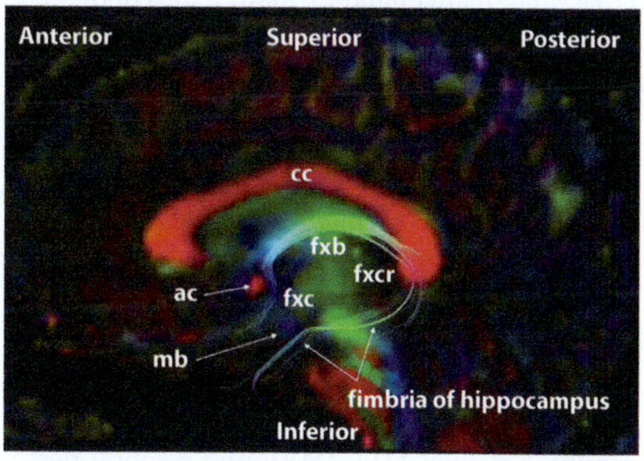

Figure 8.6 Sagittal color FA map of region of fornix. Fornix, hippocampus and mammillary body color tractography. This sagittal (viewed from the left side) plane color DTI image provides information and depiction of the major white-matter tracts in the brain. By convention, tracts oriented from anterior to posterior (front to back) are green, tracts oriented from side to side are red, and tracts oriented superior to inferior (head to toe) are blue. Fxc = columns of fornix, fxb = body of fornix, fxcr = crura of fornix, mb = mammillary body, ac = anterior commissure, cc = corpus callosum. (From Living Art Enterprises / Science Source)

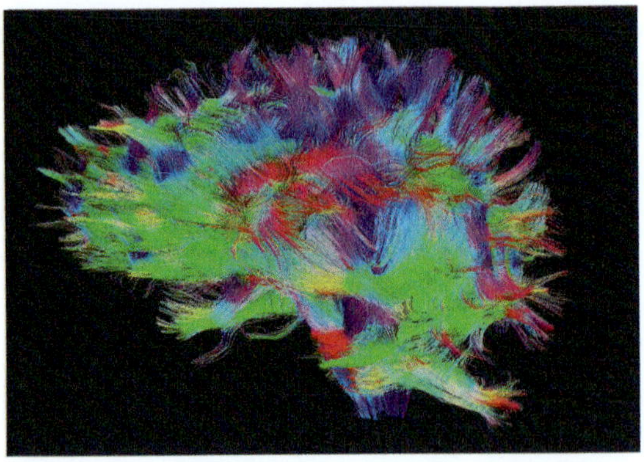

Figure 8.7 A DTI scan showing reconstructed white-matter fibers of the whole brain, from the left side. Directional color coding: left/right is red; anterior/posterior is green; superior/inferior is blue. (From DO TROMP / Science Source)

vertical occipital fasciculus (VOF); anterior commissure (AC); corpus callosum (CC); medial lemniscus (ML); optic radiation (OR); optic tract (OT); pyramidal tract (PyT); corticospinal tract (CST); thalamic radiations (TRs); and cerebellar bundles. (336) It is important to recognize that tractography and connectomes are macroscale maps focusing on large white-matter bundles. Many axons in the cerebrum are local, terminating in the same gyrus from which they originated, and may not be visualized using currently available technology. The human connectome represents a balance of complexity and simplicity. To make the images readable, efforts should be made to avoid loss of thoroughness. Functional connectivity reflects the probability of connections between two points in the brain. (375)

While brain imaging using CT and MRI scanning often shows no abnormalities in patients who have suffered concussions, more advanced scanning such as DTI, fMRI, and cerebral perfusion imaging may show insight into the neuropathology of concussion. While FA may show an increase in the acute phase after a concussion, it may show a reduced FA during the chronic phase in patients with persistent post-traumatic symptoms. Potential causes such as cytotoxic edema and acute decrease in the water content in myelin sheaths have been described in the semi-acute phase. (367) When diffusion weighted MRI was used in 44 patients, it was found that brain swelling in patients with severe brain injury appears to be cellular in both focal and diffuse brain injury. Various pathological findings of primary and secondary brain injury may be difficult to measure, and advanced models may be needed to better evaluate these. (51, 52, 78, 134)

While recognizing the great value of quantitative information that can be obtained from DTI, it must also be remembered that while a change in microscopic configuration, such as increase in intra or extracellular water content or cell loss, may result in a change in FA, this is an average of diffusing water molecule behavior over the region of the entire voxel; this model may, for this and other reasons, be oversimplified and not necessarily reflect detail at a microstructural level. The spatial resolution of a DTI scan (possibly 1–3 mm) contributes to the average signal in each voxel, whereas the diameter of an axon may be in the order of microns (1/1,000th of a mm). (7, 128, 317, 318)

DTI LITERATURE

In general, FA is often reduced in various white-matter tracts during the chronic phase after a mechanical (non-blast) TBI following a possible transient increase during the acute and subacute phases. It is difficult to make specific detailed generalizations because different methods, brain regions, and protocols of scanning and analysis (DTI, CSD, DKI, etc.) are performed in different studies. Varying techniques will manage the analysis of crossing fibers differently. In addition, parameters like FA, MD, AD, RD, and ADC have been evaluated differently in various investigations. Duration of time between injury and scan may also vary. Due to this, a number of studies will be presented next.

One general finding (although there are some differences in the literature) is that in the chronic phase after a mechanical TBI, more significant decreases in FA seen over a greater number of white-matter tracts in the brain are often associated with worsened severity of brain injury and worsened cognitive function. In the acute phase, FA is sometimes increased but there is variability in findings. Common white-matter regions of decreased FA in the chronic phase include the corpus callosum, frontal lobe, cingulum bundle, internal capsule, superior longitudinal fasciculus, and others.

The concept and ability to evaluate the cerebral white-matter tracts in both a quantitative and qualitative manner is an important one, as it gives insight into the form and function of the brain, helping us to understand the normal and diseased states of the brain. Because DTI and other white-matter imaging techniques are so important, we will review several studies on this subject. White-matter lesions and changes in white-matter microarchitecture may be the basis of significant component of cognitive impairment, as was seen in an evaluation of 50 patients with white-matter lesions in comparison to healthy controls who underwent cognitive evaluation. (330). DTI and FA provide important information in the assessment of TAI in patients who have suffered a concussion as well as more severe brain injury and may have prognostic value for neural tissue recovery. (461–463, 466, 470) Evaluation of adult mild chronic TBI patients has shown higher levels of aggression when compared to controls, and the aggression was associated with reduced white-matter integrity in the corpus callosum. DTI revealed higher RD in the corpus callosum than seen in controls, indicating decreased fiber integrity. FA was also lower in this tract, but this finding did not survive false discovery rate correction. (476)

Due to the differing nature of mild, moderate, and severe TBI, a number of DTI literature studies will be reviewed, but categorized according to the severity of TBI.

Mild, moderate, and severe TBI overview

Hulkower in a review entitled, *A decade of TBI in Traumatic Brain Injury: 10 Years and 100 Articles Later* (7), has reviewed 100 papers in the literature covering relevant articles up through 2011, and included articles pertaining to mild, mild complicated, moderate, and severe TBI, with 13 longitudinal studies covering assessments at acute, subacute, and chronic points after TBI. They found that the most commonly identified region of abnormal FA and MD was the corpus callosum, possibly because it is the largest white-matter tract in the brain and an important site of TBI pathology. Other regions of interest when studied with different methodologies, such as region of interest analysis, tractography, or whole brain analysis, were found to show differing findings, possibly due to different regions being evaluated and differing methods of analysis used. The most common areas of abnormal MD using different methods of analysis were as follows: (1) using region of interest analysis, the most common location of abnormal findings were in the corpus callosum (posterior/splenium and anterior/genu), frontal lobe, white matter, and thalamus, (2) using tractography analysis, the common locations were the corpus callosum (anterior/genu), fronto-occipital fasciculus, inferior longitudinal fasciculus, uncinate fasciculus, and cingulum bundle, and (3) using whole-brain analysis, the most common locations were the cingulum bundle, corpus callosum (total), superior longitudinal fasciculus, posterior limb of the internal capsule, fronto-occipital fasciculus, and frontal lobe. Hulkower points out in summary that the general finding, regardless of method of analysis, was that the corpus callosum, frontal lobe, internal capsule, and cingulum were among the most commonly found locations of abnormal DTI post-TBI, which may be related to their anatomic relationship to the skull and the falx cerebri. DWI, using ADC values, may look at intracellular and extracellular fluid and cytotoxic edema. (7, 114)

Importantly, based upon their extensive literature review, Hulkower stated, "despite significant variability in sample characteristics, technical aspects of imaging, and analysis approaches, the consensus is that DTI effectively differentiates patients with TBI and controls, regardless of the severity and timeframe following injury." Hulkower also importantly felt

> "a unifying theme can be deduced from this large body of research: DTI is an extremely useful and robust tool for the detection of TBI-related brain abnormalities. The overwhelming consensus of these studies is that low white-matter FA is characteristic of TBI. This finding is consistent across almost all the articles we reviewed, despite significant variability in patient demographics, modest differences in data acquisition parameters, and a multiplicity of data analysis techniques. This consistency across studies attests to the robustness of DTI as a measure of brain injury in TBI."

It was also found that in FA histograms, which pooled all white-matter voxels across the whole brain, a substantial portion of the hundreds of thousands of voxels in the image datasets were abnormal. (7)

After a TBI, a greater degree of decreased FA within different regions of the brain has been seen in association with increased severity of brain injury as well as with worsened cognitive function of patients. In a DTI study of cognition after TBI, it was found that decreased FA was seen in more regions of the brain in patients who had suffered moderate-to-severe TBI as compared to those in the mild TBI category, suggesting greater white-matter pathology is related to greater cognitive deficits. Twenty mild TBI patients, 17 moderate-to-severe TBI patients, and 18 controls were studied with DTI and neuropsychological testing. The moderate-to-severe TBI subjects showed reduced white-matter integrity in all regions of the brain that were of interest, whereas the mild TBI group showed this change in more limited regions. With cognitive testing, the moderate-to-severe TBI group was more impaired than the controls, whereas the mild TBI group was similar to the controls. Greater degrees of white-matter changes appeared to correlate with more cognitive impairment. The possibility is raised that while severe TBI may result in white-matter damage to both axons and myelin, mild TBI may involve mainly axonal but not myelin damage. (129)

DTI scans revealed a significant structural disconnection in another group of 12 subjects who suffered a mild-to-severe TBI when compared to controls, using both a region of interest technique for the corpus callosum and whole-brain assessment using tract-based spatial statistics (TBSS) (showing reduced FA throughout the brain). This generalized white-matter structural disconnection as measured by FA correlated with the severity of the TBI, suggesting that demyelinization of axonal shrinkage may occur from TBI. (377)

DTI in children: TBI analysis

When 46 children (roughly 7–17 years) were evaluated, the findings of those who suffered moderate-to-severe TBI when compared to those of 43 children who sustained orthopedic injuries revealed findings about the cingulate cortex or cingulum bundle. In children who suffered a TBI, although there were no findings of lesions in the cingulate cortex or cingulum bundle on conventional structural MRI imaging, there were injuries to the cingulum bundle seen on DTI scans (decreased FA and increased ADC, which differed from the orthopedically injured group). The cingulum bundle is an important component of neural networks involved with cognitive abilities and reaction time on measures of cognitive control was related to white-matter integrity within the region. (372)

In a meta-analysis literature study reviewing pediatric TBI (mild, moderate, and severe), while in the short term (≤4 weeks post-TBI) FA was inconsistent, in the medium-to-long term (more than four weeks), FA values were lower and both ADC and MD were higher for white-matter tracts, indicative of decreased white-matter integrity. This correlated with worse performance on a range of cognitive functions tested. DTI of the large white-matter tracts including the corpus callosum, uncinate fasciculus, and cingulate, in addition to the whole brain, correlated to the worsened cognitive function (better cognition was seen with higher FA). (239)

The uncinate fasciculus, which connects the orbitofrontal and temporal lobes, may be an early biomarker for identification of behavioral problems, as seen in a study using probabilistic diffusion tensor tractography (DTT) in a group of pediatric patients who suffered moderate-to-severe TBI. (331) Using diffusion magnetic resonance imaging in another pediatric sample of more than 500 patients suffering mild-to-severe TBI, the uncinate fasciculus was particularly vulnerable to white-matter disruption and as it is a frontolimbic tract connecting the ventral prefrontal cortex with the amygdala, it may create an increased risk for behavioral or emotional difficulties after injury. It was found that female patients had a lower uncinate fasciculus FA and higher RD compared to controls, whereas this effect of TBI was not significant in male patients. (332)

Mild TBI analysis

Although there are exceptions, review of the literature is consistent with a general observation of lower FA seen in certain white-matter tracts in the chronic phase after a mild TBI, although there may be increased FA seen in the acute phase. Rutgers found in patients who suffered mild TBIs at a median of 5.5 months post-injury that there were multiple white-matter regions and fiber bundles (cingulum, corpus callosum, cerebral lobar white matter) with abnormally reduced FA. (435)

A multicenter DTI study from Transforming Research and Clinical Knowledge in Traumatic Brain Injury (TRACK-TBI) incorporated data from 391 patients and 148 controls across 11 United States Level 1 trauma centers to study the imaging and outcome on patients who suffered a mild TBI. DTI imaging was performed two weeks and six months after the mild TBI, and outcome was evaluated using the Glasgow Outcome Scale Extended (GOSE). At both the two-week and the six-month study, the AD, MD, and RD were higher, whereas the FA was lower in the mild TBI patients when compared to controls, and these changes were present in most of the major white matter tracts of the cerebral hemispheres. The authors describe their prospective longitudinal multi-center study of DTI in mild TBI as "to our knowledge the largest to date." They found that higher AD and MD at two weeks were independently associated with better long-term clinical outcome, and these prognostic measures were strongest in long association tracts (SLF, superior fronto-occipital fasciculus and external capsule), especially of the left hemisphere. Importantly, the authors note "DTI provides reliable imaging biomarkers of dynamic white matter microstructural changes after mild TBI that have utility for patient selection and treatment response in clinical trials. Continued technological advances in the sensitivity, specificity, and precision of diffusion magnetic resonance imaging hold promise for routine clinical application in mild TBI." (690)

In a review of 121 studies of mild TBI patients, the articles were organized into four categories: acute/subacute pediatric mild TBI; acute/subacute adult mild TBI; chronic adult mild TBI; and sports-related concussion. Acute represented approximately less than seven days after injury; subacute was 8–89 days post-TBI; and chronic was more than three months post-TBI. With such a large number of studies, there will be inconsistencies between them depending upon parameters of analysis. The general findings (there were exceptions) were that in children and adolescents, there was initially a pattern of higher FA and lower ADC or MD in the acute and subacute recovery phases. In the adult acute and subacute groups, the majority had initially lower FA and higher MD and RD (there were exceptions). In the chronic adult group, lower FA was predominantly seen across tracts. (382)

Despite a normal conventional MRI brain scan, 51 patients who had suffered a mild TBI demonstrated significantly decreased white-matter findings on DTI, which correlated with cognitive impairment. A study of 51 consecutive patients who suffered a mild TBI were studied in the chronic phase (at least six months post-injury, with a mean of about 35 months), and while they had no abnormalities seen on conventional brain MRI scans, DTI scans and FA maps did reveal positive findings. Using TBSS, there were found to be significantly decreased FA values in the mild TBI group in the right superior longitudinal fasciculus, left superior frontal gyrus, right insula, and left fornix (**Figure 8.8**; 363). Cognitive examination scores positively correlated with FA values in several regions of deep brain structures, including the basal ganglia and limbic system. Wada concluded that "the regions with abnormally reduced FA values are strongly suggested to be related to chronic persistent cognitive impairments in these patients." (363)

When 30 military veterans who suffered mild TBI were studied and compared to controls, HARDI showed loss of white-matter integrity was associated with chronic mild TBI with a pattern

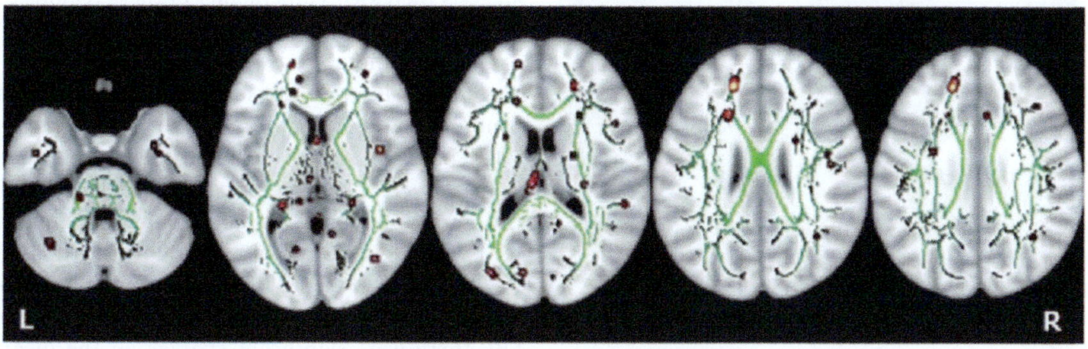

Figure 8.8 Tract-based spatial statistics analysis of the white-matter skeleton. Voxels demonstrating significantly decreased FA values for the subjects with mild TBI compared with the control group are shown in red-yellow. Voxels are thickened into local tracts and overlaid on the white-matter skeleton (green). Reproduced with permission of American Society of Neuroradiology (363)

located in the corpus callosum, forceps minor, forceps major, superior and posterior corona radiata, internal capsule, superior longitudinal fasciculus, and other areas. (544)

Sung indicated that theirs is the first original DTT-based study (published in 2022) "to assess the diagnostic sensitivity of TAI for the STT (spinothalamic tract) in patients with mild TBI." Sung cited works of Kishi, Apkarian, and Krause, in describing the spinothalamic tract (STT) as a sensory pathway that projects to several cortical regions (primary somatosensory cortex, mid-cingulate cortex, supplementary motor cortex) through various regions of the thalamus (ventro-postero-lateral nucleus, pulvinar) and transmits information related to touch, temperature, and pain. Their study included 35 patients with a mild TBI (with 30 healthy control subjects) who had no lesion observed on brain MRI (T1, T2, and FLAIR sequences). Fiber tracking, FA, and tract volume (TV) values were determined for the STT in both hemispheres. They found a high diagnostic sensitivity (100% for torn or narrowed configuration of a damaged STT) (**Figure 8.9**; 464) for TAI of the STT and ~94% (at 1 standard deviation below controls)

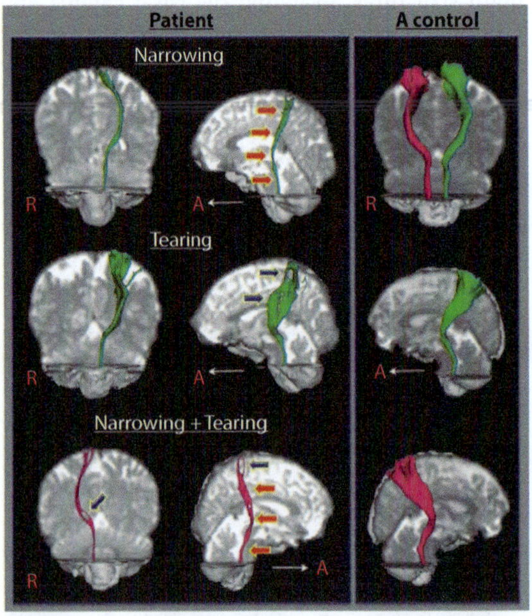

Figure 8.9 Results of diffusion tensor tractography for the spinothalamic tract (STT) in the patient group. Narrowing (red arrows) and tearing (blue arrows) of the STT are defined as abnormal compared with a normal control subject. Reproduced with permission of Wolters Kluwer Health, Inc. (464)

and ~57% (at 2 standard deviations below controls) sensitivity for FA and TV measurements. (464)

Post-mild TBI in the acute phase FA was reduced, while it was significantly reduced in the chronic phase. Sixty-one patients who suffered a mild TBI were studied with an acute DTI scan performed about 10 hours post-trauma and again at six months post-injury. Controls were also studied. There was reduced FA but increased MD and RD in the acute phase, which was thought to indicate vasogenic edema. In the chronic phase, FA was significantly reduced in comparison to the acute phase with unchanged MD and subtly increased RD across the following six tracts: (1) corona radiata, (2) anterior limb of the internal capsule, (3) cingulum, (4) superior longitudinal fasciculus, (5) optic radiation, and (6) genu of the corpus callosum. (365)

In contrast, in the acute phase of mild TBI in another study, FA was increased. In 10 adolescents who suffered a mild TBI, and who had a negative CT scan of the brain and a GCS score of 15, DTI of the brain was performed within six days of injury. Findings revealed increased FA and decreased ADC and RD. These findings suggested cytotoxic edema. They were also found to correlate with severity of post-concussion symptoms. (134)

Gardner found in seven out of eight studies of DTI in athletes who suffered sports-related concussion, DTI abnormalities were identified, although the neuro-anatomical sites varied. It was reported that the variance in location may be expected, given the heterogeneity of concussion and differences in injury to scanning time interval. The observation that the majority of findings were in the corpus callosum, internal capsule, and longitudinal fasciculus suggests increased vulnerability of these regions to concussion-related axonal injury. (139)

Cerebral microbleeds (CMBs) can affect white-matter bundles with consequences for the tracts remote from the site of the hemorrhage. Volunteers with a mild TBI were evaluated with imaging studies that were performed acutely (≤3 days after an injury) and about six months after the injury. MRI and DTI were combined to show that in 47% of TBI CMBs, when MRI/DTI scans were performed six months after subjects suffered a mild TBI, there were significant changes in the mean FA of perilesional white-matter bundles, suggesting that CMBs can result in chronic changes in the perilesional white matter even distant from the hemorrhage locations. Importantly, personalized medicine consisting of longitudinal within subject analysis of white-matter changes may be of interest for the evaluation of TBI in the future. (133)

Literature case report: Delayed neurological deterioration in mild TBI

A case report of a patient suffering a mild TBI documents the sequelae of delayed cognitive findings, with DTT also showing delayed degeneration of the left fornical crus. A 50-year-old woman was driving a car that was struck on the opposite side. Although her neck flexed and extended and she reported a "dazed feeling," she suffered no loss of consciousness or post-traumatic amnesia. One year after the injury, the patient visited the hospital with complaints of headache and dizziness, but no lesion was observed on a brain MRI with T1, T2, and FLAIR sequences. Initial memory function was normal on the Memory Assessment Scale: global memory (95th percentile), short term memory (68th percentile), verbal memory (77th percentile), and visual memory (98th percentile). Although initially not compromised, there was a progressive increased forgetfulness and decline in memory function 1.5 years after the injury, with no intercedent head trauma. By the time the difficulties progressed, she had to frequently use memory aids. At two years, there was a decrement of memory function (particularly verbal) as follows: global memory (70th percentile), short term memory (37th percentile), verbal memory (16th percentile), and visual memory (97th percentile). DTI (fiber tracking using a FA threshold of >0.2 and direction threshold <60°) was performed both one and two years after injury, with the findings of a well-preserved fornix at one year, but a discontinuation in the left fornical crus at two years post-injury (**Figure 8.10**; 444). In addition, the left fornix showed decreased FA value and fiber numbers when compared to its values at one year. The corticospinal tracts maintained their integrity. The authors concluded that "evaluation using follow up DTT would be useful for patients with delayed onset of neurological symptoms following TBI." (444)

Mild-to-moderate TBI analysis

The corpus callosum has shown decreased FA in TBI more pronounced with moderate than mild TBI. Eighty-three patients who suffered a mild-to-moderate TBI and underwent DTI imaging of the

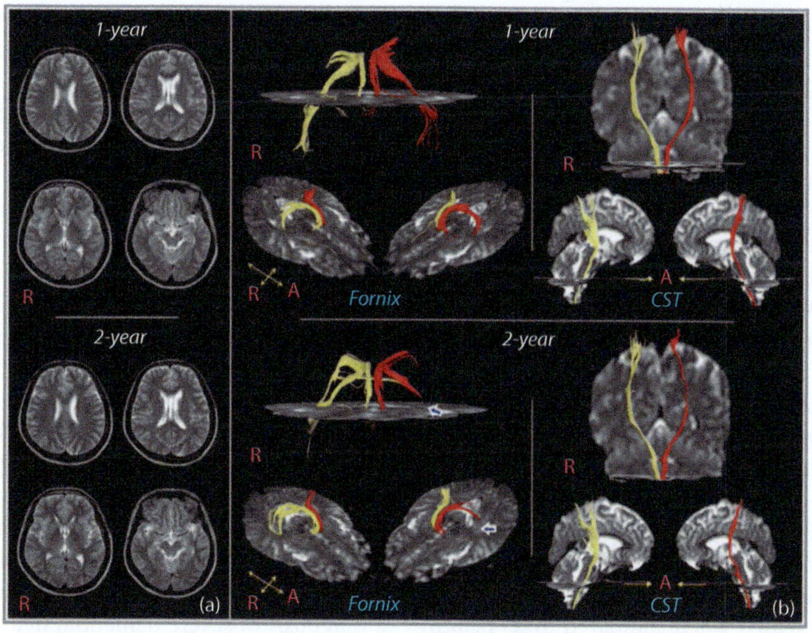

Figure 8.10 T2-weighted magnetic resonance images taken at one-year and two-years after injury showed no specific lesions (a). DTT of the fornix (b). The integrity of the fornix is well-preserved between the fornical column and fornical crus on one-year DTT. By contrast, at two-years after injury, DTT shows a discontinuation (arrows) is observed in the left fornical crus. DTT = diffusion tensor tractography, CST = corticospinal tract. Reproduced with permission of Wolters Kluwer Health, Inc. (444)

brain at six months post-injury, showed decreased FA abnormalities in the corpus callosum were more prevalent in those with moderate TBI than in those with mild TBI, also correlating with relatively poor six-month post-injury neuropsychological evaluation. (373)

Decreased FA in the anterior forceps has been seen one year after mild and moderate TBI. Fifty-three patients with a TBI (44 patients had a mild TBI and 9 had a moderate TBI) were compared to 33 controls. The TBI patients underwent an MRI DTI study roughly six days post-injury, and 23 patients had a follow up scan one year later. TBSS were used to compare DTI values. At the acute time point (early DTI scan), there were widespread increases in MD, FA, and AD in the TBI group (there were no changes in RD). At 12 months post-injury, the DTI scans showed that MD remained significantly increased, but FA was now decreased with RD increased and AD showing no differences in any location. It was felt that gliosis rather than cytotoxic edema is most consistent with the changes in metrics (increased FA and AD at six days) after acute mild TBI. In the chronic state (one-year scans) the decrease in FA and increase in MD and RD was seen principally in the anterior forceps. (364)

Moderate-to-severe TBI analysis

In patients who have suffered a moderate-to-severe TBI, CT and MRI scans of the brain will typically show hemorrhagic pathology. MRI measures of diffuse axonal injury (DAI) after moderate-to-severe TBI have a strong predictive value of post-traumatic neurodegeneration and are associated with progressive brain atrophy in both whole-brain and voxel-wise analysis. (459). Tractography confirms tract injury related to hemorrhages as well as axonal injury, and has also evaluated regions of the brain related to consciousness and the default mode network. (563, 564)

Free water within the brain following a moderate-to-severe TBI may have a negative predictive value on cognitive function. In 34 patients suffering moderate-to-severe TBI, it was found that free water volume fraction in patients was significantly increased when compared to 35 healthy controls using a measuring parameter known as a Mahalanobis distance. If was further observed that this measurement, taken from imaging studies three months post-injury, significantly predicted functional outcome as well as performance on neuropsychological testing (executive function and processing speed) measured at 12 months post-injury and significantly correlated with severity of injury. They suggested that the increase in free water seen in widespread regions of the white matter of the brain and persisting three months after injury may relate to increased extracellular water caused by atrophy, inflammation, or cellular changes. Importantly, the authors felt that their study may have been the first to utilize free water estimations in patients with moderate-to-severe TBI to predict functional and cognitive outcomes utilizing a patient-specific summary score of free water volume fraction. (135)

Literature case report: Progressive neurological deterioration after moderate/severe TBI, with DTI and pathology correlation

Kenney presents reports on two patients who developed early onset of dementia after a moderate-to-severe TBI with imaging and neuropathological correlates. The patient whose images are seen in **Figure 8.11**, suffered a concussion with brief loss of consciousness (LOC) in his second decade of life, and a second TBI with LOC of unknown duration at age 46 (presented with GCS of 11, agitated, combative). During this second TBI, his brain CT scan was negative. He had post-traumatic amnesia for 18 days, and was classified as a moderate-to-severe TBI. One month after the injury, he experienced cognitive impairment and a brain MRI showed only a single focus of increased signal in the left periventricular white matter. At 21 months after the injury, his neuropsychological evaluation was within normal range (mild cognitive deficits) and he returned to a major military command position with full active duty. At age 51, he retired and took a job in the private sector, but his performance skills had been gradually declining since one year after the injury. After age 59, the cognitive decline progressed along with behavioral and affective symptoms including depression, irritability, agitation, fatigability, and multiple cognitive and executive function issues. After his death at age 72 with a diagnosis of severe dementia, neuropathological studies were performed that found significant diffuse brain atrophy and a very thinned posterior corpus callosum, but preserved anterior corpus callosum (**Figure 8.11**; 445). Histology evaluation revealed high levels of amyloid-ß neuritic plaques

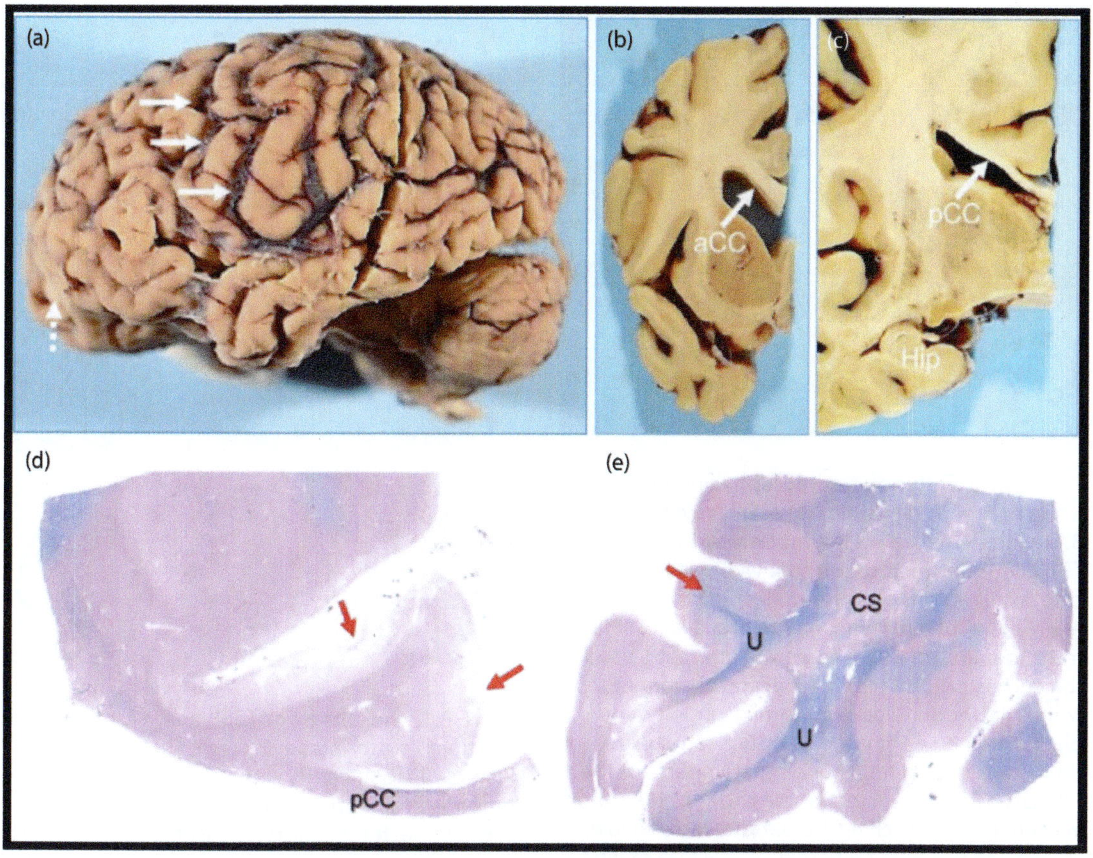

Figure 8.11 Macroscopic appearance of the brain of a subject with dementia after a moderate-to-severe TBI with thinning of the posterior corpus callosum and myelin loss. The intact brain (a) with left cerebral (contusion labeled with dashed arrows) and cerebellar hemispheres. Coronal cross-section of the left hemisphere (b) at the level of the caudate/putamen and anterior corpus callosum (aCC). Coronal large cross-section (c) of left hemisphere at the level of the hippocampus (Hip) and posterior corpus callosum (pCC). Of note, the marked intrasulcal space enlargement (as per diffuse cortical atrophy) (arrows, a) and marked thinning of the posterior corpus callosum (pCC) (arrow, c) contrasts the relatively preserved thickness of the anterior corpus callosum (aCC) (arrow, b) and the relatively normal appearance of the hippocampus (c). An LFB-hematoxylin (where LFB is luxol fast blue) stain of the left posterior corpus callosum (pCC) (d) and of the left superior temporal cortex (e). These stains demonstrate extensive loss of myelin in the pCC and adjacent centrum semiovale (CS). Of note, the patchy myelin loss in temporal lobe spares the U-fibers (U). Cortical pathology associated with contusions are indicated by red arrows in d and e. The images were obtained using a 2.5x objective. Reproduced with permission of American Association of Neuropathologists, Inc. (445)

(Aß-NP) in most regions of the brain, with neurofibrillary tangles and tau neurites seen throughout the cortical and subcortical regions. *Ex vivo* MRI imaging showed right parietal white-matter rarefaction and a thinned splenium of the corpus callosum. DTI tractography (**Figure 8.12**; 445) showed disruption of fibers traversing the corpus callosum in two regions: 1) parietal fibers traversing the splenium of the corpus callosum and 2) frontal fibers crossing the genu. (445)

Severe TBI analysis

Severe TBI may be associated with significant cortical thinning and significantly decreased FA values within the brain. Twenty-six patients who had suffered severe and diffuse TBI (GCS 5.19 ± 1.7) were compared to 22 controls. MRI imaging involved T1, diffusion weighted, FLAIR, and T2 GE scans and was performed over two years after the injury. Cortical thickness measurement was performed using the automated FreeSurfer stream

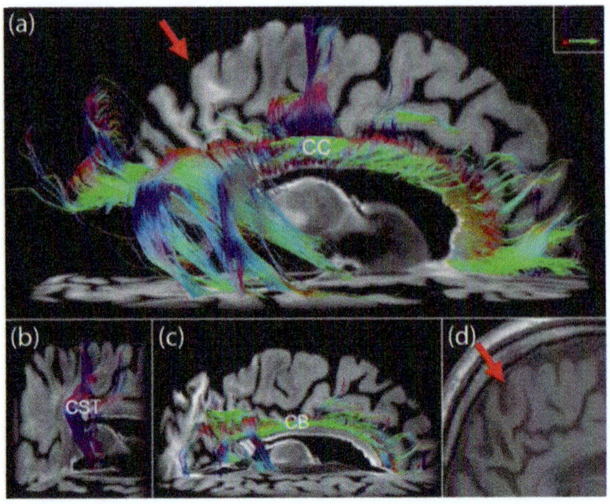

Figure 8.12 Diffusion tractography findings of white matter in same subject as in previous **Figure 8.11** with dementia after a moderate-to-severe TBI. Diffusion tractography (*ex vivo*) results indicate focal regions of white-matter injury. Right lateral view (a) of interhemispheric, transcallosal fiber tracts generated with a region of interest traced in the corpus callosum (CC). Fiber tracts from nearby white-matter bundles (e.g., fornix, cingulum bundle) have been eliminated to optimize visualization. Transcallosal tracts are intact in parts of the frontal and temporal lobes, but they are disrupted in other regions such as the parietal lobe (arrow). To exclude the possibility that global loss of white matter and/or technical artifact is responsible for the transcallosal tractography results, also shown is relative preservation of corticospinal tract (CST) fibers from a right lateral view (b) and cingulum bundle (CB) fibers from a right lateral view (c). Corresponding imaging from an MRI (d) obtained four years before patient's death does not show the extensive gliosis visible in the *ex vivo* imaging (arrow). Reproduced with permission of American Association of Neuropathologists, Inc. (445)

software. Cortical thickness analysis revealed a significant pattern of cortical atrophy in both hemispheres in the patient group with significant thinning in the following regions: rostral and middle frontal cortex, superior and middle temporal cortex (including anterior temporal lobes), superior and inferior parietal cortex, precentral and postcentral cortex, precuneus, parahippocampal cortex, lingual cortex, pericalcarine cortex, isthmus-cingulate, and anterior and posterior cingulate cortex. Of note, the preserved areas were the medial prefrontal cortex and the occipital and temporal lobes. DTI analysis using TBSS revealed widespread white-matter damage with

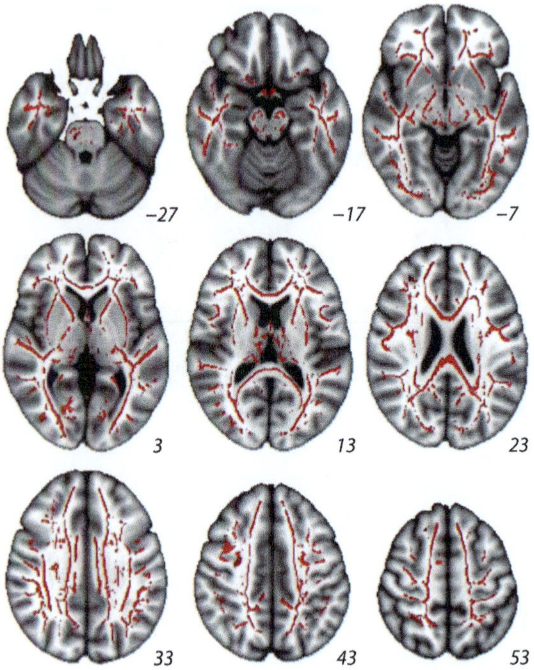

Figure 8.13 Results from TBSS analysis of FA maps in patients suffering severe TBI, showing (in red) clusters of significantly reduced FA in TBI patients compared to controls. Widespread impairment of white-matter integrity is observed. Images are displayed in radiological convention. Reproduced with permission of Elsevier. (366)

significantly decreased FA values in the following fasciculi: intra-hemispheric association fibers of the inferior and superior longitudinal fasciculi, inferior fronto-occipital fasciculi and the cingulum bundle; inter-hemispheric fibers of the corpus callosum (genu and splenium); projection fibers of the corticospinal tracts; and the anterior thalamic radiations, anterior limb of the internal capsule, and anterior corona radiata (**Figure 8.13**; 366). The study concluded that although patients had widespread gray and white-matter atrophy (**Figure 8.14**; 366), left parietal hemisphere white-matter alterations and decreased cortical thickness were the main contributors to long-term memory deficits. Although there was extensive cortical atrophy and widespread white-matter damage, FA only correlated with cortical thickness in specific regions of the frontal and parietal lobes and the cingulate cortex. It was suggested that cortical atrophy in certain regions may be a consequence of retrograde degeneration of the fasciculi connecting to them. Palacios cited Buki and Povlishock

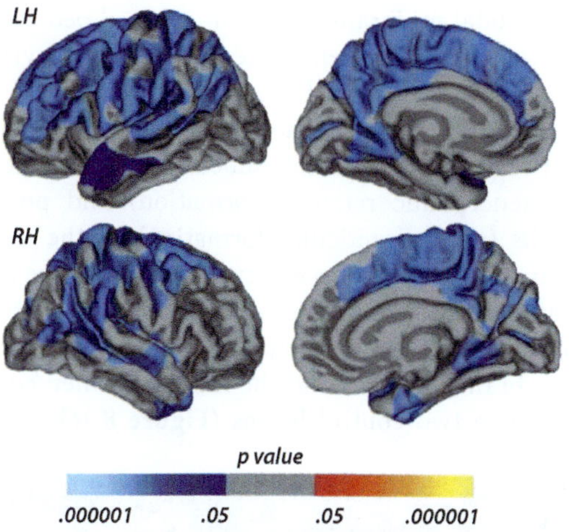

Figure 8.14 Regions of significant cortical thinning in severe TBI patients compared with controls. Regions affected were rostral and middle frontal cortex, superior and middle temporal cortex, superior and inferior parietal cortex, precentral and postcentral cortex, precuneus, parahippocampal cortex, lingual cortex, pericalcarine cortex, isthmus-cingullate, and anterior and posterior cingulate cortex. Reproduced with permission of Elsevier. (366)

in noting that general white-matter damage in the DTI analysis may reflect primary and secondary axotomy, anterograde or Wallerian degeneration, demyelinization, and other events. (366)

Literature case report #1: Severe TBI and consciousness

Edlow reported on a 29-year-old patient who suffered a severe TBI and was "comatose" upon arrival at the hospital. Shown in **Figure 8.15** (538) is a personalized connectome of the patient, which is compared to a healthy control. Although there is a paucity of tracts emanating from the ventral tegmental area (VTA) in the patient suffering from a coma, Edlow pointed out that there are still multiple preserved tracts from this area to the medical prefrontal cortex (MPFC), a node of the default mode network, and this patient recovered consciousness and functional independence by six months post-TBI. (538) Edlow evaluated the HARDI tractography with respect to the ascending reticular activating system (ARAS) and felt that this technique may be used to study human consciousness and its disorders. (561)

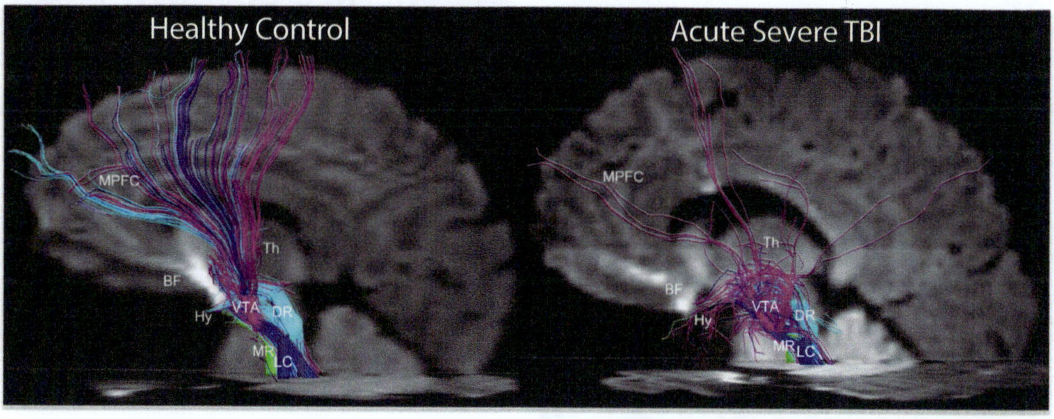

Figure 8.15 Personalized connectome mapping in the ICU reveals preserved ventral tegmental area (VTA) connections. VTA tracts are shown from a left lateral view in a 33-year-old healthy male control and a 29-year-old man with acute severe TBI. The patient was comatose on arrival to the hospital and in a minimally conscious state at the time of this scan on post-injury day 7, as determined by a Coma Recovery Scale-Revised assessment. Tractography analysis was performed using TrackVis, as Edlow previously described. (561). All tracts are color-coded by sites of VTA connectivity: Turquoise with dorsal raphe (DR), blue with locus coeruleus (LC), green with median raphe (MR), and pink with cortex, thalamus (Th), hypothalamus (Hy), or basal forebrain (BF). Multiple VTA connections are preserved in the patient, including with the medial prefrontal cortex (MPFC), which is a node of the default mode network. The patient recovered consciousness and functional independence by six months. Even in a patient with acute severe TBI, the VTA may be a hub through which multiple brainstem ascending arousal network (AAN) nodes connect with the Th, Hy, BF and cerebral cortex. (From Brian L. Edlow, MD, Massachusetts General Hospital, Harvard Medical School.) Reprinted with permission of Springer Nature. (538)

Literature case report #2: Severe TBI and ascending arousal system

Edlow, in an imaging study with pathological correlation, used HARDI tractography in a post-mortem brain (patient had suffered acute traumatic coma) to map the connectivity of arousal and awareness and demonstrated complete white-matter disruption of the pathways connecting brainstem arousal nuclei to the basal forebrain and other structures. A post-mortem tractography study was performed on a 62-year-old woman who suffered from an acute traumatic coma. Edlow cited McNab and Miller in stating that "postmortem fixation does not preclude measurement of anisotropic water diffusion or fiber tract reconstruction." Edlow felt that traumatic coma may be a subcortical disconnection syndrome involving interruption of connections between the thalamus and basal forebrain with specific brainstem arousal nuclei. The coronal CT brain scan reveals hemorrhages within the right dorsal midbrain and the left cingulum (**Figure 8.16a**; 539). Focal hemorrhagic tears were found on post-mortem macroscopic evaluation in the right dorsolateral quadrant of the rostral pons and caudal midbrain, left dorsolateral quadrant of the caudal midbrain, and right cerebral peduncle, as well as in the left posterior cingulate gyrus, body of the corpus callosum, and other locations. Using HARDI tractography analysis, connectivity between the cuneiformis/subcuneiformis nucleus (mesencephalic reticular formation) and pontis oralis (pontine reticular formation) in the midbrain and rostral pons was evaluated and there was found to be symmetric and bilateral disruption of the white-matter connections between these two brainstem sites and the thalamus when compared to two control brains (**Figure 8.16b**; 539).

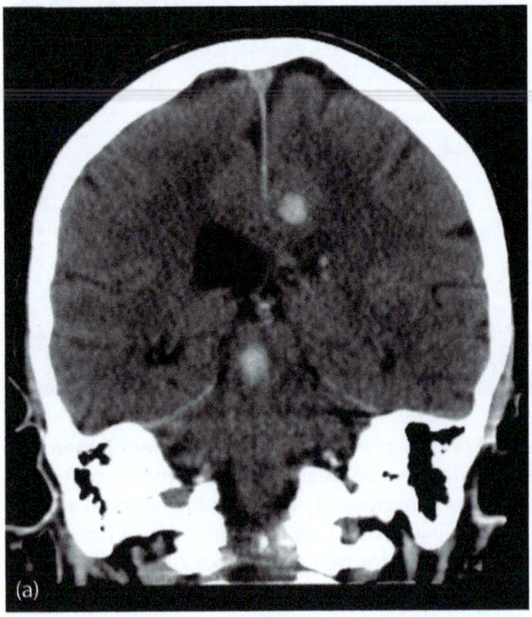

Figure 8.16a Coronal head CT reveals hemorrhages within the right dorsal midbrain and left cingulum. (From Brian L. Edlow, M.D., Massachusetts General Hospital, Harvard Medical School.) Source image [B] reproduced with permission of American Association of Neuropathologists, Inc. (539)

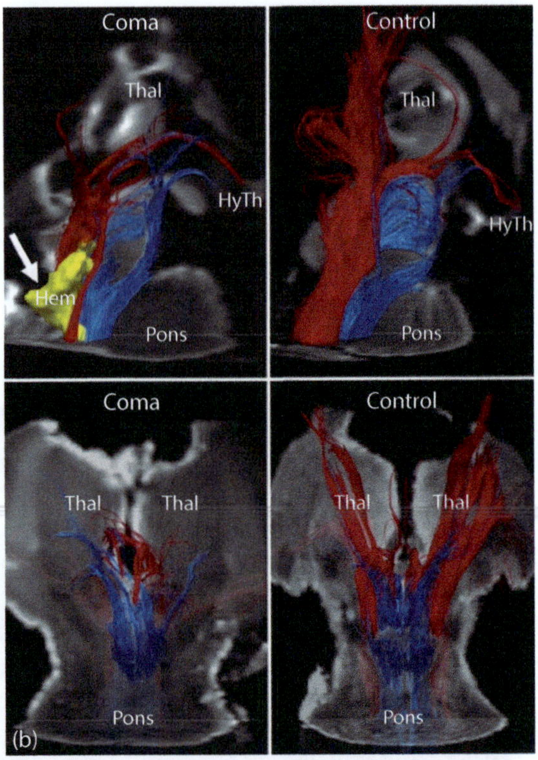

Figure 8.16b Brainstem arousal network disruption in traumatic coma. Right lateral view (top two images) and ventral perspective (bottom two images) of patient's thalamus and brainstem regions, showing fiber tracts (red and blue) as well as location of a midbrain hemorrhage (yellow) and images from a control. The patient who had suffered a coma (left) was found to have disruption of thalamic (Thal) connectivity but partial preservation of hypothalamic (HyTh) connections. Tracts are superimposed on diffusion-weighted images. The right caudal midbrain hemorrhage (Hem) is rendered in three dimensions (solid yellow with arrow). Source images [C, D, E, F] reproduced with permission of American Association of Neuropathologists, Inc. (539)

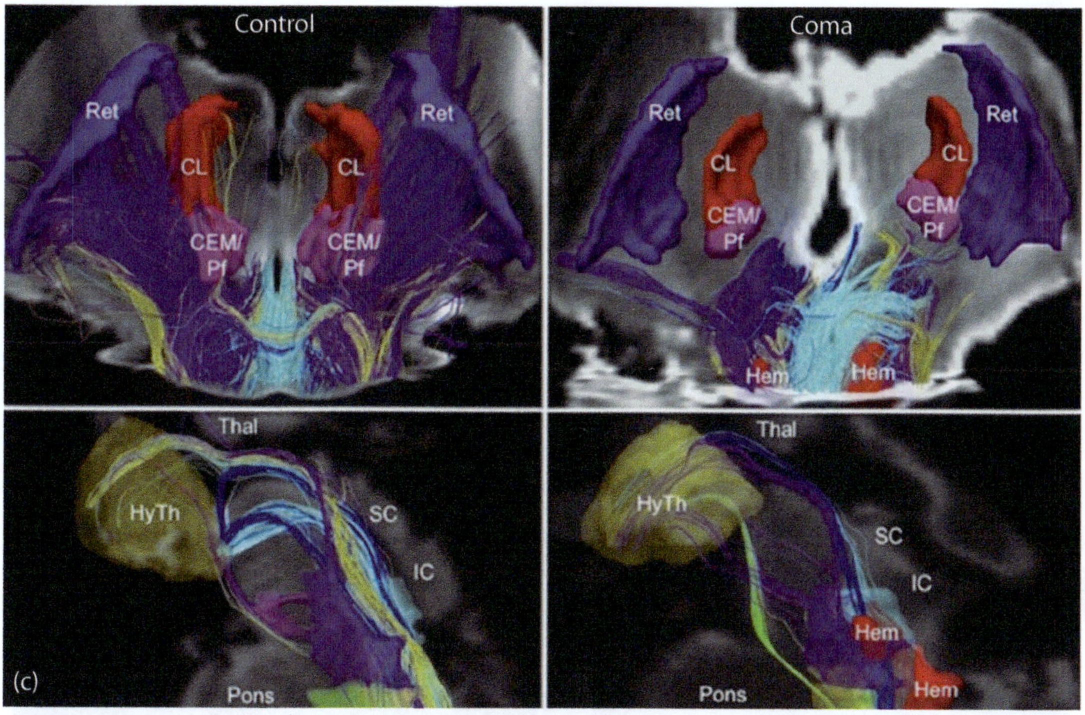

Figure 8.16c Connectivity of the brainstem arousal network, showing tracts in control and traumatic coma patient, is seen from both dorsal and side views. Tracts shown are color-coded according to the brainstem nucleus from which they originate: Pedunculopontine nucleus (cholinergic: purple); parabrachial complex (glutamatergic: yellow); dorsal raphe (serotonergic: turquoise); locus coeruleus (noradrenergic: dark blue); median raphe (serotonergic: green); ventral tegmental area (dopaminergic: pink). Fiber tracts in the control, but not in the traumatic coma patient, connect with the reticular nuclei (Ret) of the thalamus (thal) and intralaminar nuclei (central lateral nuclei [CL]; centromedian/parafascicular complex [CEM/Pf]). Significant tract disruption occurs rostral to the hemorrhages (Hem, red) and is likely caused by non-hemorrhagic axonal injury in the rostral midbrain. In the traumatic coma patient, fiber tracts to the hypothalamus (HyTh) are partially preserved. Also seen are the inferior colliculus (IC) and superior colliculus (SC). Source images [A, B, C, D] reproduced with permission of American Association of Neuropathologists, Inc. (539)

Additional tractography analysis of the brainstem nuclei of the ARAS revealed bilateral and symmetric disruption of multiple pathways between this region and the basal forebrain. The only remaining partially preserved fiber pathways connecting the thalamus and brainstem arousal nuclei were those to the lateral geniculate nucleus from the mesencephalic reticular formation, pedunculopontine nucleus, and dorsal raphe (**Figure 8.16c**; 539). There was disruption of thalamocortical tracts, especially in areas where hemorrhages were seen, in the patient who was in a coma, as compared to a control patient. There were also disconnected transcallosal fibers in the traumatic coma patient (**Figure 8.16d**; 539). Both HARDI tractography (**Figure 8.16e**; 539) and histologic examination revealed no axons passing through the center of the left cingulate hemorrhage.

Whole-brain FA histogram analysis

FA histogram whole-brain analysis shows that global white-matter analysis correlates with injury severity. Benson reported on a study of 20 patients with mild to severe TBI (who had a mean duration to scan of 35.3 months) and 14 controls, on which DTI imaging of the brain was performed, and a white-matter FA histogram-based method of analysis was used to compare persons with TBI to healthy controls. This analysis revealed a global decrease in FA in white

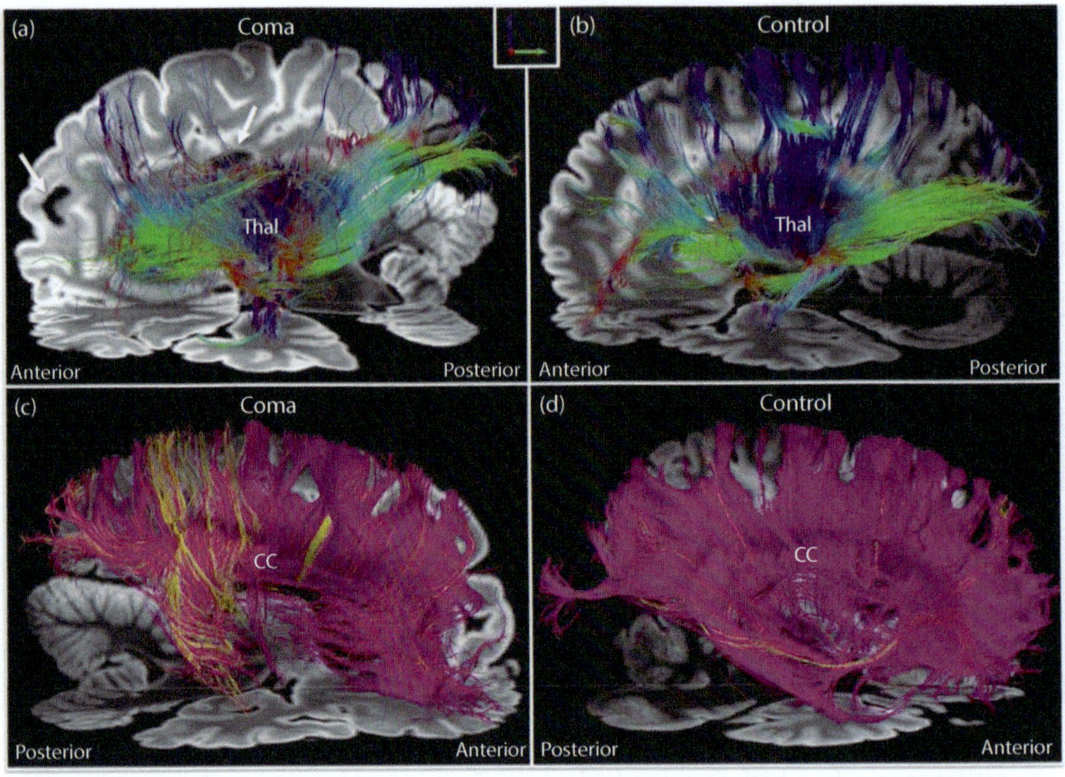

Figure 8.16d Connectivity of thalamocortical and transcallosal fiber pathways. Left lateral views (a and b) of traumatic coma patient (a) and control (b) with thalamocortical fiber tracts that are color-coded by direction (inset). Thalamocortical tracts are disrupted in the patient, especially in regions with hemorrhages (arrows), but tracts can be seen connecting with the frontal, temporal, parietal, and occipital lobes. Right lateral views (c and d) of traumatic coma patient (c) and control (d) transcallosal fiber tracts (pink). Tracts that terminate within the corpus callosum (CC) are dissected using the DISCONNECT segmentation technique and color-coded yellow. More disconnected yellow fibers are seen in the traumatic coma patient than in the control, but many transcallosal fiber tracts remain intact in the traumatic coma patient. All fiber tracts in (a–d) are superimposed on diffusion-weighted images. Reproduced with permission of American Association of Neuropathologists, Inc. (539) (From Brian L. Edlow, M.D., Massachusetts General Hospital, Harvard Medical School.)

matter in TBI patients versus controls. In addition, the histogram shape (**Figure 8.17**; 362) revealed a leftward shift with greater kurtosis on the curve, which, along with mean FA, suggests a common mechanism (axonal injury) was responsible. They indicated that this likely results from increased radial diffusion and decreased axial diffusion, and Benson cited the works of Grady and Christman with respect to axotomy and impaired axoplasmic transport as contributing to this. Benson also cited the work of Povlishock and Pettus regarding myelin breakdown, axonal swellings, retraction balls, and increased membrane permeability, which may lead to increased radial diffusion. Importantly, after analyzing histogram parameters such as skew, kurtosis, FA mean and peak FA, Benson felt that FA mean was a "better predictor of clinical scores than the other parameters, while PTA showed a greater correlation with histogram parameters than did admission GCS." In this study, "comparison of single subject images revealed differences in FA maps, where conventional imaging was often unrevealing." (362)

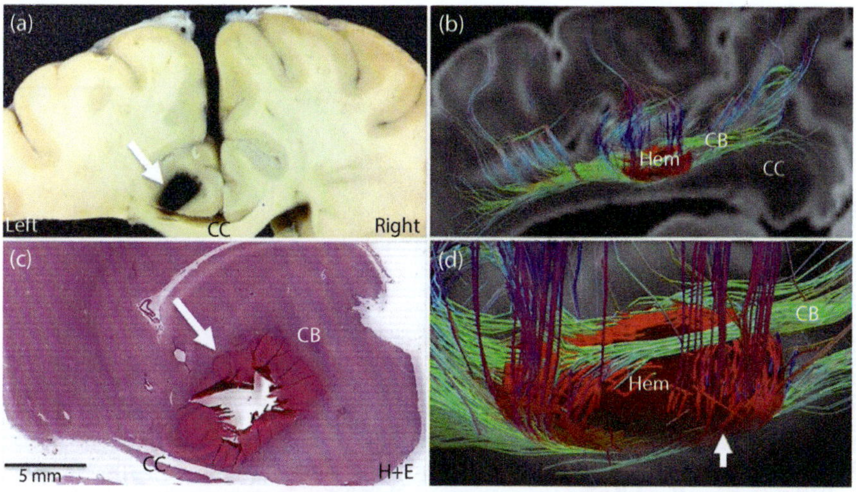

Figure 8.16e Tractography-histopathology analysis of a hemorrhage-related axonal injury in the left cingulum bundle (CB). Coronal section of gross pathologic specimen showing the left CB hemorrhage (arrow, a). Left lateral view (b) of fiber tracts generated using the left CB hemorrhage as a seed region of interest; this is rendered as a three-dimensional semitransparent object (red, Hem) superimposed on a sagittal diffusion-weighted image at the midline. Tracts are color coded according to their direction (green, anterior-posterior; blue, superior-inferior; red, medial-lateral). Hematoxylin and eosin (H&E) stain of CB hemorrhage demonstrates complete destruction of tissue within the hemorrhage (arrow, c), as indicated by the loss of tissue integrity at the center of the hemorrhage. Zoomed left lateral view (d) of tractography analysis from (B) demonstrates the presence of green (anterior-to-posterior) CB fiber tracts and blue (superior-to-inferior) transcallosal fiber tracts (arrow, d) passing along the borders of the hemorrhage (Hem) but not through its center. Source images [A, B, C, D] reproduced with permission of American Association of Neuropathologists, Inc. (539) (From Brian L. Edlow, M.D., Massachusetts General Hospital, Harvard Medical School.)

Laboratory TBI studies

DTI (measuring FA, MD, AD, RD) in rats exposed to a single blast injury was utilized to evaluate three major white-matter brain structures: the corpus callosum (largest commissural white-matter bundle in the brain); the cingulum bundle (prominent white-matter longitudinal tract above the corpus callosum and within the limbic system); and fimbria (covers a portion of the hippocampus). Acutely after injury, all three white-matter bundles showed imaging evidence of axonal injury, vasogenic edema and demyelination. In the subacute phase, the corpus callosum showed persistent axonal pathology with cytotoxic edema and demyelination (confirmed on ultrastructural analysis), whereas the cingulum showed cytotoxic edema. Of interest, even though only the right side of the rat head was exposed to the blast wave, the changes in diffusion were almost identical on both sides of the brain. In addition, greater diffusion metric change was seen in the medial corpus callosum fibers when compared to the lateral fibers, suggesting that the regions closer to the midline suffered greater damage than the lateral regions. (137) Another DTI study in rats showed white-matter vulnerability and chronic microstructural abnormalities following mild TBI. (436)

DTI OF BLAST INJURY

After blast injuries, differing results were seen with respect to imaging studies. Although FA is often increased in certain white-matter tracts in the chronic phase, there are also studies that find inconclusive or opposite results with FA decreased in the chronic phase.

Among 202 military service members with PCS six months after a blast-related mild TBI, there was an association with reduced FA in the pathways within the fronto-limbic, fronto-striatal circuits, and, in particular, the parasagittal cortical white-matter fibers (cingulum-angular bundle, anterior thalamic radiations, superior longitudinal

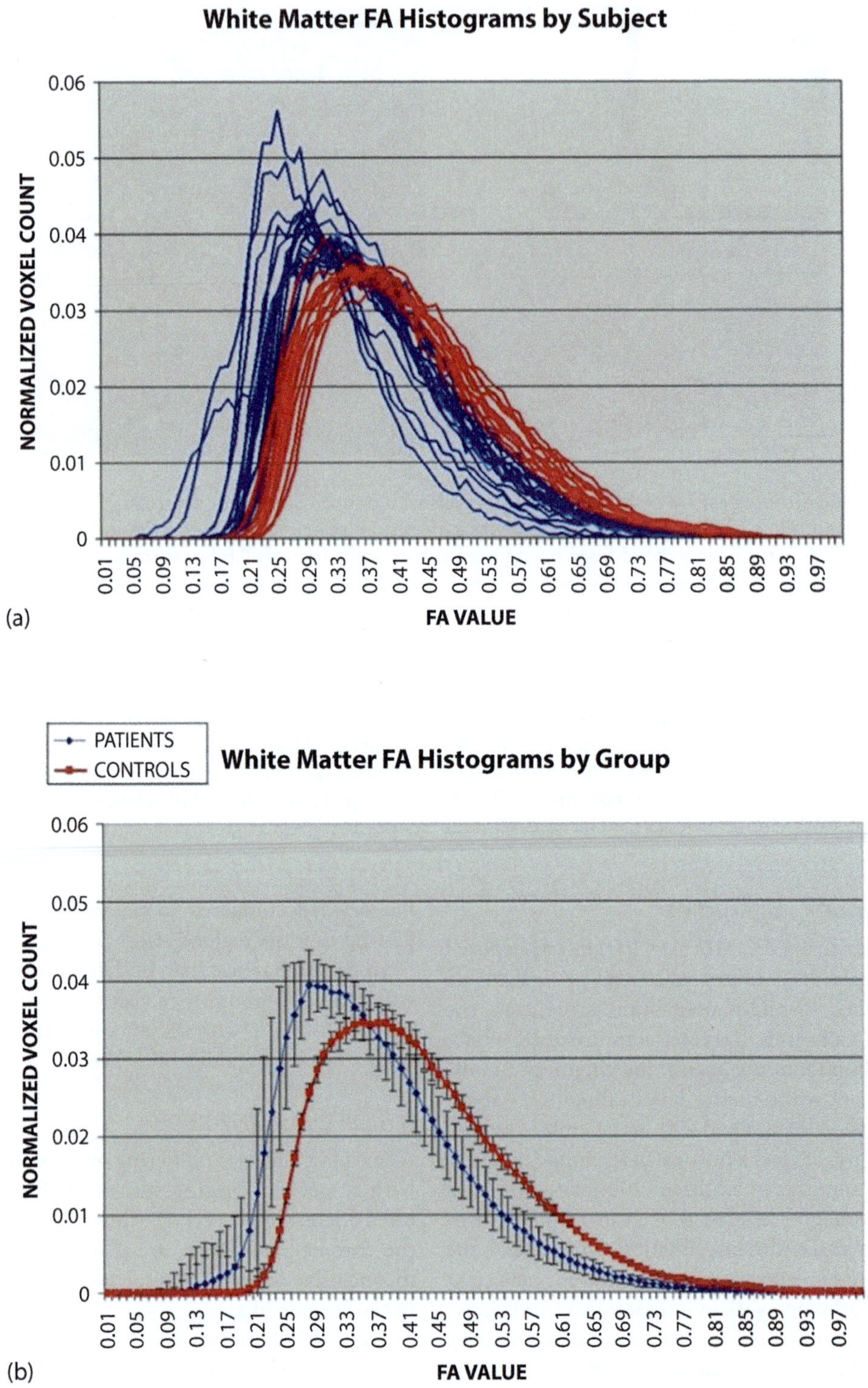

Figure 8.17 White-matter FA histograms for all subjects (a). Healthy volunteers shown in red, TBI patients in blue. Two histograms are group-averaged histograms, respectively, where each data point is the mean voxel number for the FA bin range (b). FA total range was divided into 100 equally spaced bins with marker (closed circle) at the center of the bin range. Error bars show standard deviations. The publisher for this copyrighted material is Mary Ann Liebert, Inc. publishers. Reproduced with permission. (362)

fasciculus, and inferior fronto-occipital fasciculus). Injured fiber tracts with reduced FA are associated with increased PCS, post-traumatic stress disorder (PTSD) symptoms, and neuropsychological function findings. There was a negative association between FA and time since the most severe blast exposure in a subset of the multiple-blast exposed group. Blast exposure also correlated with lower FA of the bilateral cingulum bundles as the age of the patient increased. In addition, high frequency of blast exposures may negatively impact the aging trajectory of white-matter integrity. (447) A greater number of blast exposures is associated with lower white-matter integrity and FA, regardless of the presence of clinical TBI, and may be related to changes of FA in the bilateral cingulum. (449)

After blast injury and a mild TBI, FA was reduced in the acute phase 6–12 months after injury. Sixty-three U.S. military personnel, who suffered blast-related and other trauma to the head with a mild uncomplicated TBI, were evaluated with DTI scanning performed within 90 days of the injury and were compared to 21 controls with blast exposure but no clinical diagnosis of TBI. Although there were no abnormalities on CT brain scans, many in the TBI group had abnormalities on DTI imaging. Follow-up DTI studies in 6–12 months on 47 individuals showed persistent abnormalities consistent with evolving injuries. The DTI pattern in the initial scans were consistent with axonal injury (decreased FA, increased radial and mean diffusivity) in addition to a cellular inflammatory response and edema, whereas on the follow-up scans (6–12 months post-injury), the findings were consistent with persistent axonal injury (decreased FA, decreased AD) with resolution of edema and cellular inflammation. Importantly, it was felt that the evolution of findings over time confirmed that they were unlikely to have been preexisting. The authors point out that only 18 of the 63 subjects with TBI had definitely abnormal DTI scans. Importantly, the authors find that normal DTI findings do not rule out a TBI, and that DTI findings in isolation are not sufficient to make a TBI diagnosis with certainty. (115)

Five years after suffering a concussive blast TBI, 50 injured military personnel were compared to 44 combat-deployed controls. While cross-sectional analysis of white matter on DTI images did not reveal significant differences, single-subject analysis showed 74% of the concussive blast TBI cohort to have reductions in FA compared to the controls, indicating chronic brain injury. (663)

Another group of 34 veterans with a blast/impact mild TBI were found to have reduced FA in the corpus callosum compared to controls as well as reduced macromolecular proton fraction in sybgyral, longitudinal, and cortical/subcortical white-matter and gray-matter regions. (546)

When 23 veterans exposed to a primary blast without TBI symptoms and 6 with mild TBI were compared to controls and studied with DTI, those not reporting TBI symptoms had similar white-matter abnormalities to those who did, which were consistent with the white-matter abnormalities seen with repetitive subconcussive events in elite sports participants. Notably, Taber concluded that the lack of TBI symptoms after a blast exposure should not be cause for assumption that there is little or no effect on the nervous system, but noted that their results are preliminary and suggested larger sample sizes. (547)

White-matter changes were seen in a study of blast injury veterans. Ninety veterans who had been exposed to a blast within 100 meters were subdivided into groups depending upon severity and, after undergoing DTI scanning and cluster FA analysis, were found to have heterogeneous white-matter abnormalities associated with blast-related mild TBI (especially when there was a loss of consciousness). There were correlations between white-matter abnormalities and PCS. PTSD symptoms were not related to white-matter abnormalities, but were associated with severity of PCS in all three domains (physical, emotional, cognitive). The mild TBI group that experienced loss of consciousness had more spatially heterogeneous white-matter abnormalities than the group exposed to a blast but without TBI. (545)

In contrast with the above studies, other studies have found no significant findings on DTI imaging. Levin evaluated veterans who suffered mild-to-moderate TBIs, and found no significant imaging differences (DTI, FA, and ADC) between those suffering a mild-to-moderate blast injury and controls despite residual symptoms and difficulty with verbal memory. (450)

Opposite findings with increased FA were seen in another study of blast TBI. Harrington, who studied military service members or veterans who suffered a blast mild TBI, compared them to controls using imaging performed 130–758 days post-injury. The researchers found increased FA and decreased RD in the mild blast TBI group, mostly in the anterior tracts. Harrington cited Browne and Povlishock in explaining that increased FA in the presence of decreased RD is likely due to the stretching and twisting of axons caused by blast-related deformation of the microstructural white-matter regions. Harrington noted the discrepancy of their findings from other studies in the literature and cited Davenport, Isaac, Miller, Browne, Morey, Petrie, and Taber in noting that for people who have suffered a blast-related mild TBI, imaging studies performed longer than two years later typically show decreased FA. Harrington also noted that for imaging studies performed sooner, discrepant findings may be seen and cited Povlishock and Johnson regarding possible explanations of different fiber recovery stages and axonal degeneration. (446)

In a laboratory study of blast TBI, rats exposed to a blast mild TBI showed a biphasic response to FA analysis in the corpus callosum with a decrease on days 2 and 12, and increase on day 5, which they noted was similar to FA dynamics in humans. (548)

IMAGING OF INTRACORTICAL MYELIN

While DTI is useful for evaluating damage to the deep white matter of the brain, it is less helpful for evaluating axonal injury and demyelination that may occur in the cortical regions of the brain. To evaluate cortical myelination, a T1 weighted (T1-w) and T2 weighted (T2-w) ratio method can be used at each voxel, thus creating a myelin map. In essentially all cases, the entire cerebral cortex showed some negative association between the cortical myelin contrast and the number of lifetime TBIs a patient experienced. Blast injury was not found to have any effect on intracortical myelin. The study concluded that the intracortical myelin ratio may be a biomarker for TBI, which is complementary to diffusion MRI. (371)

DTT/CONNECTOME

Quantifying fiber tracts in the brain evaluates the data produced by DTI and uses assumptions to define likely fiber tracts, incorporating thresholds of FA and turning angles. Two methods may be used to try to define the tracts: 1) region of interest (ROI) method, and 2) tract-based for the long association tracts. (467) Tract-based analysis appears to provide a reproducible tool to perform core analysis. (468) Tractography can be made more difficult due to the analysis of crossing fibers. Reid described an approach to determine the most probable trajectory of white-matter projection between two ROIs. They performed probabilistic tractography twice, seeding in one region and terminating in another. They arrived at directed probability distributions, which were averaged to yield a bidirectional probability average, and thresholds identified a set of inter-region continuous voxels. This technique is used to identify the most likely geometry of a path between two regions. (469)

Sung reported that more studies have used the ROI method than the DTT method, but the ROI approach can produce false results due to individual variability in neural tract anatomy, possibly leading to measurements in an incorrect location or the ROI being placed within a lesion itself. An advantage of DTT over DTI is that the entire tract can be evaluated for DTT parameters (FA, MD, TV), in addition to the appearance of reconstructed tracts that may show tearing, narrowing, or discontinuation (potentially detecting TAI in a mild TBI patient). (467)

In a group of 25 patients who suffered a severe TBI, diffusion MRI tractography was performed (median of ten days post-injury), revealing a significant relationship between early (within 30 days of injury) command-following and integrity of the thalamic connections with the prefrontal cortex (PFC), medial PFC (mPFC), anterior cingulate cortex (ACC), and orbitofrontal cortex (OFC). Cosgrove stated, "our data show that PFC (prefrontal cortex), more specifically its medial subregions, is important for recovery after TBI." (475) (**Figure 8.18**)

DKI AND DSI

Tractography based on DTI has difficulty at imaging multiple fiber orientations within a single voxel. (550) Both DKI and diffusion spectrum imaging are better with handling the challenge of imaging crossing fibers. The directionality of multimodal diffusion in regions of the brain that possess complex fiber architecture can be described with an orientation distribution function (ODF). (443) Kurtosis is a measure that reflects the deviation of a water diffusion profile from a Gaussian distribution. This technique may be used to better image anatomical barriers not detected by standard DTI. DKI provides a b-value (diffusion weighting strength)

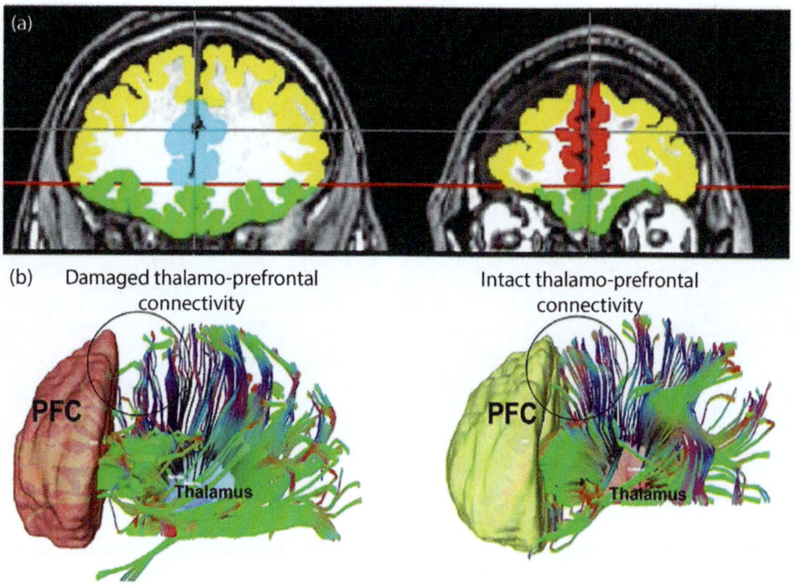

Figure 8.18 Connections between the prefrontal cortex and thalamus. An example of prefrontal cortex (PFC) regions of interest with colors representing each one (coronal view) (a). Yellow = dlPFC; green = OFC; teal = ACC; red = mPFC. Thalamo-prefrontal tractography from two representative patients (sagittal view from left side of brain) (b): One with damage to thalamo-prefrontal projections and one without. An area of decreased thalamo-prefrontal projections in the patient with damage to these connections is represented by a circle. This same area in the patient with intact projections is circled as well. DlPFC = dorsolateral prefrontal cortex, ACC = anterior cingulate cortex, mPFC = medial prefrontal cortex, OFC = orbitofrontal cortex. From (475) https://creativecommons.org/licenses/by/4.0/legalcode

independent estimation of diffusion tensor parameters. (441) Using DKI, the ODF is broken down into both Gaussian and non-Gaussian diffusion contributions, with the non-Gaussian being most sensitive for the purpose of defining the directions of fibers. DKI also uses low b-values, yielding a higher signal-to-noise ratio than other techniques. (443) Paydar has cited Veraart, Jensen, Lu, and De Santis in stating "the DKI technique is a clinically feasible extension of the traditional DTI model while maintaining the ability to estimate all the standard diffusion tensor metrics, including axial diffusivity, radial diffusivity, and FA, but with improved accuracy." Paydar further cites Veraart and Jensen in noting that DKI requires a greater number of b-values and diffusion gradient directions than does DTI, resulting in a higher angle resolution of diffusion acquisitions. There was also found to be higher sensitivity for the evaluation of crossing fibers with DKI than with DTI (**Figure 8.19**; 438). As with DTI, the analogous metrics obtained from DKI are axial kurtosis, radial kurtosis, and mean kurtosis. (438)

DSI also addresses the limitations of DTI for imaging of multiple fiber orientations within a single voxel and shows characteristic local heterogeneities of fiber architecture, including angular dispersion and intersection. (552) DSI provides for delineation of crossing and touching fibers and can reveal transcallosal fibers better than DTI. (551) DSI provides better fiber bundle orientation estimates than does DTI, which can significantly affect tractography. DSI has been found to be qualitatively similar to DKI in terms of tractography obtained, but DKI uses shorter scan times. Both are superior to DTI for resolving crossing fibers on tractography (**Figure 8.20**; 549).

FIXEL-BASED ANALYSIS (FBA)

FBA is intended to address the difficulties of analyzing crossing white-matter fibers. Dhollander cites Raffelt as proposing a statistical analysis framework, FBA, in which a fixel refers to an individual fiber population within a voxel. Fixels relate to the white-matter anatomy. Dhollander cites Tournier, Jeurissen, and Dhollander in stating that

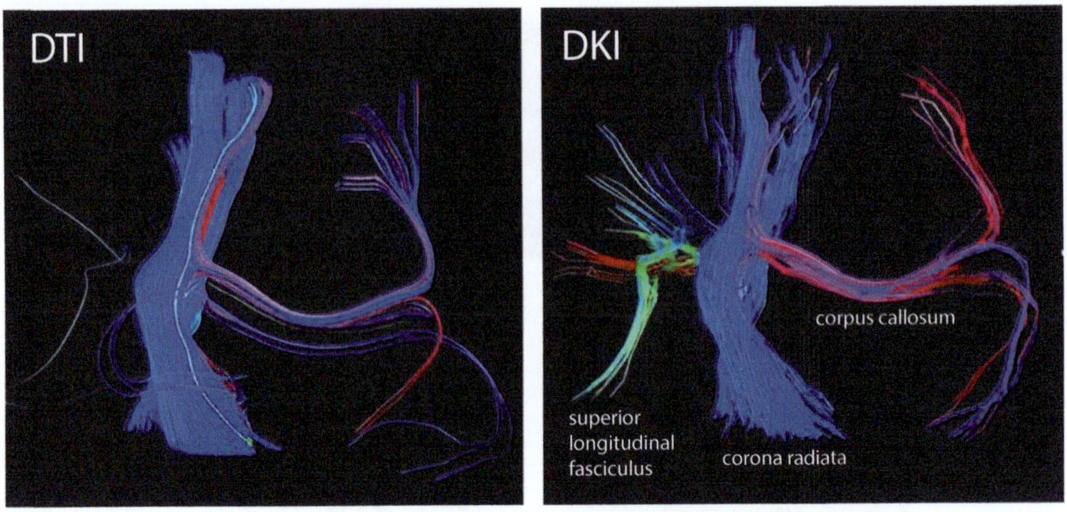

Figure 8.19 DTI and DKI tractographies performed on a normal brain illustrate the difference in sensitivity for the detection of tiny crossing fibers between DTI and DKI fiber-tracking techniques. Reproduced with permission American Society of Neuroradiology. (438)

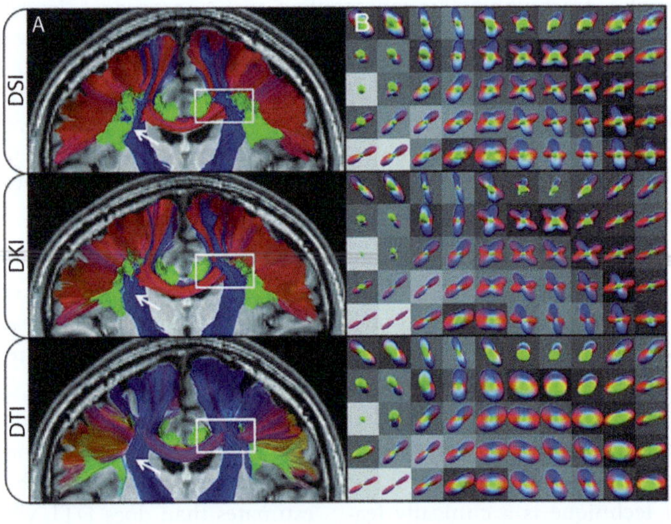

Figure 8.20 Effects of the diffusion orientation distribution function (dODF) reconstructions on white-matter tractography. Column A shows a coronal cross-section through the fiber tracts identified with DSI, DKI, and DTI, respectively, overlaid on the corresponding section from the magnetization-prepared rapid gradient-echo sequence (MP RAGE) image for anatomic reference. The color encoding is used to represent the overall displacement of the end points of each tract with one color being applied per tract, where red represents a left-right orientation, blue represents an inferior-superior orientation, and green represents an anterior-posterior orientation. DSI is the most sensitive technique for detecting fibers (white arrows); however, DSI and DKI are fairly similar in both the color, which illustrates the overall trajectory, and distribution of fibers identified. Column B shows selected dODFs with the same coloring scheme as the fibers in column A, overlaid on the corresponding FA image from the DTI scan. The region shown in column B is demarcated by the white box in the corresponding images in column A. DTI fibers are conspicuously affected in this region because the dODFs cannot detect crossing fibers; this feature causes fibers to prematurely terminate or for anatomically distinct tracts to meld. This cross-section was chosen to demonstrate interactions that occur among the corpus callosum, corona radiata, superior longitudinal fasciculus, and cingulum bundle and their effect on dODFs and subsequent tractography. Reproduced with permission American Society of Neuroradiology. (549)

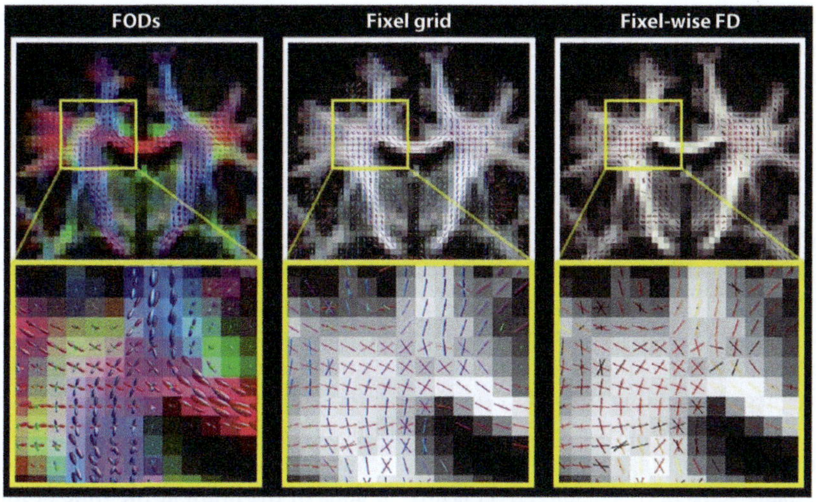

Figure 8.21 Derivation of a fixel grid and fixel-wise apparent fiber density (FD). (Left) Voxel-wise white matter (WM) fiber orientation distributions (FODs) (here obtained from three-tissue CSD) serve as the source from which both the fixel grid and fixel-wise apparent FD metric are computed. In this image, WM FODs in a coronal slice are overlaid on an FOD-based directionally-encoded color map) (red = right to left, green = anteroposterior, blue = superoinferior). (Middle) The fixels are obtained by segmenting the FODs into their individual "peaks." Unlike the regular lattice structure of the underlying voxel grid, the fixel grid's presence and orientations are tied to the WM anatomy itself. (Right) Apparent FD is computed as the integral of each FOD lobe (hot color scale). The underlying voxel intensities show the total voxel-wise apparent FD (gray color scale). Both fixel-wise and voxel-wise apparent FDs are expressed in arbitrary units. From (570) https://creativecommons.org/licenses/by/4.0/legalcode

"fixels are derived from WM (white matter) fiber orientation distributions (FODs) as computed by constrained spherical deconvolution (CSD) techniques" (**Figure 8.21**; 570). Fixel-based analysis measures apparent fiber density (FD). (570)

FLAIR

FLAIR is an MRI sequence which suppresses the signal from CSF and can significantly improve the image quality of brain lesions adjacent to CSF. Since many traumatic lesions of the brain, such as DAI, cortical contusions, brainstem injuries, and subdural hematomas occur close to CSF, they may be difficult to see on conventional T2-w images, but are better seen on FLAIR images. (568)

In the subacute and chronic phase of TBI evaluation, MRI scanning has advantages, as it can detect subacute and chronic subarachnoid hemorrhage. It is also more sensitive than CT scanning for the detection of blood products 24–48 hours after injury as well as for the detection of axonal injuries. MRI may be indicated in patients who have a normal CT scan of the brain, but experience persistent neurologic findings that cannot be explained. FLAIR sequence images performed 18–45 days after a subarachnoid hemorrhage were able, in all cases, to detect blood in the sylvian fissures and cerebral sulci. It was concluded that FLAIR images are useful in detecting small areas of subarachnoid hemorrhage diluted by CSF, which are not detected on conventional MRI or CT scans. (110, 111)

In a study of 128 patients who suffered moderate and severe TBI, brain MRI imaging was performed about eight days after injury as well as in 47 healthy controls and outcomes 12 months later were assessed using the GOSE. In patients who suffered severe TBI, the magnitude of diffusion-weighted imaging (DWI) and FLAIR lesions in the corpus callosum, brainstem, and thalamus were correlated inversely with outcome. In the moderate TBI group, the number of cortical contusions predicted outcome. The study concluded that in severe TBI, lesions in the corpus callosum were most predictive of outcome, but in moderate TBI, it is the number of cortical contusions that are predictive. (136) FLAIR imaging has also been used in evaluating TAI, where it was found that lesion burden calculated from the volume of contusions on FLAIR imaging, was strongly associated with GCS scores. (569)

SWI

SWI is a sensitive imaging study for detecting microhemorrhages within the brain, (525) which are a biomarker of DAI/TAI (369). CMBs (471) may appear as ovoid, hypointense lesions on SWI (**Figure 8.22**; 471). They may be temporarily less detectable for 24–72 hours after a TBI, possibly leading to false-negative finding if an SWI scan is performed during that time period. (473) In addition to visualizing hemorrhage well, SWI is also used for visualizing veins in tissue. (589) SWI is an MRI sequence that utilizes differences in magnetic susceptibilities among different tissues, and its sensitivity increases with the magnetic field strength. (589) The disturbances to a homogeneous magnetic field, which may be caused by paramagnetic or

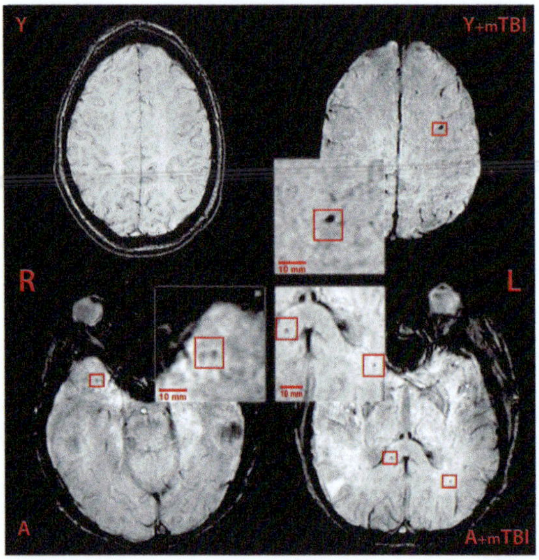

Figure 8.22 Axial susceptibility weighted imaging (SWI) MRI (three Tesla) of a young control patient (Y, 38-year-old, male), a young patient following mild TBI (Y + mTBI, 36-year-old male, GCS: 15), an aged control patient (A, 67-year-old male), and a 65-year-old patient with a mild TBI (A + mTBI, 65-year-old male, GCS: 15). Cerebral microbleeds (CMBs) appear as ovoid, hypointense lesions and are indicated by the red squares, showing magnified regions of the brain. R = right, L = left. From (471) https://creativecommons.org/licenses/by/4.0/legalcode

diamagnetic substances (such as iron-laden tissues, clots, partially deoxygenated blood, calcium), are used to enhance contrast in the brain. As blood products (deoxyhemoglobin, methemoglobin, hemosiderin) have their paramagnetic properties accentuated by SWI, this technique is useful for detecting intravascular venous deoxygenated blood and extravascular blood products. (112) MRI imaging methods utilizing SWI can evaluate hemorrhagic DAI. SWI provides good contrast between gray matter, whiter matter, iron-laden tissues, venous blood vessels, and other tissue. Information about magnetic field and chemical shift of tissues is provided by phase images. SWI scans have shown that the number and volume of lesions in the brain at the time of injury are moderately correlated in a negative manner with intellectual and neuropsychological scores one to four years later. In a study of 18 children who suffered a TBI, SWI scans two to ten days after injury found that lesion volume explained a 32.9% variance in Full Scale IQ (intellectual function) and 44.3% variance in neuropsychologic function when measured one to four years after the injury (112–114). MRI/CT multimodal imaging data acquisition using SWI and DWI have been utilized to find changes to the human connectome that are related to CMBs within the brain. (132)

Sixteen patients who suffered traumatic hemorrhagic contusions in the brain and an average admission GCS score of 7.9 underwent neuropsychological evaluations at six months post-injury, which revealed that outcome is related to lesion size in the temporal lobe, whereas frontal-lobe lesion volume did not correlate with neuropsychological outcome. On average, more than 50% of the initial intracerebral blood volume was present on MRI brain scans six months after injury, where the hemorrhage and iron deposits may be an important factor in secondary brain injury. (286)

Dahl raised an interesting point in a paper that evaluates CMBs and structural white matter in patients with TBI. The researchers evaluated 20 patients who suffered a TBI and had CMBs, 34 patients with TBI but without CMBs, and 11 controls with orthopedic injuries using SWI imaging two months post-injury to detect CMBs. At eight months post-TBI, DTI and clinical outcome assessment using the GOSE was performed. Patients with TBI and CMBs had lower FA and higher MD values (altered white matter) than those with TBI but without CMBs, as seen with

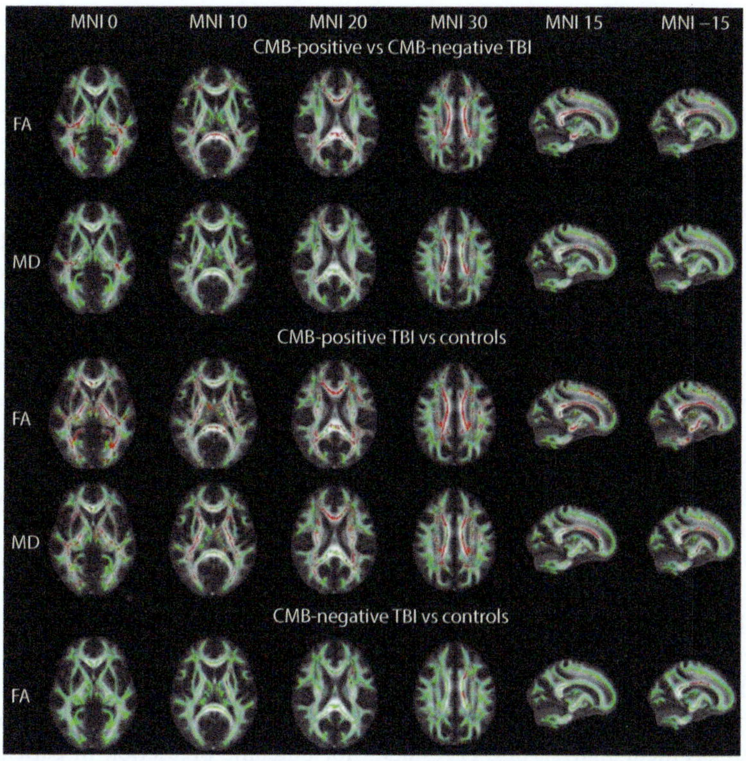

Figure 8.23 TBSS comparison of the following groups: CMB positive versus CMB negative, CMB positive versus controls, CMB negative versus controls. TBSS images show fractional anisotropy (FA) and mean diffusivity (MD) with statistically significant voxels (shown in red) indicating brain regions with differences between two compared groups overlaid on a mean FA skeleton template (shown in green) on a brain MRI (Oxford Center for Functional MRI of the Brain). CMB = cerebral microbleed, TBI = traumatic brain injury. MRI is in Montreal Neurological Institute (MNI) 152 space. From (472) https://creativecommons.org/licenses/by/4.0/legalcode

TBSS results. (**Figure 8.23**; 472) CMBs were associated with worse clinical outcomes. The researchers found that in TBI patients although increased CMB total lesion load was associated with lower FA and worse clinical outcomes, after adjusting for severity of TBI, CMBs were not associated with microstructural white-matter alterations. This finding may reflect the worsened trauma causing increased white-matter injury and CMBs as well. They note that "the effect of CMBs on WM (white matter) alterations was not independent and was strongly related to clinical severity." (472)

fMRI (BOLD)

fMRI utilizes blood oxygen level dependent (BOLD) imaging to evaluate for changes in local blood flow within the brain to assess brain function. The principle behind fMRI involves the detection of increased blood flow to areas of the brain that experience increased neuronal activity. fMRI can be performed during the resting state as well as when performing a task (task-based). (657) During a task-based study, while in the MRI machine, the patient repeatedly either carries out a specific task or is presented with a stimulus (such as a visual stimulus). The scan takes advantage of the differences in magnetic susceptibility of deoxyhemoglobin (paramagnetic with small positive susceptibility to magnetic fields) and oxyhemoglobin (diamagnetic with weak negative susceptibility to magnetic fields). (370, 432) Machine learning methods have been applied to resting state fMRI interpretation to identify diagnostic network features to predict mild TBI severity. (657)

In a study of 10 patients who suffered subacute/chronic severe TBI, fMRI revealed poor problem-solving as related to impaired function of the dorsolateral prefrontal cortex and the anterior cingulate cortex. (376)

Of 24 patients who suffered TBI and were admitted to a neurointensive care unit, serum S100B levels were taken 12–36 hours post-injury and were found to have a negative relationship with resting-state brain connectivity as well as visual, auditory, sensory and fronto-parietal networks as evaluated on a resting state fMRI. It was suggested that resting-state brain fMRI brain connectivity may potentially predict long-term outcome in TBI patients. (378)

Twelve patients who suffered a mild-to-severe TBI with significant white-matter disruptions seen on DTI were evaluated with resting state fMRI. Despite decreased white-matter connectivity, the resting fMRI showed an increase in connectivity in various regions of the default mode network, possibly due to functional compensation in which the neurons work harder to accomplish the same task. (377)

A meta-analysis of functional MRI results in patients with mild TBI found that there is decreased signal within the prefrontal cortex when compared to controls, demonstrating a frontal vulnerability to injury. A meta-analysis of DTI results showed elevated anisotropy in the acute phase of mild TBI, but decreased anisotropy in the chronic phase. Immediately after injury, poor neuropsychological performance was associated with high anisotropy scores but with low anisotropy scores in the chronic phase. (117)

MR spectroscopy

MRI uses the strong signals from protons in water and fat molecules to create anatomical images. MR spectroscopy (MRS) looks at the signals from metabolites, which are very weak, to identify and quantify these substances in the tissue. MRS allows the evaluation of certain metabolites within the brain, such as the neuronal metabolite *N*-acetylaspartate (NAA), membrane-related choline, and glial metabolite myo-inositol, as well as creatine (Cr), glutamine (Glu), and lactate. Following a TBI, cellular injury with altered neuronal viability, cell membrane damage, and gliosis can be evaluated with MRS. (118, 138) MRS has the potential to detect tissue pathology prior to anatomical imaging because after a mild TBI, biochemical changes often occur before anatomical changes do. (589)

In a literature review, Gardner found that 9 of 11 studies of athletes who suffered sports-related concussions were found to show proton MRS abnormalities consistent with an alteration in neurochemistry. The authors conclude that MRS abnormalities may reveal neurophysiological changes even after clinical post-concussive symptoms (balance and cognitive problems) have resolved. (118, 138, 432) A study utilizing single-voxel proton MRI and proton MRS imaging found that changes in creatine-phosphocreatine (Cr) and glutamate (Glu) may occur after a mild TBI. Cr is a critical component of brain energy metabolism and Glu is a major neurotransmitter. In mild TBI patients, Cr was elevated in the supraventricular white matter and the splenium whereas Glu was reduced. (381) In an MRS and DTI study of 18 patients who suffered a range of TBI severities, structural injury and metabolic disruption were detected within hours of injury. MRS evidence of neuronal injury in the posterior cingulate cortex was seen within 24 hours of trauma, reflecting disruption in markers of axon coherence in the associated corpus callosum and cingulum bundle. (379)

MRS has been used in conjunction with DTI for outcome prediction in patients who have suffered severe TBI. MRS evaluations of the *N*-acetylaspartate/creatine (NAA/Cr) ratio in the pons, thalamus, and insula, in conjunction with DTI evaluation of FA in the supratentorial and infratentorial regions, was found to have a predictive value of an unfavorable (86% sensitivity and 97% specificity) versus favorable outcome. (463)

Volume segmentation/brain volume

After suffering a TBI, brain volume is often decreased in the chronic phase. Analysis of volumes of regional portions of the brain is used to gain insight into various brain diseases. Automated segmentation procedures have been developed, but it is important that they are reliable and reproducible. Some of the algorithms utilize freely available automated segmentation tools such as FreeSurfer (https://surfer.nmr.mgh.harvard.edu/). (451) NeuroQuant (452) and Neuroreader (Brainreader) (453, 454) are also available.

NeuroQuant, a computer-automated method for measuring brain MRI volume, was introduced in 2007 and received approval from the U.S. Food and Drug Administration (FDA) for routine brain volume measurements in humans. In a study in which the results of NeuroQuant were compared to those of radiologists, it was found that Neuroquant was more sensitive in finding brain atrophy than the traditional radiologist approach. (452) Neuroquant has been used to study hippocampal atrophy after TBI. (455)

3 Tesla (3T) MRI brain imaging was performed with both automated FreeSurfer 5.3 segmentation and manual correction and the results compared using an interclass correlation coefficient. When 86 former NFL players were evaluated, it was found that there were excellent correlations between both techniques regarding volume measurements of the corpus callosum and lateral ventricles, but correlation was not as good for the amygdala, hippocampus, and cingulate gyrus. The correlations are improved when the amygdala and hippocampus are combined into one unit (amygdala–hippocampal complex). (451)

In a study of white-matter integrity after pediatric TBI, it was found that manual tracings on imaging studies were more conservative in identifying white-matter hyperintensities than was NeuroQuant, which was found to be much more liberal or inclusive of these lesions in all patients. (457)

Volume measurements using FreeSurfer showed that one to two years after suffering a severe TBI, adolescents showed global atrophy and white-matter loss, reflected by an increase in ventricle-to-brain ratio and a reduction in the cross-sectional area of the corpus callosum on MRI when compared to controls. Both of these findings correlated with worsened intellectual performance. (456)

Fully automatic segmentation of MRI of the brain, called "Multi-Atlas Label Propagation with Expectation-Maximisation based refinement" (MALP-EM) (**Figure 8.24**; 131) has been able to differentiate favorable from non-favorable outcomes in TBI cases with a 64.7% accuracy using acute-phase (0–8 days after injury) MRI images, and 66.8% using follow-up (3–17 months after injury) images. Subcortical structures including the thalamus, putamen, and hippocampus had potential to predict clinical outcome. (131)

A study of 157 patients who suffered a moderate-to-severe TBI were evaluated at the time of injury as well as six months later with MRI scans of the brain, GCS scores, GOSE scores, and, in some patients, neuropsychological testing. Based upon imaging, the functional outcome of patients was found to be associated with acute thalamic atrophy, as well as the degree of secondary atrophy in the left thalamus, which connects to the prefrontal, temporal, and posterior parietal cortices.

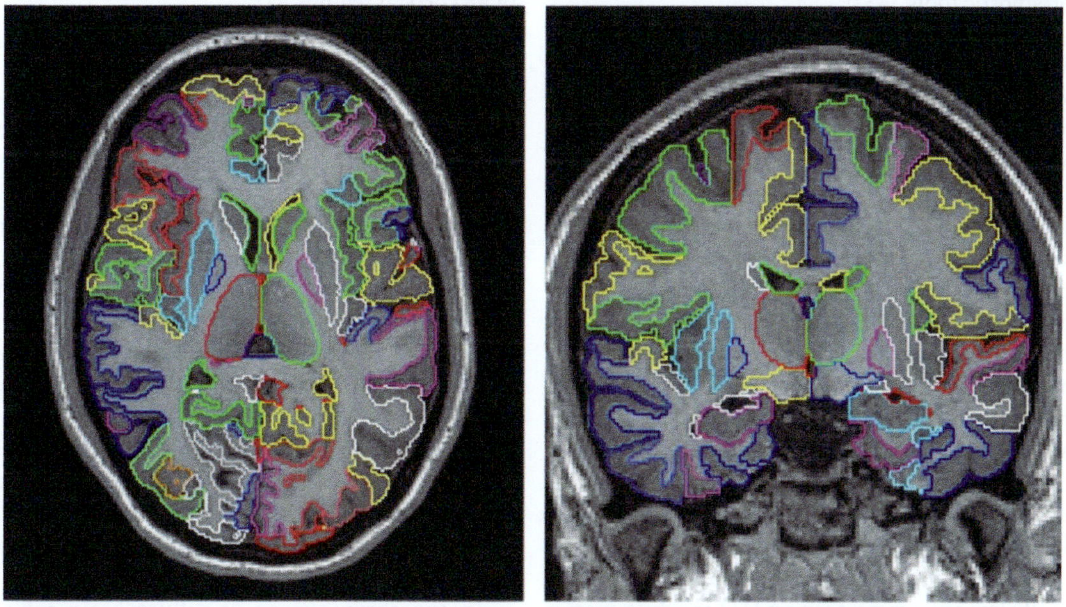

Figure 8.24 Segmentation result obtained using MALP-EM (maximization based refinement) of a subject with a close-to-normal brain configuration (female, age 17, GOS = 5, follow up MRI taken nine months after injury). Axial (left) and coronal (right) views. From (131) https://creativecommons.org/licenses/by/4.0/legalcode

The authors found that during the six months after injury, most of the cortex and subcortical areas (bilateral thalamus, left pallidum, caudate) experience atrophy and thinning, but it is this pattern of damage to the subcortical areas that correlates with functional and cognitive performance at six months. Maximal atrophy was seen in the left thalamus. (285)

Emerging imaging technology

Emerging imaging techniques for the study of TBI include QuickBrain MRI, dynamic susceptibility-weighted contrast enhanced perfusion MRI, MR arterial spin labeling, perfusion CT, and MR elastography. MR elastography may hold promise in the future for the evaluation of mechanical properties of the brain through non-invasive scans, although more research is needed. (432) ASL is a noninvasive MRI technique which can quantify cerebral blood flow through the use of magnetically labeled water protons from arterial blood. (718) These labeled water protons serve as an endogenous diffusible tracer, and have been used to evaluate cerebral perfusion changes after TBI. (717) The next 50 years of neuroimaging of TBI appear poised for significant growth and understanding, including deep machine learning, leading to better diagnostic and prognostic tools. (432)

MEG

MEG is a technique which measures neuronal activity generated electrical fields from the brain. (658) MEG may be more sensitive in diagnosing mild TBI than DTI is, as it has been found in some cases that abnormal delta waves were found despite DTI imaging showing no abnormality. The delta waves (1–4 Hz), which may be generated by neurons that have suffered de-afferentation from axonal injury in the brain, can be localized and measured by MEG. (658) Ten subjects who suffered a mild TBI and underwent MRI and CT scans of the brain (nine patients showed no visible lesion), also underwent MEG and DTI imaging. Axonal injury following a mild TBI caused both abnormal MEG slow waves in the cortical gray matter and abnormally low anisotropy seen on DTI in white-matter fiber tracts. The abnormal cortical delta waves may arise from gray-matter neurons, which experience de-afferentation due to axonal injury in the white-matter fiber tracts seen on DTI. Abnormal MEG slow waves were consistent in all 10 mild TBI patients with post-concussive symptoms. In three cases, MEG showed abnormal delta waves despite no obvious white-matter abnormality on DTI. At times, MEG showed more areas of the brain with abnormal delta waves than were shown on DTI, suggesting that MEG may have greater sensitivity in detecting subtle injury after a mild TBI. (119) MEG, due to a higher temporal resolution, can be used to supplement a resting state fMRI. (657)

When MEG was used to evaluate 45 patients with a mild TBI and 10 patients with a moderate TBI (subacute and chronic phases between four weeks and three years post-injury), and who had persistent post-concussive symptoms, abnormalities were detected in 87% for the mild TBI group, and 100% for the moderate TBI group. The mild TBI group had patients who suffered blast injuries (military personnel) as well as those with non-blast injuries (motor vehicle collisions, falls, etc.) and the moderate TBI group were not blast related. Blast-injured mild TBI patients had abnormal scans in 96% of cases, while in the non-blast mild TBI group had abnormal scans in 77% of cases. The authors felt that the high positive finding rate was partly due to an automated imaging approach in which comparison is made with a control database of 96 cortical regions. (117)

PET

PET scanning evaluates gamma rays which are emitted from radiopharmaceutical agents such as ^{18}F-fluorodeoxyglucose (FDG) and ^{11}carbon. (659) PET, which evaluates metabolism in the brain, has been utilized extensively for the imaging and evaluation of metabolism in brain tumors compared to the surrounding brain and may be a prognostic tool for histological grading and survival in patients with gliomas. Positron emitting isotopes such as FDG can also yield information about changes in brain metabolism following TBI because it evaluates the utilization of glucose in the brain. For days to months after a mild TBI, brain hypometabolism may be seen in consistent regions of the brain. (121–125)

In the chronic stage of diffuse brain injury, FDG PET scanning revealed bilateral hypometabolism in the medial prefrontal regions, the medial frontobasal regions, the cingulate gyrus, and the thalamus. It was felt that this may result from a cortical disconnection due to white-matter tract disruptions (rather than from direct cerebral focal contusion), resulting in cognitive decline and consciousness disturbance. These findings were seen in a study of 52 patients who suffered a high-velocity, high-impact motor vehicle collision, who did not have large focal lesions but did have disturbance of consciousness for more than six hours not due to mass lesions or ischemia in the acute or subacute stages. Three groups of patients were evaluated: 1) those with a higher brain dysfunction but could communicate, 2) those with a minimally conscious state, and 3) those in a vegetative state. (316)

In a study on rats exposed to a mild lateral fluid percussion, FDG PET imaging revealed depressed glucose uptake in both ipsilateral and contralateral hemispheres in comparison to controls, although there was no measurable change in neuronal loss or gross tissue damage. It was felt that the decrease in metabolism was related to glial activation and axonal damage. (315)

SPECT

SPECT utilizes a radioactive isotope such as technetium-99, thallium-201, iodine-123, iodine-125, and xenon-133, which emits gamma rays. SPECT perfusion imaging looks at regional blood flow in the brain, which is a biomarker for neuronal activity since under most neurophysiologic circumstances, it is coupled to neuronal metabolism. (659) In a review study using SPECT, it was found to be better than CT and MRI in evaluating the brain in both the acute and chronic phase of mild TBI. It was found that SPECT has a near 100% negative predictive value for TBI patients in the subacute and chronic settings with respect to psychiatric sequelae and is useful for distinguishing between mild TBI and psychological response to head injury when the brain CT and MRI scans are normal. An abnormal perfusion SPECT scan is more sensitive than CT or MRI, with respect to association with abnormal neuropsychological or neurological tests, and may be used as a baseline study in patients with subclinical TBI and evaluated for possible progression if a patient clinically worsens months or years after the injury. In a literature review, it was found that SPECT abnormalities correlated with abnormal neurology or neuropsychology outcomes in 93% of studies. When mild, moderate, and severe TBI patients were reviewed, lesion localization was found most commonly in the frontal and temporal lobes, followed by the parietal lobes, occipital lobes, and cerebellum. (126)

A group of 161 retired and active National Football League (NFL) players were compared to 124 healthy controls and assessed using SPECT. The players on average showed decreased cerebral perfusion in 36 brain regions, with 90% sensitivity, 86% specificity, and 94% accuracy. (660)

9

Acute neurosurgical management of brain injury

Upon arrival in an emergency room, a brain injured patient will be assessed. Depending upon whether the patient has suffered a mild, moderate, or severe traumatic brain injury (TBI), their treatment course may vary significantly. While patients with a mild TBI might be discharged home, those with a severe TBI may undergo emergent surgery on the brain. After an initial clinical assessment, a computed tomography (CT) scan of the brain may be performed to assess for acute findings such as a fracture, hematoma (epidural, subdural, intracerebral, etc.), brain contusion, and any shift of the midline of the brain.

SURGICAL MANAGEMENT OF HEMATOMAS

Bullock et al. have recommended that regardless of a patient's Glasgow Coma Scale (GCS) score, an epidural hematoma should be surgically evacuated if it is greater than 30 cm^3. Smaller lesions may be monitored with neurological evaluations and follow-up CT scans of the brain. Time from neurological deterioration to surgery is more important than the time from trauma to surgery. (105) They also suggested that patients with intracerebral parenchymal hemorrhages with associated neurological deterioration, elevated intracranial pressure (ICP) not responding to medical treatment, or brain CT signs of mass effect, should be treated operatively. They also make recommendations for surgery on patients with GCS scores of 6–8 and parenchymal hemorrhages meeting certain criteria (frontal or temporal contusions greater than 20 cm^2), midline shift of 5 mm or greater, and/or cisternal compression. Those patients, if treated non-surgically, will likely have a poor outcome. (106) In addition, regardless of their GCS scores, patients with an acute subdural hematoma of greater than 10 mm thickness or a midline shift greater than 5 mm, should undergo craniotomy for evacuation of the blood clot. Those with a GCS less than 9 and less clot thickness or midline shift, no pupillary dilatation, no raised ICP, and treated non-surgically should have ICP monitored and neurological functions evaluated. (107) Elevated ICP may occur after a severe TBI, frequently leading to disability and death. With additional clinical research, recommendations (see review of Guidelines 4th edition) have been made to check which measures should be incorporated in order to control elevated ICP. Historically, they involve intubation, sedation, hyperventilation and hypocapnia (may not be currently recommended

DOI: 10.1201/9781003354154-9

as discussed in review of Guidelines 4th edition (87) below), intravenous mannitol (hyperosmolar therapy, mixed conclusions as to current recommendations, see Guidelines 4th edition), ventriculostomy for cerebrospinal fluid (CSF) drainage, hypothermia (not currently recommended, see Guidelines 4th edition), and decompressive craniectomy. (97) It was felt that there is no high-quality evidence that hypothermia is beneficial in the treatment of patients with TBI. (579) Additional research is needed.

Cerebral perfusion pressure (CPP), which is the difference between the mean arterial blood pressure and the ICP, must be sufficient to keep the brain perfused with blood. If ICP is elevated, and insufficient blood flow and oxygen can reach the brain, an intravenous-induced barbiturate coma and hypothermia (data on hypothermia is not conclusive (579)) may be induced in an effort to protect the brain. (273) Treatment should be aimed at keeping ICP at or below 22 mm Hg. (578)

After the initial traumatic insult to the brain, secondary brain injury may set in and measures must be implemented to try to minimize the consequences of this secondary insult and maintain proper cerebral perfusion. Causes of raised ICP and cerebral ischemia are cell death, microvascular occlusion, and injury to mitochondria, all of which may create a downward spiral of further secondary injury events and worsening intracranial hypertension and cerebral ischemia. (98, 274)

In a study from Norway of 2,151 patients who had pathological findings on head CT, 27% (3.9/100,000 person-years) required at least one emergency neurosurgical procedure (most frequently the placement of an ICP monitor and possibly craniotomy for a mass lesion). This translated to a worldwide statistic of 3.3 patients per 100,000 person-years who required an emergency procedure. The emergency neurosurgery rate was low in children, but peaked in the 60- to 70-year age group, and was more likely in those with CT findings of midline shift ≥5 mm and compressed or absent basal cisterns. Twenty-six percent of patients with a GCS score of 9–12 received an ICP monitor. (25)

Children aged 15 or younger, who have suffered a severe TBI, have a better functional outcome and lower mortality rate than adults. The authors felt that children who suffer a severe TBI have a GCS score of 3, and bilaterally fixed and dilated pupils should be treated aggressively. (26)

The fourth edition of *Guidelines for the Management of Severe Traumatic Brain Injury* published in 2016, which has been endorsed by the American Association of Neurological Surgeons and the Congress of Neurological Surgeons, discusses the following treatment measures for the treatment of severe TBI, which is reviewed below:

- Decompressive craniectomy
- Prophylactic hypothermia
- Hyperosmolar therapy
- CSF drainage
- Ventilation therapies
- Anesthetics, analgesics, and sedatives
- Steroids
- Nutrition
- Infection prophylaxis
- Deep vein thrombosis prophylaxis
- Seizure prophylaxis (87)

DECOMPRESSIVE CRANIECTOMY

In situations where there is significant brain swelling, herniation may result in death or disability. When medical therapies have failed, a decompressive craniectomy may be considered, removing a large portion of the skull to give the brain additional room in which to expand. According to the Guidelines 4th edition mentioned previously, "a large frontotemporoparietal DC (decompressive craniectomy) (not less than 12 × 15 cm or 15 cm diameter) is recommended over a small frontotemporoparietal DC for reduced mortality and improved neurological outcomes in patients with severe TBI." (87) Updated research has shown that secondary decompressive craniectomy for late refractory elevated ICP is recommended to improve mortality and favorable outcomes. Secondary decompressive craniectomy for early or late refractory ICP elevation is suggested to reduce ICP and the duration of intensive care (relationship between this and favorable outcome is uncertain). (577)

PROPHYLACTIC HYPOTHERMIA

In situations where ICP is elevated, depending upon the mean arterial blood pressure, the CPP may also be reduced. Hypothermia may reduce the metabolic requirements of brain tissue, and may also reduce ICP. According to the Guidelines 4th edition, "hypothermia is not recommended to improve outcomes within the first 48 hours, in patients with diffuse injury." (87) Another review found no high-quality evidence that hypothermia is of benefit in the treatment of patients with TBI. (579)

HYPEROSMOLAR THERAPY

Mannitol and hyperosmolar infusion therapy, such as hypertonic saline, have been routinely used to reduce ICP through objectives involving brain dehydration, and reducing blood viscosity, leading to improved blood flow within the brain. Hyperosmolar intravenous agents may also lead to decreases in systemic arterial blood pressure. According to the Guidelines 4th edition, it is mentioned that the 3rd edition of the Guidelines did support the use of intravenous mannitol at 1 g/kg body weight, but recognized that more research is needed for more specific recommendations. The Guidelines 4th edition confirmed that there is general belief that hyperosmolar agents are useful in the care of patients with TBI, but the literature does not support recommendations that meet strict criteria for their evidence-based approaches for guideline development. (87) Although it may be helpful in reducing elevated ICP or cerebral edema, hyperosmolar therapy may not affect neurological outcomes. (259)

CEREBROSPINAL FLUID DRAINAGE

A commonly utilized method to attempt to reduce ICP, is the use of drainage of CSF from the ventricles. A ventricular catheter can be placed, often at the bedside in the ICU or emergency department, and spinal fluid can be drained from the brain along with ICP being able to be easily monitored. A fiberoptic pressure monitor may be placed within the ventricular catheter to allow for the measuring of ICP. The catheter can be left in a closed position, and only opened intermittently to allow the drainage of CSF, or it may be left open continuously, allowing for the constant drainage of CSF.

According to the Guidelines 4th edition, an external ventricular drainage system "zeroed at the midbrain with continuous drainage of CSF may be considered to lower ICP burden more effectively than intermittent use." The Guidelines 4th edition further states "use of CSF drainage to lower ICP in patients with an initial Glasgow Coma Scale (GCS) <6 during the first 12 hours after injury may be considered." (87)

According to the Guidelines 4th edition, "management of severe TBI patients using information from ICP monitoring is recommended to reduce in-hospital and 2 week post-injury mortality." (87)

A study that evaluated CPP management in treatment of patients with severe TBIs compared the outcomes of three groups of patients and found that patients had the best clinical outcomes and fewer complications when the CPP was kept above 60 mm Hg, as compared to the group in whom CPP was kept above 70 mm Hg. Both of these groups did better than the group in which only management of ICP was performed. (99)

VENTILATION THERAPIES

Patients suffering from severe TBI are typically placed on a ventilator to assist with breathing and to protect their airway. Normally, the amount of carbon dioxide (CO_2) in the blood is an important factor in determining blood flow to the brain. As one increases the rate of breathing and the tidal volume on a ventilator, more CO_2 is exhaled, and the level of CO_2 in the arterial blood decreases, while the opposite occurs if the rate of ventilation is decreased, causing arterial CO_2 to consequently rise. Normally, when the brain is autoregulating, a lower arterial CO_2 level will result in decreased cerebral blood flow and the opposite with higher arterial CO_2 levels. Historically, hyperventilation was recommended in patients suffering TBI and raised ICP. This may, however, reduce blood flow to the brain, and cerebral ischemia has been seen after severe TBI, resulting in a change to ventilation recommendations, as Guidelines 4th edition cites the works of Liu, Tawil, Carrera, and Stein. (87)

According to Guidelines 4th edition, "prolonged prophylactic hyperventilation with partial pressure of carbon-dioxide in arterial blood of 25 mm Hg or less is not recommended." (87)

While hyperventilation may be used for emergency cases when no other medical treatments, such as mannitol hyperosmolar treatment, may be effective, it is no longer an initially recommended therapy. A study of 36 patients suffering from severe TBI suggested that mannitol may be better than hyperventilation, which was believed may possibly worsen cerebral blood flow. (104, 249)

ANESTHETICS, ANALGESICS, AND SEDATIVES

Intravenous barbiturates have been used in the treatment of raised ICP with the aim of decreasing straining and coughing, straining against the endotracheal tube, and, most importantly, decreasing cerebral metabolism requirements and, thus, protecting brain tissue. Adverse side effects include hypotension, which might offset the benefits of cerebral protection. When a patient is placed on intravenous barbiturates with the intention of cerebral protection, because of the sedative effects, an accurate neurological examination to follow the GCS score will no longer be possible. In this case, continuous electroencephalographic (EEG) monitoring and evaluation of burst suppression will be required.

According to the Guidelines 4th edition, "administration of barbiturates to induce burst suppression measured by EEG as prophylaxis against the development of intracranial hypertension is not recommended. High-dose barbiturate administration is recommended to control elevated ICP refractory to maximum standard medical and surgical treatment. Hemodynamic stability is essential before and during barbiturate therapy." In addition, the Guidelines 4th edition state "although propofol is recommended for the control of ICP, it is not recommended for improvement in mortality or 6 month outcomes. Caution is required as high-dose propofol can produce significant morbidity." (87)

STEROIDS

Historically, the use of intravenous steroids to treat edema in patients with brain tumors in the perioperative period has been common. This practice was extended to the treatment of patients suffering severe TBI. In the Corticosteroid Randomization After Significant Head Injury (CRASH) randomized control trial of the use of corticosteroids in 10,008 patients with TBI and a GCS score of 14 or less, it was concluded that corticosteroids should not be routinely used in the treatment of head injury. (89) According to the Guidelines 4th edition, "the use of steroids is not recommended for improving outcome or reducing ICP. In patients with severe TBI, high-dose methylprednisolone was associated with increased mortality and is contraindicated." (87)

NUTRITION

After a TBI, the body goes into a hypermetabolic state and there is an increase in cerebral as well as systemic energy requirements. In a study of 797 patients with severe TBI and a GCS less than 9, it was found that in the first five to seven days after the injury, every decrease of 10 kcal/kg body weight of caloric intake was associated with a 30%–40% increase in mortality rate within the first two weeks. Within the first five days of a TBI, any nutrition given was associated with a lower mortality rate. It was concluded that good early nutrition is important in improving outcome after severe TBI. (90) According to Guidelines 4th edition, "feeding patients to attain basal caloric replacement at least by the fifth day and, at most, by the seventh day post injury is recommended to decrease mortality. Transgastric jejunal feeding is recommended to reduce the incidence of ventilator-associated pneumonia." (87)

INFECTION PROPHYLAXIS

Due to the need for mechanical ventilator support in patients who have suffered severe TBI, their susceptibility to infection also increases. In addition, ventricular brain catheters, central venous lines, arterial lines, urinary bladder catheters, and lack of physical activity also increase risks of infection.

In a study of 24,525 patients who suffered TBI and required mechanical ventilator support, there was an additional risk of pneumonia at the rate of 7% for each additional day a patient was on a ventilator. Although often life-saving and necessary, mechanical ventilation was the primary factor related to increased incidence of pneumonia in patients who have suffered a TBI. It was suggested that in patients suffering TBI, every effort must be made to try to get the patient independent of ventilator dependence as quickly as possible. (696)

According to the Guidelines 4th edition, "early tracheostomy is recommended to reduce mechanical ventilation days when the overall benefit is felt to outweigh the complications associated with such a procedure. However, there is no evidence that early tracheostomy reduces mortality or the rate of nosocomial pneumonia." In addition, the Guidelines 4th edition suggest "antimicrobial-impregnated catheters may be considered to prevent catheter related infections during EVD (external-ventricular drainage)." (87)

DEEP VENOUS THROMBOSIS

TBI poses an increased risk to patients for developing a venous thromboembolism (VTE). In a study of 5,787 patients, 25% of 88 patients with an isolated TBI suffered a VTE, with 59% of those occurring in the veins of the thigh (which may be related to femoral central venous access) and 22% below the knee. (91) In another study of 716 patients admitted to a trauma unit, 49 of 91 patients (54%) with major head injuries suffered a deep venous thrombosis (DVT), with proximal DVT in 18%, yet less than 2% of patients with DVT had symptoms of such (the confirmation was made with venography). (92)

The Guidelines 4th edition state "low molecular weight heparin or low-dose unfractionated heparin may be used in combination with mechanical prophylaxis. However, there is an increased risk for expansion of intracranial hemorrhage. In addition to compression stockings, pharmacological prophylaxis may be considered if the brain injury is stable and the benefit is considered to outweigh the risk of increased intracranial hemorrhage. There is insufficient evidence to support recommendations regarding the preferred agent, dosage, or timing of pharmacological prophylaxis for deep vein thrombosis." (87)

SEIZURE PROPHYLAXIS

Posttraumatic seizures (PTS), when they occur within seven days after a TBI, are referred to as early and when the occurrence is after seven days, they are referred to as late. Of 275,000 people in the United States who are hospitalized due to TBI each year, PTS occurred in roughly 5%–7%. (93)

The Guidelines 4th edition state "prophylactic use of phenytoin or valproate is not recommended for preventing late PTS. Phenytoin is recommended to decrease the incidence of early PTS (within 7 days of injury), when the overall benefit is felt to outweigh the complications associated with such treatment. However, early PTS have not been associated with worse outcomes." (87)

It has been suggested that early PTS occur in more than 20% of TBI patients in the intensive care unit and that since most are nonconvulsive, continuous EEG monitoring be implemented initially for patients with moderate or severe TBI. (95)

BRAIN TISSUE OXYGEN MONITORING

To evaluate oxygen delivery to the brain, evaluation of the differences in arterio-jugular venous oxygen ($AVDO_2$) extraction may be measured. This method evaluates whole-brain blood oxygen saturation, but is less sensitive to regional cerebral ischemia and hypoxia. Alternatively, brain-tissue oxygen partial pressure monitoring may be clinically useful and may be placed in the frontal lobe. The measurements should not be used alone, but in conjunction with ICP and CPP monitoring. (100, 275)

Less beneficial results of oxygen monitoring have also been seen. In a study of 74 patients hospitalized with severe TBI and a GCS score of less than 8, brain-tissue oxygen monitoring and ICP/CPP monitoring was not found to improve survival or functional status at discharge as compared to treatment management aimed solely at controlling ICP and CPP. It was noted that the group with brain-tissue oxygen monitoring were also more likely to undergo craniectomy and did have more subdural and epidural hematomas. (101)

TRANSCRANIAL DOPPLER (TCD)

The role of Transcranial Doppler (TCD) in the evaluation of TBI was examined in a patient database study and it was found that when compared to patients with normal TCD blood flows, patients who had an abnormally elevated intracranial blood flow of more than 120 cm/second had a threefold higher likelihood of suffering poor clinical outcomes and a ninefold higher likelihood of mortality. Some patients may not be able to be evaluated with TCD due to a poor temporal window. (102)

In another TCD study of 255 patients with severe TBI and a GCS score of less than 8, a higher incidence of mortality and severe disability was seen in those patients who showed vasospasm on TCD. When patients had normal TCD measurements, more than 80% will have a good outcome with a Glasgow Outcome Scale score of 4–5. (103)

10

Recovery and rehabilitation

Following traumatic brain injury (TBI), depending upon the severity of the injury, a number of scenarios may occur. If a patient has suffered a mild TBI, they might be seen in an emergency department, or they may have gone home directly after the injury. For moderate and severe TBIs, patients would likely be seen at an emergency department, and may have been admitted to a hospital. A neurosurgical procedure on the brain may have taken place, and the patient may have spent a short or long amount of time in a neurosurgical intensive care unit. After being discharged from a hospital, the patients may return home, or may be cared for at inpatient rehabilitation facility, long-term acute care hospital, skilled nursing facility, or have therapy performed on an outpatient basis. Patients can also receive treatment as an outpatient through outpatient rehabilitation programs or with home health care and rehabilitation. TBI has significant ramifications on patients and those around them. As medicine and technology improve, so does our understanding of TBI and the ability to treat patients who have suffered a TBI in the acute, subacute, and chronic settings.

Because the effects of TBI, depending upon severity, may have significant and long-lasting consequences for patients and their families and caregivers, and the patients may experience significant neuropsychological, psychiatric, and physical difficulties (cognitive, behavioral, emotional, medical, interpersonal, financial, vocational), a team of individuals in various specialties will help with the rehabilitation process. Team members may include neurosurgeons, neurologists, neuropsychologists, psychiatrists, neurotologists, neuro-ophthalmologists, endocrinologists, nurses, physical therapists, nutritionists, respiratory therapists, occupational therapists, vocational counselors, speech pathologists, social workers, psychologists, psychotherapists, case managers, marriage counselors, and others.

After a TBI, life for a patient may instantly change in dramatic ways. Activities of daily living, such as going shopping, balancing a checkbook, preparing a meal, and dialing a phone number, may become difficult or impossible to accomplish. Swallowing and speaking may be difficult as well as remembering any new information or names of people. Apathy, aggressiveness, depression, and anger may be seen. A patient's feeling of self, and who they are, may be altered.

Medical, neurological, cognitive, neuropsychological and psychiatric problems, as well as post-concussion syndrome may also play a role in the patient's daily life. Early educational intervention

DOI: 10.1201/9781003354154-10

may provide some benefit. Neuropsychological evaluation may be implemented. Exercise, good nutrition, and a positive and stimulating environment are to be encouraged. Other types of cognitive therapy may be implemented.

Since the brain either directly or indirectly affects almost every aspect of a person's body, damage to the brain can also eventually impact every part of the body. Since almost every organ system may eventually be impacted, recovery and rehabilitation after a TBI involves not only treating problems which might arise in any part of the body but also anticipating and preventing likely difficulties before they arise.

We will review many of the different issues which may arise and challenge a patient who has suffered TBI. It is beyond the scope of this book to provide an exhaustive list.

POST-CONCUSSION SYNDROME/ MILD NEUROCOGNITIVE DISORDER

Patients who have suffered a mild TBI may experience post-concussion symptoms, which, if they persist for a period of time, may be termed post-concussion syndrome (PCS). The symptoms may include somatic symptoms (fatigue, imbalance, headache, dizziness, etc.), cognitive symptoms (difficulty with cognition, memory, and executive function, etc.), and emotional or behavioral problems (depression, irritability, etc.). There has been inconsistency in the literature regarding the definition of PCS as well as a differing consensus as to the criteria for the syndrome. Overlapping symptoms from comorbidities such as depression, post-traumatic stress disorder (PTSD), amnesia, and other issues may have a complex interaction with post-concussion symptoms. Social factors, such as family and other support networks, coping strategies, and other issues may also interact with post-concussion symptoms. Polinder suggested that standardization of the multidimensional comprehensive diagnostics, treatment interventions, and follow-up assessments may improve reliability and validity of research comparisons and refine personalized treatment. (158)

The clinician evaluating a TBI patient must do their best to try to determine whether any of the symptoms were present prior to the injury. Symptoms may be new or they could be pre-existing symptoms, which may be stable or may have worsened.

There have been inconsistencies in the literature regarding the definition of post-concussion symptoms and syndrome, both in terms of classification, nomenclature, types, and length of symptoms. With respect to definitions, the Diagn*ostic and Statistical Manual of the American Psychiatric Association* 5th edition (DSM-5) no longer uses the term "post-concussional disorder" (which was used in the *Diagnostic and Statistical Manual of the American Psychiatric Association* 4th edition (DSM-IV), but has replaced it with "major or mild neurocognitive disorder due to traumatic brain injury."

To understand the important changes in criteria as defined by DSM-5 (published in 2013) and (DSM-IV) (published in 1994), it is best to review the criteria of each.

DSM-5 criteria of major or mild neurocognitive disorder due to TBI

According to the DSM-5 (277), the diagnostic criteria of major or mild neurocognitive disorder due to TBI are as follows:

- The criteria are met for major or mild neurocognitive disorder.
- There is evidence of a TBI—that is, an impact to the head or other mechanisms of rapid movement or displacement of the brain within the skull, with one or more of the following:
  - Loss of consciousness.
  - Post-traumatic amnesia.
  - Disorientation and confusion.
  - Neurological signs (e.g., neuroimaging demonstrating injury; a new onset of seizures; a marked worsening of a pre-existing seizure disorder; visual field cuts; anosmia; hemiparesis).
- The neurocognitive disorder presents immediately after the occurrence of the TBI or immediately after recovery of consciousness and persists past the acute post-injury period.

The DSM-5 (277) defines a major or mild neurocognitive disorder with the following diagnostic criteria:

Major neurocognitive disorder:

- Evidence of significant cognitive decline from a previous level of performance in one or more cognitive domains (complex attention,

executive function, learning and memory, language, perceptual-motor, or social cognition) based on:
  - Concern of the individual, a knowledgeable informant, or the clinician that there has been a significant decline in cognitive function; and
  - A substantial impairment in cognitive performance, preferably documented by standardized neuropsychological testing or, in its absence, another quantified clinical assessment.
- The cognitive deficits interfere with independence in everyday activities (i.e., at a minimum, requiring assistance with complex instrumental activities of daily living such as paying bills or managing medications).
- The cognitive deficits do not occur exclusively in the context of a delirium.
- The cognitive deficits are not better explained by another mental disorder (e.g., major depressive disorder, schizophrenia).

Mild neurocognitive disorder:

- Evidence of modest cognitive decline from a previous level of performance in one or more cognitive domains (complex attention, executive function, learning and memory, language, perceptual-motor, or social cognition) based on:
  - Concern of the individual, a knowledgeable informant, or the clinician that there has been a mild decline in cognitive function; and
  - A modest impairment in cognitive performance, preferably documented by standardized neuropsychological testing or, in its absence, another quantified clinical assessment.
- The cognitive deficits do not interfere with capacity for independence in everyday activities (i.e., complex instrumental activities of daily living such as paying bills or managing medications are preserved, but greater effort, compensatory strategies, or accommodation may be required).
- The cognitive deficits do not occur exclusively in the context of a delirium.
- The cognitive deficits are not better explained by another mental disorder (e.g., major depressive disorder, schizophrenia). (277)

As noted above, this definition reflects a change when compared to DSM-IV, where it was stated "post-concussional disorder can be differentiated from mild neurocognitive disorder by the specific pattern of cognitive, somatic, and behavioral symptoms and the presence of a specific etiology (i.e., closed head injury)." In DSM-IV, the terms "post-concussional disorder" and "mild neurocognitive disorder" were included in Appendix B entitled "Criteria sets and axes provided for further study."

DSM-IV research criteria for post-concussional disorder

The DSM-IV (278) includes research criteria for post-concussional disorder as follows:

- A history of head trauma that has caused significant cerebral concussion.

  Note: The manifestations of concussion include loss of consciousness, post-traumatic amnesia, and, less commonly, post-traumatic onset of seizures. The specific method of defining this criterion needs to be established by further research.
- Evidence from neuropsychological testing or quantified cognitive assessment of difficulty in attention (concentrating, shifting focus of attention, performing simultaneous cognitive tasks) or memory (learning or recalling information).
- Three (or more) of the following occur shortly after the trauma and last at least three months:
  - Becoming fatigued easily.
  - Disordered sleep.
  - Headache.
  - Vertigo or dizziness.
  - Irritability or aggression on little or no provocation.
  - Anxiety, depression, or affective lability.
  - Changes in personality (e.g., social or sexual inappropriateness).
  - Apathy or lack of spontaneity.
- The symptoms in Criteria B and C have their onset following head trauma or else represent a substantial worsening of pre-existing symptoms.
- The disturbance causes significant impairment in social or occupational functioning and represents a significant decline from a previous level of functioning. In school-age children, the impairment may be manifested by a significant worsening in school or academic performance dating from the trauma.

- The symptoms do not meet criteria for Dementia Due to Head Trauma and are not better accounted for by another mental disorder (e.g., Amnestic Disorder Due to Head Trauma, Personality Change Due to Head Trauma).

The DSM-IV research criteria for mild neurocognitive disorder are as follows:

- The presence of two (or more) of the following impairments in cognitive functioning, lasting most of the time for a period of at least two weeks (as reported by the individual or a reliable informant):
  - Memory impairment as identified by a reduced ability to learn or recall information.
  - Disturbance in executive functioning (i.e., planning, organizing, sequencing, abstracting).
  - Disturbance in attention or speed of information processing.
  - Impairment in perceptual-motor abilities.
  - Impairment in language (e.g., comprehension, word finding).
- There is objective evidence from physical examination or laboratory findings (including neuroimaging techniques) of a neurological or general medical condition that is judged to be etiologically related to the cognitive disturbance.
- There is evidence from neuropsychological testing or quantified cognitive assessment of an abnormality or decline in performance.
- The cognitive deficits cause marked distress or impairment in social, occupational, or other important areas of functioning and represent a decline from a previous level of functioning.
- The cognitive disturbance does not meet criteria for a delirium, a dementia, or an amnestic disorder and is not better accounted for by another mental disorder (e.g., a Substance-Related Disorder, Major Depressive Disorder). (278)

Tator, in a paper published in 2016 on PCS, points out that this recategorization of criteria of PCS provides a lack of unanimity. In their study of 284 consecutive concussed patients, 221 (78%) had PCS, which they classified as having at least three symptoms persisting at least one month (they shortened the interval from three months to one month as per the criteria of the 4th International Consensus on Concussion in Sport) and excluded patients with intracranial lesions (hemorrhages, contusions). The most common symptoms were headache (89.1%), memory deficits (61.5%), concentration difficulties (56.1%), imbalance (52%), dizziness (51.6%), fatigue (45.7%), nausea (43%), sensitivity to light (38.9%), sleeping disturbance (difficulty falling or staying asleep) (32.6%), irritability (31.7%), depression (30.8%), visual changes (blurry or double vision, etc) (28.5%), anxiety (23.1%), mental fogginess (such as feeling not quite right or dazed) (22.6%), sensitivity to noise (22.2%), as well as neck pain, tinnitus, increased emotionality, pressure in the head, lightheadedness, personality changes, vertigo, confusion, numbness, feeling slowed down, learning difficulties, loss of appetite, vomiting, panic attacks, increased thinking time, frustration, increased sensitivity to alcohol, speech problems, seizures, aggression, problem-solving difficulties, slowed response speed, restlessness, stomach ache, and apathy. The individuals had suffered an average of 3.3 (range of 1–12; 23.1% of individuals had 1 concussion) concussions, with a median duration of PCS of seven months, with 11.8% lasting more than two years. PCS was found to be commonly associated with multiple concussions. Notably, the authors used the DSM-IV (and not the more current DSM-5) criteria, as well as the International Statistical Classification of Diseases and Related Health Problems (ICD-10) for PCS criteria. (116)

Additional ways in which patients might report post-concussion symptoms may include changes in taste or smell, the feeling of being overwhelmed, reading difficulties, poor coordination / clumsiness, hearing difficulties, changes in appetite, forgetfulness, difficulty with information processing and with decision making, slowed thinking, inability to complete tasks, irritability, and lack of motivation or interest in things.

Post-concussion symptoms, cognitive and psychiatric changes

After a TBI, cognitive and psychiatric disorders may contribute to each other, and may be mistaken for each other. Cognitive changes that may occur after a TBI might affect processing speed, reaction time, memory, and be related to aphasia, spatial neglect, changes in alertness, sleep cycle changes, and other findings. Treatment has included cognitive rehabilitation, pharmacological interventions, and external aids (notebooks, tablet computers, mobile phones, etc.). (276)

Emotional and behavioral disorders may be present after a TBI, possibly contributed to by a loss of control due to physical and cognitive dependence. Medical conditions that may need to be addressed, and which may cause these disorders, include electrolyte disturbance, endocrine disorders, hydrocephalus, epilepsy, and infection. Treatment may include cognitive behavioral therapy (CBT) among other therapies, social support, and pharmacological intervention. Social support and reintegration into the community are important. Families and caregivers of patients with TBI may also experience significant emotional stress. (276)

In a study of 731 patients who suffered a mild TBI, PCS (considered when symptoms persisted more than three months post-injury) was present in 11.4–38.7% of cases at six months post-injury, depending upon the method of classification used. Assault was significantly associated with six-month PCS, but acute lesions on the head CT were not. Female gender and lower education were associated with PCS. At six months post-injury, 27.1% of patients were functionally impaired and had a GOSE score ≤6. PCS was associated with functional impairment and with more severe symptoms having a higher relationship with impairment. During the first few weeks after a mild TBI, many patients will experience post-concussion symptoms including "physical symptoms (e.g., headaches, dizziness, blurred vision, fatigue, and sleep disturbances), cognitive deficits (e.g., poor memory, and attention and executive difficulties), and behavioral/emotional symptoms (e.g., depression, irritability, anxiety-related disorders, and emotional lability)." (140)

Interventions to improve PCS/mild neurocognitive disorder

Treatment of post-PCS following a mild TBI consists mainly of education, reassurance, and education as to the cause of a patient's symptoms. Early brief psychological treatment may help to protect against protracted PCS. A single session of treatment early on may be sufficient. Pain may be treated with nonsteroidal anti-inflammatory medications and antidepressants may be utilized for depression. Psychological consultation may be needed in 40% of cases. (174)

A study of 202 adults with mild TBI was performed in which they were assigned to two groups, one with intervention involving an information booklet (outlined symptoms and coping strategies) given one week after injury, and the other that did not receive any intervention. At three months post-injury, the group that underwent intervention had less anxiety. The group that did not receive the booklet reported more symptoms, including sleep disturbances and psychological distress at three months post-injury. (142)

Early psychological intervention was also seen to be beneficial in a study of 58 patients who suffered persistent PCS, half of which met with a therapist and were given a printed manual prior to discharge (the treated group), and half of which did not (the control group). Six months after injury, those who were treated had a significantly shorter duration of symptoms and experienced fewer symptoms. The conclusion was that early psychological intervention may decrease the incidence of PCS. Informing patients of possible symptoms and reattributing them to benign causes may reduce anxiety. (175) In another study of 20 patients suffering symptoms after mild and moderate TBI, cognitive behavioral psychotherapy and cognitive remediation given for 11 weeks appeared to improve cognitive functioning and decrease psychologic distress, depression, and anxiety. (176)

In contrast, another study found the educational intervention did not appear to improve outcomes. A randomized study of patients suffering minimal, mild, and moderate head injury compared patients who had undergone early educational intervention (cognitive-oriented counseling and additional information and reassuring two weeks after the injury) with those controls who did not and found no difference in outcome at three and six months after injury. Although a significant number of patients who had post-concussion symptoms improved from 3 to 12 months post-injury, there was no effect on outcomes from an educational intervention given two weeks post-injury. The authors concluded that a more extensive intervention may be more effective, but evidence on this is conflicting. (144)

NEUROPSYCHOLOGICAL TESTING/ASSESSMENT

Objective neuropsychological evaluation and testing is performed to be able to quantify deficits, predict current and future outcomes as they pertain to and impact real-world measures, and help neuropsychologists to guide recommendations regarding life and treatment planning. As the skills and capabilities required in the real world are extremely varied and complex, growth in the field of neuropsychological testing and adding performance-based activities of daily living will help to refine this method of analysis, leading to better assessment of a patient's current capabilities and serving as a better prognosticator for future improvement. As technology (including imaging of the brain and biomarkers in the serum, cerebrospinal fluid, etc.) and our understanding of the brain improves, objective tools for assessment will improve as well, with the goal of detecting brain changes at the earliest possible point after an injury. (288)

After a TBI, the quality of life, productivity, and outcome of an individual is in large part dependent upon the impact on cognition. Although the Glasgow Outcome Scale Extended (GOSE) remains the standard for clinical trials, it is dependent upon the interviewer who is assessing the patient. Neuropsychological tests that are patient performance based may provide more detail into cognition impairment. The external manifestation of improvement in cognition is seen by increased independence, improvement in therapy and rehabilitation, return to employment, and participation in one's community. Discussion with family, friends, employers, and anyone else who may have known the injured patient before and after their injury may provide insight into the patient's condition and evaluation.

Neuropsychological testing is used to evaluate functioning in patients who have suffered a TBI. Testing can be used to evaluate the following domains: cognition, neurobehavior, psychological health, life participation, and physical function. Within each of these domains are subdomains, including:

- *Cognition:* Memory, executive function, language, intelligence, attention, processing speed, visual-spatial function.
- *Neurobehavioral:* Judgment, anger, social behavior, insight, impulsivity, disinhibition, apathy.
- *Psychological health:* Mood, PTSD, personality, resilience, anxiety, psychosis, PCS symptoms.
- *Life participation:* Social, recreational, financial, living situation, vocational, sexual function, transport.
- *Physical function:* Motor, perceptual, pain, endurance, sensory, mobility, sleep. (162)

There are many neuropsychological tests available and the design of the test may impact what the outcomes are and which conclusions are drawn. Testing should meet several criteria. It should be **sensitive**, meaning that if an individual has a disorder, it should be picked up and confirmed by testing and those results should differentiate between clinical patients and normal controls. Testing should be **specific**, meaning that if a test shows positive results for a finding, the conclusions drawn should reflect the pathology it indicates and not be confused with the pathology of another disease process, resulting in an incorrect conclusion due to confounding variables. The test should be **reliable**, and if the test is given several times, the results should be repeatable (test-retest reliability). There should be minimal practice effects. The test should be **valid**, testing what it is intended to test. Are there confounding variables? The test should be sensitive to impairment in individuals with known deficits. (144, 279)

There has been controversy in the utilization of neuropsychological testing in cases of mild TBI, with studies and data to support differing opinions. Additional research will help further improve analysis. Individuals may also underreport symptoms, leading to difficulty in analyzing and interpreting correlating neuropsychological tests.

Neuropsychological testing was implemented initially with pencil-and-paper tests and more recently has advanced to computerized tests. Computerized neurocognitive assessment tools (NCATs) have logistical advantages (ease of use, time efficiency, automatic scoring) over traditional neuropsychological tests. The assessment of cognitive function appears to be important in the assessment and management of concussion.

Traditional pencil and paper neurocognitive tests include:

- Hopkins Verbal Learning Test; brief Visuospatial Memory Test; WAIS-III Digit Symbol subtest; Symbol Digit Modalities Test; Trail Making Test; Controlled Oral Word Association Test; Stroop Color and Word Test; WAIS-III Digit Span Test; WAIS-III Letter-Number Sequencing Test; Paced Auditory Serial Addition Test; and Repeatable Battery for the Assessment of Neuropsychological Status. (144) (as Randolph cited Shapiro, Benedict, Wechsler, Smith, Reitan, Benton, Golden, Gronwall and Randolph)

Computerized neurocognitive tests include:

- Automated Neuropsychological Assessment Metrics (ANAM); CNS Vital Signs (CNS VS); CogSport; CogState; HeadMinder Concussion

Resolution Index (HeadMinder CRI); and Immediate Post-Concussion and Cognitive Testing (ImPACT). (144, 146) (as Randolph cited Reeves, Makdissi, Lovell and Concussion Resolution Index)

Jones noted that cognitive functioning is critical for daily activities of military personnel and assessing cognitive function is important for management and treatment of mild TBIs. Jones referenced Ivins in stating that computerized automated neurocognitive assessment tools (NCATs) should be used only in combination with information from other clinical tools and observations. (145)

Arrieux reviewed existing literature regarding the four commonly used computerized NCATs (ANAM, CNS VS, CogState, and ImPACT). The ANAM is commonly used to assess cognitive functioning in U.S. Military service members. ImPACT is the most widely used NCAT in U.S. athletes and it has Food and Drug Administration approval for post-concussion assessments. ANAM correlated best with traditional neuropsychological tests of processing speed and was found to have moderate sensitivity and specificity for concussion and post-concussive symptoms during the acute injury period. ImPACT appears to measure cognition in a similar manner to traditional neuropsychological tests, as well as possibly detecting cognitive decline during the acute injury period. It was felt that future investigation should focus on cognitive impairment as well as return-to-play (sports) and return-to-duty (military) decisions. (145, 146)

Broglio utilized the ImPACT concussion assessment test to evaluate 21 National Collegiate Athletic Association (NCAA) Division I athletes at baseline within 72 hours after a concussion and after their symptoms resolved. After symptoms resolved, as assessed on the Symptom Assessment Scale (SAS), there were positive findings on the ImPACT test showing neurocognitive impairment in 38% of concussed athletes. They concluded that cognitive deficits may persist after symptoms have resolved. Based upon this, it was felt that players should not return to activity based upon symptoms alone, as it may place them at risk for further injury. Neurocognitive testing may help with guidance for return-to-play timing, and should be undertaken in all athletes who have suffered concussions, in conjunction with symptom inventory assessment. Symptoms on the SAS included "headache, nausea, difficulty balancing, fatigue, drowsiness, sleep disturbances, difficulty concentrating, feeling 'in a fog,' feeling 'slowed down,' sensitivity to light, sadness, vomiting, sensitivity to noise, nervousness, difficulty remembering, numbness, tingling, dizziness, neck pain, irritable, depression, blurred vision." (147)

Schwartz also found evidence to support the use of ImPACT testing in athletes who suffered a concussion. In a study of 72 high school athletes who had ImPACT testing and Post-Concussion Symptom Scale (PCSS) scores evaluated within 72 of suffering a concussion, the sensitivity of ImPACT was 81.9% and the specificity 89.4% when matched with controls. It was felt that ImPACT is both a sensitive and a specific tool for the assessment of neurocognitive and neurobehavioral sequelae of concussion and is helpful for assisting with decisions on return-to-play as it offers a thorough assessment of changes in cognitive functioning and symptom status after a concussion. (148)

Erlanger also supported neuropsychological testing for return to play decisions. Using an online assessment tool, the Concussion Resolution Index was found to reliably measure cognitive performance in athletes. The test was felt to be a valid and reliable method of evaluating changes in psychomotor speed and speed of information processing after sports related concussions. (149)

Having a baseline neuropsychological level of function is very helpful in determining levels of changes in function following a TBI and for assessing timing of return to activities. Baseline neuropsychological testing is routinely performed for athletes and pre-deployment for those entering the military. Since 1997, the National Hockey League has had its players who had a contract to play undergo baseline neuropsychological testing, mostly in pre-season training camp. (156)

In 2008, Congress directed the United States Department of Defense to have the ANAM given across all branches for those who are deploying to certain areas of operation. The intent is to be able to evaluate a soldier's function before and after they are deployed. This baseline exam, which takes 20–30 minutes to complete, assesses attention, concentration, reaction time, processing speed, and decision-making. This baseline study allows a comparison to subsequent neuropsychological evaluations should a soldier suffer a TBI as a result of an explosion, motor vehicle collision, fall, or other cause. As described in a paper published by Meyers in 2020, ANAM data was collected for 1,067,899 active duty service members representing all branches and the

Coast Guard; this represented the largest representative set of data for military personnel. (151, 152).

Additional detail regarding neuropsychological testing in the military is provided in Chapter 11.

BALANCE DIFFICULTIES

Balance difficulties after concussion are likely the result of improper processing of vestibular and visual information. Athletes who have sustained concussions and experienced postural stability deficits, often recovered their stability by day 3 post-injury. A study of 11 Division I athletes concluded that athletes who suffered a mild head injury may have decreased stability until three days after the insult. The postural instability may be due to a sensory interaction problem, with difficulty appropriately integrating sensory input, possibly from the vestibular and visual systems. Neurocognitive deficits are more difficult to identify acutely after a concussion. (167, 170)

Postural control is the ability of a subject to maintain a desired postural orientation at rest or in movement in response to perturbations from internal or external sources. Postural control is affected following a concussion. In a study of NCAA Division I athletes, it was found that athletes who have normal postural stability after a concussion may demonstrate subtle changes in postural control. (168)

The American Medical Society for Sports Medicine indicated in their position statement that, "balance disturbance is a specific indicator of a concussion, but not very sensitive." They recommend that any athlete who is suspected of having a concussion be stopped from playing and undergo a cognitive evaluation, balance tests, and a neurological physical examination. (169)

BRAIN HEALING AND PLASTICITY

It ain't what you don't know that gets you in trouble. It's what you know for sure that just ain't so.

Mark Twain

The capacity of neurons and neural networks to change, structurally and functionally, in response to environmental changes and stimulation is referred to as brain plasticity or neuroplasticity. This plasticity allows the central nervous system (CNS) to attempt to recover from injury. Evidence of plasticity in the brain can be seen after the brain has suffered a lesion from stroke, (590, 595) tumor, (591) as well as injury. (605) Neural plasticity may be structural (neurogenesis, synaptogenesis, changes in axons or dendrites) and functional (activity-dependent synaptic plasticity and biochemical mechanisms related to synaptic efficacy) as Tonti cited Fernandez-Espejo. (593, 594)

Dendritic spines, first described by Santiago Ramón y Cajal more than a century ago, are specialized structures on neuronal processes where most excitatory synapses are located. These spines are highly dynamic and are influenced by synaptic activity, which is important for experience-dependent development of the brain, storage of information within the brain circuitry, and for adaptive function of the brain. (609) Depolarization of neurons, modulated by neural stimulation, may trigger activity associated neuronal plasticity. (610) Interestingly, when a brain lesion develops slowly (as in a slow-growing tumor versus an acute stroke), recruitment of brain activity in remote areas of the ipsi- and contralesional hemispheres is more efficient. (597) It is not possible to predict how normal areas of the brain will react to injury elsewhere. (605) Plasticity may also be a target to treat diseases such as epilepsy, stroke, and dementia. (620)

Neuroplasticity occurs at both microscopic and macroscopic levels. The microscopic level involves neurogenesis, synaptic activity modifications, modulation of neural circuits thru glia and extracellular matrix (ECM), as well as changes in synaptic activity. Macroscopic changes involve cross-modality plasticity that can even occur in mature brains in which a modality-specific region of the brain has been deprived of its typical sensory input changes, becoming responsive to stimulation of other modalities. (593, 604) This has been seen when the occipital cortex of a blind patient is activated by sound changes. In addition, transcranial magnetic stimulation of the occipital cortex in these patients may result in distortions and omissions of letters in Braille text read by the subject. (600) Visual system neuroplasticity may be elicited in adulthood. (593) In cats who were deprived binocularly (of vision), auditory localization abilities increased, resulting in an increased sharpening of auditory spatial tuning as a result of visual deprivation, known as compensatory plasticity. (602) In proficient Braille readers, there has been found to be an expansion of the sensorimotor cortical representation of the reading finger. (603) In addition to experience-dependent plasticity allowing neurons to refine connections, astrocytes may also play a role in brain plasticity. Astrocytes are partners of neurons with respect to mechanisms of coding and homeostatic plasticity, as they ensheathe synapses and are in close contact with presynaptic and postsynaptic elements. (618, 404)

Traditionally, treatments for functional recovery after a TBI have been related to neurorehabilitation. Sanes and Jessell cited that the generally recognized central dogma of dead neurons not being able to regenerate may not be correct and that there is evidence that neurogenesis does occur in some regions of the adult mammalian brain; however, the work is preliminary and somewhat controversial. Sanes indicated that through better cell labeling technologies and work in non-human primates, in the dentate gyrus of the hippocampus, precursor cells divide throughout life and new neurons are added to the olfactory bulb as well. Sanes further stated, "in both cases the new neurons extend axons and dendrites, form synapses, and become integrated into functional circuits." The neurons appear to arise from multipotential progenitor stem cells, which is leading to research in this area. Embryonic stem cells, derived from early blastocyst stage embryos, can give rise to any cell in the body. Research into stimulation of neurogenesis in regions of injury are also being studied. Neuron generation can be stimulated by traumatic or ischemic injury, even in the cerebral cortex, but Sanes pointed out that "the fact that recovery after stroke and injury is poor demonstrates that spontaneous compensatory neurogenesis is insufficient for tissue repair." Embryonic stem cells may also potentially develop into oligodendrocytes and possibly help in the future with remyelination of damaged brain tissue. (499)

At this time, regenerative approaches for the treatment of TBI, including the use of mesenchymal stem cells appears to be promising for the future, although much research needs to be done. (540)

Stem cells that reside in certain regions within the adult mammalian brain can divide *in-situ* and give rise to new neurons, a process known as adult neurogenesis. The functional consequences of new neurons and their synaptic function and plasticity arise from interactions of glial cells, the ECM, as well as presynaptic and postsynaptic neurons that together form the "tetrapartite synapse." (614, 615) In the adult mammalian hippocampus, neurogenesis produces the dentate gyrus granule cell. New cells produced within the adult dentate gyrus can generate action potentials within a week after undergoing mitosis. (614) To contribute to hippocampal function, adult-generated dentate granule cells must not only survive but also integrate into the existing network. As Chancey cited Biebl, Dayer, and Sierra, most of these cells undergo apoptosis within the first few weeks of maturation, with only a fraction of newly generated granule cells surviving. Importantly, Chancey cited Kee, Tashiro, Kitamura, and Anderson in recognizing that environmental enrichment, learning tasks, and electrical stimulation increase the survival rate of these neurons during their first one to three weeks after mitosis. It is also during this important time period that an animal's experience may control the fate of each newborn cell. (616) During post-natal development, the formation and refinement of neural networks is affected by the environment surrounding an individual, resulting in an experience-dependent shaping of neuronal connections, allowing adaptation to a world around them. During critical periods of post-natal development, plasticity is high and the onset and closure of critical periods is controlled by a number of molecular and cellular mechanisms. Termination of a critical period may be related to perineural nets (PNNs, first discovered by Camillo Golgi in 1898), which are aggregates of ECM surrounding the cell body, dendrites, and axon initial segments of several neurons in the adult CNS. In the adult brain, the dynamic expression of PNNs may change the plasticity-associated conditions of the brain, including memory processes. PNNs contribute to the end of critical periods for development of sensory systems as well as memory systems. They appear to have a dual role, and can inhibit new learning by restricting plasticity, but can protect memories by stabilizing synaptic connections. As brain aging is associated with a decrease in sensory, motor and cognitive functions, and a progressive reduction in neural plasticity, and it is expected that there is an increase in PNN expression during aging. Carulli cited Gogolla, Tsien, and Duncan in noting that PNNs in the adult brain may be important in understanding how memories are encoded in the brain. In addition, Carulli indicated "developing molecular tools (vectors, antibodies, peptides, antagonists, etc.) to specifically interfere with PNN components would be beneficial to further our understanding of PNN functions and, in view of designing therapeutic tools, to improve certain CNS conditions." (617)

During development, experience-dependent synaptic plasticity plays a role in forming brain circuits, and 83 candidate plasticity proteins have been identified that may have a role in this process. They may be involved with RNA splicing and protein translation, regulated at the level of protein synthesis by sensory experience, which Liu states had not been reported prior to their study. (619)

Regions of the brain such as the hippocampus that retain plastic capabilities throughout life are also targets of neurodegeneration. (606) The ability of the hippocampus (which is often affected in Alzheimer's disease) to add neurons throughout life, called adult hippocampal neurogenesis, yields unparalleled plasticity to the entire hippocampal circuitry. (607) Weerasinghe-Mudiyanselage cited Mateus-Pinheiro, Dioli, Sun, Zhu, Moodley, and Herzog in noting that the hippocampus experiences neuronal remodeling during a number of neurodegenerative diseases including Alzheimer's disease, Parkinson's disease, Huntington's disease, multiple sclerosis, vascular dementia, frontotemporal dementia, and amyotrophic lateral sclerosis. The remodeling of neurons occurs mainly through structural changes in the dendrites and spines of hippocampal neurons. (608) In the adult hippocampus, aberrant adult neurogenesis may contribute to brain disorders including epilepsy, mental disorders, and neurodevelopmental disorders. The potential of using adult neural stem cells therapeutically as a regenerative source for neural repair, while very exciting, also has potential adverse consequences, especially if neuron generation occurs under pathological conditions. The impact of the surrounding neuronal circuitry and neuronal integration must be considered and future research should take this into consideration. (621)

Using positron emission tomography (PET) scans, it was found that in patients with slow-growing tumors occupying the hand region of the motor cortex there was a shift of the activation region in the brain by 9–43 mm. (591) Interestingly, in patients who had suffered strokes, there was a dynamic bihemispheric reorganization of motor networks, with activation in the sensorimotor cortex and posterior parietal regions ipsilateral to the paretic hand as well as in the bilateral prefrontal regions. Contralateral function increased as paresis diminished. (592) In patients who have suffered a stroke in the hand area of the primary motor cortex or a deep lesion sparing the motor cortex, it was found that recruitment occurred, in which extension of activation into areas not activated by movements of the unaffected hand (ipsilateral sensorimotor cortex, supplementary motor area, and frontal premotor and superior parietal areas) occurred. It was considered that this recruitment may be due to a disinhibition caused by a lesion in the primary motor cortex and the underlying reciprocal corticocortical connections from the motor region, resulting in ipsilateral and contralateral activation. Over time, in some patients, this recruitment decreased and focusing of activation returned to the contralateral supplementary motor cortex. This focusing may result from inhibition from the motor cortex. (590) Similar findings of language reorganization after a stroke have been seen. Functional MRI (fMRI) studies have shown that patients with aphasia due to an infarct in the left middle cerebral artery territory were found in the subacute phase to have a large increase in the bilateral language network with peak activation in the right Broca-homologue, which normalized back to the left-hemisphere language area in the chronic phase. (599)

Preclinical studies show that stem-cell based interventions may have a potential future in the treatment of TBI, but the risks and benefits need to be further investigated. Enriched environment intervention through neurorehabilitation is important in helping TBI patients return into a functional lifestyle. A positive environment is important, as many TBI patient suffer from depression. (498)

Brain-derived neurotrophic factor in the brain and spinal cord, which appears to be a critical mediator of activity-associated plasticity, may be modulated through physical rehabilitation (passive or active exercise), possibly resulting in cortical plasticity commensurate with functional recovery. Other types of activity patterns may be achieved through electrical and magnetic stimulation. (610) Neuritin, a novel glycosylphosphatidylinositol-anchored protein expressed on the surface of developing and mature neurons, has been found to be expressed in postmitotic-differentiating neurons of the developing nervous system associated with plasticity in the adult and may be a downstream effector of activity-induced neurite outgrowth in hippocampal and cortical neurons. (611) Immediate early genes may have a role in plasticity by driving rapid and transient neuronal responses, which might initiate specific transcription programs in response to neural activity patterns. (610) Hundreds of genes contribute to activity-related transcription in CNS neurons. Plasticity of the nervous system may be related to experience-driven synaptic activity, which causes membrane depolarization and calcium influx into the certain neurons, initiating cellular changes that alter synaptic connectivity. Remodeling of synapses may be related to activation of new gene transcription. The gene expression may result in neuronal development including dendritic branching and synapse maturation as well as elimination. (612)

Repetitive transcranial magnetic stimulation and transcranial direct current stimulation (tDCS) may inhibit or facilitate excitability of the cortex and may induce plastic changes within the cortical sensorimotor areas and networks, possibly improving function of an affected hand after a stroke. A literature review found tDCS to be a safe non-invasive neuromodulatory technique best combined with other therapies, such as cognitive rehabilitation and physical therapy, to improve cognitive and motor outcomes in TBI patients. Zaninotto stated that an injured brain attempts to form new cortical and subcortical connections and reorganize neural networks, and that non-invasive brain stimulation techniques aim to utilize these neuroplastic mechanisms. (497) Another study showed that neuromodulation through tDCS may potentially have benefit to TBI patients through the potential to promote motor recovery. The authors suggest a clinical trial in the future. (493) Experimental use of transcranial magnetic stimulation and other methods of brain stimulation have been implemented to increase brain plasticity and recovery. (594, 601, 610) Epidural stimulation has also been used. (598)

In patients who have suffered TBI, deep brain stimulation may potentially offer a means to "jump-start" dormant brain networks or modulate aberrant or desynchronized brain activity to facilitate brain function. Targets for the stimulation may include the ascending reticular activating system and areas of the thalamus, as well as the frontal and prefrontal cortex, internal capsule, thalamus, and other regions. (496)

C-C chemokine receptor 5 (CCR5) is a translational target for neural repair in TBI and stroke. Neuronal knockdown of CCR5 has been shown to promote early motor recovery after a TBI. (490)

In a study on rats, it was found that focal TBI may influence CNS regions distant from the brain lesion and, through alterations in expression of molecular regulators/markers of spinal plasticity, changes may occur in this region remote from the focal TBI, contributing to motor recovery or maladaptive motor responses. (492) Monkeys were studied with multi-modal MRI to determine the time course of plasticity after hippocampal lesions, where both functional and structural changes were found to occur dynamically over time. During the acute stage (three months after injury), regions of the brain that were highly connected to the hippocampus before the lesion experienced a drop in network participation and in the chronic stage (12 months after injury), they suffered a loss of gray-matter volume. Interestingly, during the chronic stage, they also increased functional connectivity with other areas in the same module. Froudist-Walsh also noted "neuronal density was associated with a greater loss of within-module functional connectivity during the chronic stage, while non-neuronal cell density was associated with increases in network participation over the same stage." In addition, network hubs are likely more vulnerable to effects of a lesion, with greater reduction in functional connectivity at both acute and chronic stages. The authors concluded that, to their knowledge, theirs was the "first study to show quantitatively that post-lesion plasticity patterns depend on pre-lesion functional connectivity." (605)

After a TBI, diffuse axonal injury may result in significant cognitive and other deficits. In a study of 23 TBI patients who were compared to controls, MRI studies along with the application of graph theory and regression analysis suggested that network reorganization and changes in structural brain connectivity may be related to recovery of impaired cognitive function in the first year post-injury. (489)

Neural plasticity may involve cellular elements (neuronal and glial cells) and subcellular compartments (synaptic, dendritic, axonal, neuromuscular plasticity). (481) Experience-dependent white-matter plasticity can involve the alteration of structural properties of an axon, leading to changes in function of the axon. Changes in properties of the axon (changes in myelin, axonal diameter, internode length) may affect nerve conduction velocity and other properties, which may affect behavior. The possibility that myelin can be regulated by functional activity and lead to nervous system plasticity is a shift from the traditional paradigm in which myelin was viewed as being static. (404) Fields cited the works of Fields, Yakovlev, Mabbott, Nagy, Kraft, Pujol, Liston, and Giedd in stating that myelination of certain brain regions coincides with the development of certain cognitive functions (reading, vocabulary development, executive decision-making proficiency). Myelination in the human brain continues for decades and, similar to synaptogenesis and synapse elimination, allows for learning and neural circuit plasticity to be influenced by functional activity. In addition to the formation and breakage of connections, the speed and timing of information transmission is important. Fields also cited Zatorre, Bengtsson, Carreiras, Scholz, and Fields in stating that white-matter structure can change after learning and functional experience in complex tasks (learning complex skills such as playing piano, learning to read, mastering juggling and others), but they do not confirm myelin changes due to the brain imaging voxel size resolution limits. (405) Synaptic plasticity may involve localization of receptors and proteins in different loci of the synaptic compartment, enabling effective plastic conversions. (562)

In a study of 59 four-year-old children, 20 were included in a word learning group, 19 in an active control group, and 20 in a passive control group. Upon MRI diffusion weighted imaging, there was found to be an increase in fractional anisotropy (FA) in the left precentral white matter (dorsal precentral gyrus) in the word learning group as compared to the active and passive controls. The authors refer to the possibility that myelination is responsible for the increase in FA. (407)

Other concepts related to brain plasticity may also relate to oligodendrocyte precursor cells in the adult brain, formation of new myelin during adulthood, activity-dependent modulation of myelin, axonal sprouting, and changes in nodes of Ranvier. (404)

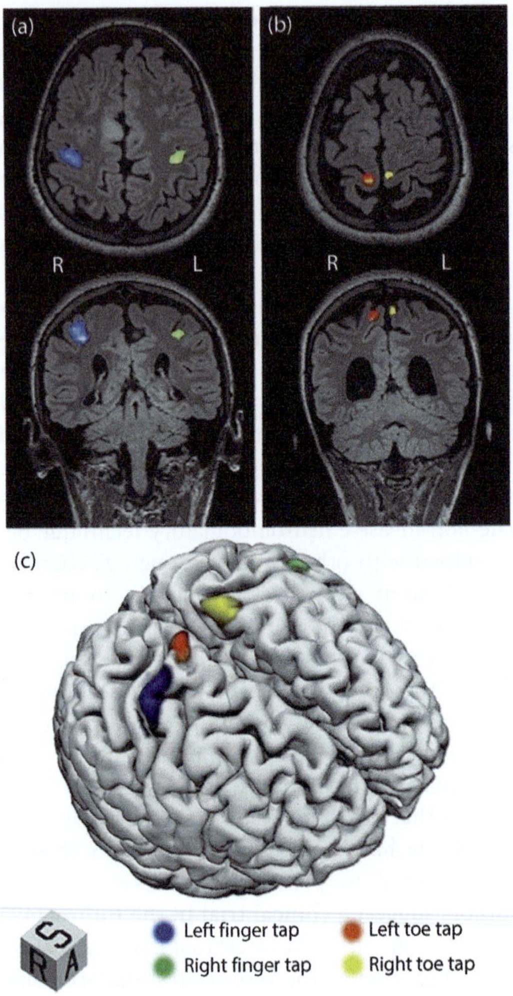

Figure 10.1 Preoperative brain axial and coronal T2 weighting of FLAIR MRI and motor task-based functional MRI (fMRI). Seen in (A) and (B) are axial and coronal fMRI showing blood-oxygen-level-dependent (BOLD) activations of the middle portion of the contralateral primary sensorimotor cortex during finger tapping (A) and the superior aspect of the contralateral primary motor cortex during toe tapping (B). A T1 surface–based three-dimensional reconstruction (C) with superimposed regions activated during motor tasks revealed anatomically concordant functional areas. Cube shows orientation: S=superior; R=right; A=anterior. Source images [B, C, D] reproduced with permission of Wolters Kluwer Health, Inc. (559).

Literature Case Report: Neural plasticity and functional reorganization

An example of neural plasticity and functional reorganization is well demonstrated in a 16-year-old patient with complete agenesis of the corpus callosum, who had undergone surgery for resection of a right-sided low-grade glioma located within the right supplementary motor area (SMA). Preoperatively, the patient had a fMRI showing locations of finger- and toe-tapping activation within the expected contralateral sensorimotor cortex (**Figure 10.1**; 559). Surgery was performed to achieve a gross total resection utilizing cortical stimulation. Post-operatively, the patient experienced left-sided 3 out of 5 weakness and significant hemiapraxia, consistent with a supplementary

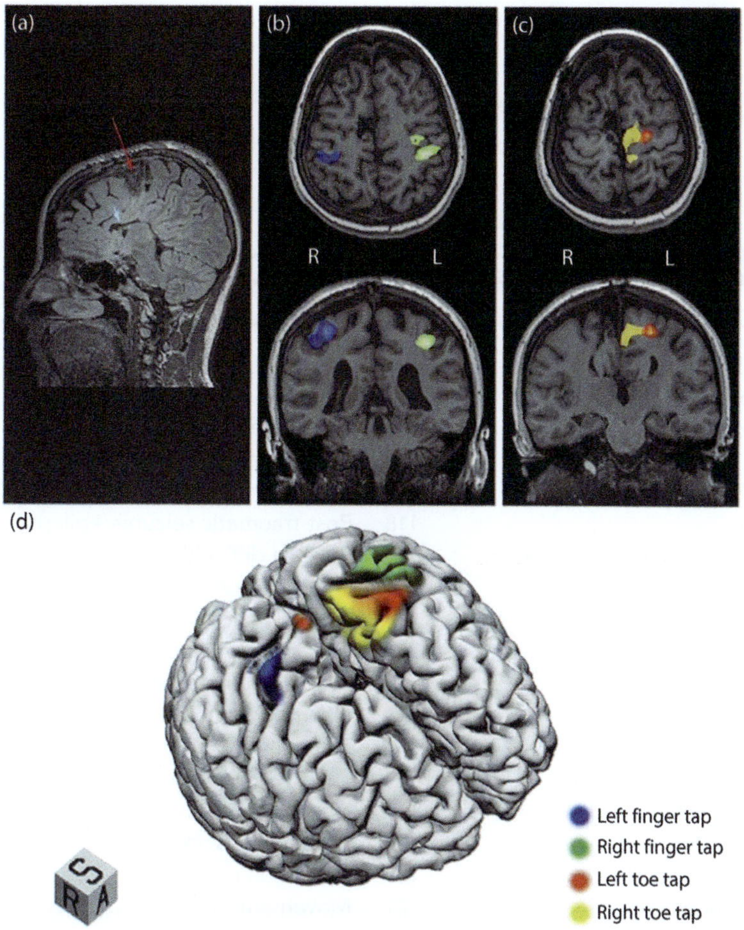

Figure 10.2 Postoperative brain T2 weighting of FLAIR MRI and functional MRI (fMRI) performed three months after surgery with the patient having fully recovered from any left-sided weakness due to supplementary motor syndrome. There is gross total resection of the tumor-infiltrated supplementary motor area with sparing of the paracentral lobule (red arrow) seen in sagittal T2 weighting of FLAIR MRI images (A). Absence of the corpus callosum (CC) is notable above the frontal horn and body of the lateral ventricle (short cyan arrow, A). In (B) and (C) are seen fMRI (axial and coronal views). Image (B) shows blood-oxygen-level-dependent (BOLD) signals matched the location of the preoperative activations during finger tapping. In (C), activation maps revealed the anterior expansion of the right toe-tapping area (now incorporating most of the SMA) and the contralateral transfer of a major part of the area activated by left toe-tapping to the left paracentral lobule and SMA. Seen in (D) is a T1 surface-based three-dimensional reconstruction with overlaid task-activated regions highlighting the expansion of right toe-tapping function and the contralateral transfer of the left toe-tapping area. The resection cavity is discernible at the medial aspect of the right premotor cortex. Cube shows orientation: S=superior; R=right; A=anterior. Reproduced with permission of Wolters Kluwer Health, Inc. (559)

motor area syndrome. Importantly, the patient fully recovered from this deficit by three months post-surgery and repeat task-based fMRI revealed that there was reorganization of brain function with the expected brain regions responsible for right finger tapping and right toe tapping continuing their function, but surprisingly, a portion of the area activated by left toe tapping had shifted to the left paracentral lobule and the adjacent supplementary motor area (**Figure 10.2**; 559). This demonstrated that there was a transfer of function from one hemisphere to the contralateral side. (559)

11

Long-term outcome: Prognosis

It is important to recognize the long-term effects of traumatic brain injury (TBI) not only on the brain and its associated neurological, psychological, cognitive, and psychiatric function, but also the tremendous impact it has on all parts of a patient's body. Some of the adverse impacts may be immediately apparent, and they may also escalate and impact other organ systems in the future. At other times, the symptoms of a TBI may be very subtle or unnoticeable, and although it may take years for their harmful impact to reveal itself, future complications and adverse outcomes may become severe. In addition, TBI may "weaken" the brain, predisposing it to more significant harm should a patient suffer another TBI in the future. This is well documented in cases of repetitive head injury

DOI: 10.1201/9781003354154-11

and chronic traumatic encephalopathy (CTE). The complications of TBI with respect to the brain and body may act in concert with each other and have profound effects in which the net sum of all the negative impacts taken as a whole exceeds the sum of the individual negative impacts. Individual body systems and organs may suffer, causing an escalating negative cascade of events that impact other body systems, and this downward spiral may have a significant influence on every aspect of a patient's life. Their quality of life may be significantly impaired and their life expectancy may be shortened as a result of these deleterious events. TBI and its sequelae can accelerate the aging process. This chapter will review many of the life-altering impacts of TBI and their prognosis.

TBI is a chronic disease process, as it increases morbidity, reduces life expectancy, and can precipitate conditions that may lead to long-term impairment and disability with reduced quality of life and functional limitations. Every organ system in the body may be affected. TBI impacts survivors in many ways and has been related to cognitive impairment, neurodegenerative diseases, Alzheimer's disease, CTE, Parkinson's disease, sleep disorders, seizures, psychiatric diseases, neuroendocrine dysfunction, mood disorders, and depression as well as non-neurological disorders including sexual dysfunction, incontinence, metabolic dysfunction, and other systemic concerns. (6, 47, 276) Patients may experience weight gain or loss, possibly related to a behavioral dysexecutive syndrome. (613)

According to a study by Thurman, of roughly 1.5 million Americans who suffer a TBI yearly, about 50,000 will die, 230,000 survive after being hospitalized, and 80,000–90,000 will have a long-term disability. (257)

Depending upon which classification method was used, the prevalence of post-concussion syndrome (PCS) has been found to vary significantly. Of all TBI cases, 70–80% of cases (depending on which study is referenced) are considered mild TBI. While the symptoms of mild TBI decrease spontaneously for most patients, they may last much longer in 5–43% (as Voormolen cited Binder, Leddy, Spinos, King, Ruff, and Hiploylee) of patients. (140) If lasting longer than three months, they may be known as PCS, although there is controversy and inconsistency in the literature regarding this classification, as described in Chapter 10 (section titled "Post-Concussion Syndrome/Mild Neurocognitive Disorder"). Part of the difficulty in determining more precisely which patients have developed PCS is the lack of consensus as to which symptoms and criteria should be included in the diagnosis of PCS (as described previously). As has also been pointed out, in the DSM-5, PCS has been replaced with the term "mild neurocognitive impairment." These changes create difficulties in comparing data and studies. Because of the inconsistencies in diagnostic criteria, some studies may have included patients in the category of mild TBI (as Voormolen cited Cassidy, De Kruijt, Williams, and Culotta), who might not have met the diagnostic criteria of other studies. (140)

In a study of 10,008 patients with TBI, it was seen that a poor prognosis was associated with a low Glasgow Coma Scale (GCS) score with absent pupil reactivity and findings of major extracranial injury. After the age of 40, increasing age was associated with worse outcomes. Computed tomography (CT) findings of the loss of the third ventricle or basal cisterns was associated with the worst prognosis at 14 days post-injury. Patients in high-income countries did better than those from low-to-middle income countries. (61)

EPIDURAL HEMATOMA

Epidural hematomas and subdural hematomas in the brain are very different with respect to epidemiology, clinical presentation, and outcome. While patients with epidural hematomas tend to have favorable outcomes, those with acute subdural hematomas tend to have a high mortality and a difficult functional recovery. The prognosis for patients with a subdural hematoma is much worse, with significantly higher mortality rates. These patients may have also suffered cortical contusions, lacerations, depressed bone fractures, brainstem injury, and diffuse axonal injury (DAI), with secondary edema, intracranial hypertension, and ischemia. (63) Epidural hematomas have been found to occur in 2% of head injuries. Those patients with a pure epidural hematoma who undergo rapid detection and surgical evacuation have an excellent prognosis. (31)

In a study of epidural hematomas, 5,189 admissions were identified in the United States between 2003 and 2010. Of these, 97–98% were discharged from the hospital to home and the median length of stay in the hospital was about four days. The mortality rate in the hospital was 3.5% and the complication rate 2.9%. The authors felt that increased availability and use of resources, as well as advances in technology and surgical capabilities, reduced mortality and adverse discharge disposition. (62)

SUBDURAL HEMATOMA

Of 1,150 patients who suffered severe head injuries with a GCS scale score of 3–7, the 101 patients who suffered subdural hematomas had an overall mortality rate of 66%, with only 19% having a functional recovery. (32) When 102 patients with a GCS score of 4–8 and an acute subdural hematoma were evaluated, there was found to be no difference in complications and outcomes in the 42 patients who were treated with a craniotomy (with evacuation of the subdural hematoma) versus the 60 who were treated with removal of the subdural hematoma and a decompressive craniectomy (removal of a 12 cm × 10 cm or larger portion of frontotemporoparietal skull which was placed in a tissue bank, and replaced with a cranioplasty two to three months later), but the decompressive craniectomy group had a higher mortality rate. The authors concluded that either method could be used to surgically treat patients with an acute subdural hematoma who sustained a severe head injury with a low GCS score. (88) This study was from 2011, and updated research included in the *Brain Trauma Foundation TBI Guidelines* (2020) has shown that secondary decompressive craniectomy for late refractory elevated intracranial pressure (ICP) is recommended to improve mortality and favorable outcomes. (577)

MILD TBI

When 122 consecutive patients with mild TBI were evaluated, 86% reported symptoms on day 1, but this improved to 49% at three months post-injury, with fatigue, sleep disturbance, and poor memory being most reported. There were four symptom domains: somatic, cognitive, affective, and vision-related. The initial three months post-injury saw mainly somatic symptoms, but at three months, somatic, cognitive, and affective had similar weight and fewer individuals reported vision-related problems. Patients with a higher number of symptoms early post-injury are more likely to develop persistent complaints. (180)

Of 3,514 patients suffering a TBI in Germany, while most were considered to have suffered mild TBI, one-third of patients were found after three months and after one year to have symptoms (per a telephone interview) related to TBI, with being female, having a GCS of 13–14, or suffering an intracranial hemorrhage as negative predictors. (22)

Another study of 421 adults who were assessed one year after suffering a mild TBI showed that 25% of patients may still experience three or more symptoms associated with mild TBI, although the study showed no significant difference (except for episodic memory measure) on neuropsychological testing or Glasgow Outcome Scale (GOS) when compared to trauma controls without a TBI. (255)

In a prospective cohort of 375 mild TBI patients in a Transforming Research and Clinical Knowledge in Traumatic Brain Injury (TRACK-TBI) study at 6 and 12 months after the injury, 82% of patients reported at least one PCS symptom, with approximately 40% having significantly reduced satisfaction with life scores at 12 months post-injury. There were 22.4% of patients at one year post-injury who were below full functional status. It was felt that recovery from a mild TBI is a nonlinear process and the time to full recovery may, for some patients, be protracted. Importantly, McMahon stated, "what is becoming clear though, is that 'mild' is indeed a misnomer for this disease, because many patients experience significant and persistent symptoms. For these patients, mTBI (mild TBI) is anything but mild." (324)

Of 182 children with mild TBI of which 32 had complicated mild TBI (positive findings on brain scans), upon comparison to 99 orthopedic injury controls, it was found that ratings of post-concussive symptoms were higher in those with more severe brain injuries and in those with lower cognitive ability. Children with low cognitive ability and a complicated mild TBI reported more post-concussive symptoms initially. Lower cognitive ability correlated with higher PCS. The conclusion was that higher cognitive ability appears to be protective. (178)

MODERATE AND SEVERE TBI

When 131 patients who had suffered a severe TBI and underwent a decompressive craniectomy were reviewed, 48.1% died during their hospital stay,

20.6% were in a vegetative state upon hospital discharge, 24.4% had severe disability, and 6.9% had moderate disability. At follow-up of at least one year, 67.7% were dead or in a vegetative state. Thirty patients who survived had major depression and neurologic deficits, yet reported only modestly reduced 36-Item Short-Form Health Survey (SF-36) scores, with high functional activities of daily living. (294)

In a study of 39 patients who had suffered a severe TBI, undergone a decompressive craniectomy, and survived but were in a severely disabled or vegetative state at 18 months after the craniectomy, subsequent reevaluation three years after the injury revealed that 7 patients died, 12 were lost to follow-up, but 20 survived. Of the survivors, 5 who were in a vegetative state at 18 months, remained so after three years post-injury, and the other 15 patients remained in a severely disabled state at about five years post-injury. The authors concluded that there was no substantial recovery for severe TBI patients beyond 18 months post-decompressive craniectomy, but patients had a reasonably high SF-36 score, reflecting an acceptance of their quality of life. (45)

In adults with severe TBI, in which ICP is elevated (over 25 mm Hg) and not responding to medical management attempts to control it, surgical decompressive craniectomy increased survival but was unlikely to decrease risk of an unfavorable functional outcome. (97)

In a study of 155 adults with severe diffuse TBI and elevated intracranial hypertension that was not manageable with medical management, those who underwent bifrontotemporoparietal decompressive craniotomy had worse outcomes than those who underwent medical management, although they had decreased ICP and decreased length of stay in the intensive care unit (ICU). The authors point out that this finding differed from those of other studies, and is contrary to what they expected, which is that a craniectomy would decrease ICP and improve functional outcome. (108)

A literature study evaluated long-term outcome of patients who had suffered a severe TBI, and when long-term outcomes over two years after injury were evaluated, approximately 46% (range of 18–75%) of patients died, 29–100% had unfavorable outcomes, and 21–27% had a favorable outcome or full recovery. SF-36 scores of survivors were lower than those of the general population. Factors associated with worse long-term outcomes were lower Glasgow Outcome Scale Extended (GOSE) scores at discharge from the hospital, increased length of hospital stay, and older age. (293)

A study of 300 patients who had suffered a severe TBI revealed that the one-year GOS score and neuropsychological performance correlated with the lowest post-resuscitation GCS score and pupillary reactivity. It was also found one year after the injury, that while cognitive function involving memory and information processing were often impaired and slowed, visuospatial and language ability often improved to a normal range. The authors note that in contrast to other studies, ICP and features of the CT scan (swelling, hemorrhage) were unrelated to neurobehavioral outcome one year post-injury. (183)

In a retrospective analysis of 213 patients with a severe TBI and a hospital admission GCS score of ≤ 8, outcome at six months with good recovery (based on the GOS) was present in 29.1%, moderate disability in 29.6%, severe disability in 13.6%, vegetative status in 8%, and death in 19.7%. (99)

Eighty-six patients who suffered a severe TBI were evaluated eight years later using the GOSE, a functional independence assessment of employment, mood, other life factors, and neuropsychological tests. It was found that cognitive measures including processing speed were important factors of long-term post-injury functional outcome. Injury severity and other demographics such as age and education were less important with respect to functional outcome. (290)

An imaging and cognitive function study revealed interesting findings at one year post-trauma, with cognitive improvement correlating with dynamic changes in diffusion tensor imaging (DTI). A group of 20 patients who had suffered moderate and severe TBI were followed for one year, and received imaging studies at 2, 6, and 12 months post-injury. They were found on imaging studies to have lower fractional anisotropy (FA) and higher mean diffusivity in all evaluated segments (genu, body, and splenium of corpus callosum; right and left superior longitudinal fasciculus). The corpus callosum, which initially had a decrease in FA, subsequently showed a rise, and the superior longitudinal fasciculi also showed a progressive rise. FA values in the genu of the corpus callosum were found to correlate with cognitive attention and FA values in both superior longitudinal fasciculi correlated with IQ. The authors felt that DTI as a noninvasive tool, may be helpful in monitoring progression of DAI and may help to monitor targeted therapies in the future. The authors also felt that DTI metrics looking at specific sites of the brain could play a role in evaluating microstructural reorganization and neuroplasticity. (460)

BLAST-RELATED TBI

The magnitude of TBI that results from a blast injury is affected by the blast energy and the distance from the center of the blast. Resulting TBI may range from a mild concussion to severe penetrating injury. The acute clinical findings are similar in blast-related and nonblast-related mild TBI, but in the military population, it is more common in the blast-injured group to find PCS, posttraumatic stress disorder (PTSD), depression, and chronic pain. Psychological factors such as PTSD and depression may lead to chronic impairment. (40)

In a review of blast injury in U.S. military service members, publications up to April 2017 included 2,290 references identified by search and 106 studies reviewed, representing 37,515 participants who suffered blast-related mild TBI. With such a large study, while there are inconsistencies in methods used to confirm criteria for diagnosis, the most frequently reported disorders were hearing disturbances, headaches, and frequent comorbidities were PTSD, cognitive difficulties, sleep disorders, depression, and attention disorders. Impairment in sensory and neurocognitive function, including neurological, psychological and perceptual may be associated with mild TBI related to blasts. In a review of headaches, more than 60% of participants with a mild TBI reported headache. The review reported, related to imaging of the brain after blast injury and citing works of Hayes, MacDonald, Miller, Morey, Nathan, Riedy, Robinson, Stout, and Vakhtin, "the most commonly reported neurological abnormalities were white matter irregularities, cerebellar damage, thalamic network architectural differences, metabolic activation, diffuse axonal injury (DAI), and sensorimotor impairment." (262)

Of 89 cases of blast injury in a domestic setting (private dwelling explosions, industrial gas explosions, military training explosion, home explosive device, fireworks explosion), 32 people suffered a head injury, and 4 suffered a tympanic membrane injury. The majority of those head injured patients had an initial GCS score of 15, and of those tested, 50% had a positive CT brain scan, with the most common finding being cerebral contusion, followed by subdural hematoma. The blast injury was missed in 36% of patients with a GCS score of 15 and the disease process may evolve over time. The authors recommend that those treating acute blast injury victims should maintain a high index of suspicion for TBI despite a normal GCS score or minimal evidence of external trauma to avoid missing patients with clinically significant injury. They note that as a result of a blast, injury to the brain may initially appear subtle, but the TBI is a dynamic process which may continue to evolve well after the injury, resulting in cognitive deficits. (39)

17 veterans who suffered a blast-related TBI were compared to 15 control veterans without a blast exposure, and functional connectivity of the globus pallidus was found to be altered in the blast exposure group when evaluated roughly 5.5 years after the injury. (716)

SOMATIC, NEUROPSYCHOLOGICAL, PSYCHIATRIC, COGNITIVE AND BEHAVIORAL CHANGES, AND PTSD

TBI-induced neuro-sequelae can be divided into two general categories, neuropsychiatric and somatic/physical, and the neuropsychiatric can be further divided into cognitive and behavioral disorders. A variety of changes can be seen after TBI. There may be interaction of disorders, which can have compounding effects upon each other and with a patient's interaction with other individuals.

Post-concussion syndrome and somatic changes

After a mild TBI, patients may suffer PCS with a wide variety or cluster of possible symptoms including somatic/physical (headache, dizziness, fatigue, imbalance, sleep disruption, visual disturbances, light and noise sensitivity [photo- and phonophobia]), cognitive (memory, attention/concentration and executive deficits), and emotional/behavioral (depression, anxiety, irritability). With a mild TBI, symptoms often resolve within one month after injury, but they may also last many months or years and eventually become permanent. When post-concussion symptoms persist, they are known as persistent post-concussion symptoms, or PCS. (49, 662)

Of 110 patients who sustained a concussion, and suffered with post-concussion symptoms lasting more than three months, only 27% recovered, of which 67% did so in the first year. Of those with symptoms lasting more than three years, there was no further recovery. In all of these patients, the CT and magnetic resonance imaging (MRI) scans of the brain were negative. The recovery rate dropped by 20% for each additional post-concussion symptom the patient experienced, showing a strong association between the total number of symptoms reported and the time to recovery. Those who experience post-concussion symptoms for over three years may have permanent difficulties. Hiployee states, "the finding that PCS may be permanent if it lasts longer than three years suggests that it may be critical to treat PCS appropriately in the early stages." The authors indicated this may be the first study to look at duration of post-concussion symptoms beyond which recovery has not occurred. (159)

A study in which 196 patients with head injury were evaluated one year post-injury, revealed about 40% had three or more symptoms including irritability (35%), lack of initiative (15%), and social disinhibition (3%). Severity of head injury associated with a low GCS score correlated with more difficulties, suggesting an organic etiology for the symptoms. (179, 302)

Cognitive changes

A meta-analysis of 39 cross sectional studies on 1,716 TBI patients was compared to 1,164 controls and found that cognitive function after moderate-to-severe TBI was adversely impacted more than three times more than the function of mild TBI-injured patients. With respect to mild TBI, cognitive function improved the most during the first few weeks and was, for the most part, back to baseline within one to three months. When moderate-to-severe TBI patients are examined, while cognitive function improves during the first two years, significant impairments remain after two years. It was felt that moderate-to-severe TBI causes more significant and more persistent impairment of cognitive function than does mild TBI. (163)

Post-traumatic amnesia (PTA) duration following TBI has been shown in a meta-analysis study of 854 patients from 21 peer reviewed papers to correlate well with intelligence impairment in the subacute (less than six months) and the chronic (more than six months) time periods following TBI. Age at the time of injury was not found to be a factor. (192)

Psychiatric disorders

Psychiatric and behavioral disorders are a serious concern for individuals who have suffered TBI. Disorders of anxiety, PTSD, mood changes (depression), impulsivity, and aggression may occur. TBI also appears to be related to post-traumatic psychiatric disorders including delusional disorders and personality disturbances. Any disorders that may have existed prior to the injury must also be considered and any accentuations should be noted. Attempts should be made to determine which issues can be treated to diminish stress to the patient and their caregivers.

Major depressive disorders and post-traumatic stress disorders are increased after TBI, most likely manifesting within the first year post-injury with depressive disorders becoming more persistent post-injury. Much of this may result from the impact of TBI on the frontolimbic structures, potentially leading to organically based psychiatric disorders. (20) Mood disorders are frequent complications of TBI, and are often overlooked and not adequately treated. They may be exacerbated by a previous psychiatric history or poor social support and have a negative impact on a patient's recovery. (202)

In a study of 28 patients with moderate-to-severe TBI and 27 controls, those with TBI showed a significant increase in urgency, lack of premeditation, and lack of perseverance, showing an increase in impulsivity after moderate-to-severe TBI. The results suggest that the decreased ability to inhibit rash actions in some situations results from the lower prepotent response inhibition, as opposed to being a result of general cognitive impairment. (208)

Neuropsychiatric difficulties are a major cause of disability after a TBI, and injuries to the frontal and temporal lobes may cause problems with cognition, memory, attention, executive function, mood disorders, depression, and behavior issues. While improvements can occur as late as five to ten years after the injury, most improvement occurs within the first two years. (305) Deficits in self-awareness after a TBI appear to be related to the severity of the injury, IQ, mood state, and executive functions. (307)

There was found to be a higher rate of psychiatric diagnosis in adults with a TBI than in the general population. Of 164 patients studied one year after TBI, of those aged 18–64 years, 27.1% had a psychiatric illness while that of the general population was 16.4%. A breakdown showed that depression was present in 13.9% of the TBI group (2.1% in the general population) and panic disorder in 9% (0.8% in the general population). Lower initial GCS scores and fewer years of pre-injury education were associated with greater findings. Occurrence of psychiatric illness after a TBI depends on an interaction between psychosocial and organic factors. (303)

Behavioral disorders after a TBI may include psychiatric disorders, such as mood disorders and anxiety, and personality disorders. In a study of 89 patients with TBI and 26 patients without TBI but with multiple trauma, it was found, during the initial six months post-injury, that aggressive behavior was seen in 33.7% of TBI patients, but in only 11.5% of non-TBI patients and the aggressive traits were associated with the presence of frontal lobe lesions, major depression, and poor pre-injury social functioning. Factors associated with aggression following TBI include major depression, substance abuse, and impaired social functioning. In TBI patients, both aggression and depressive disorders were associated with poor social functioning. (204)

In a study of 40 patients who suffered very severe blunt head trauma, with PTA for more than one month, evaluations were performed about four to five months after the injury, and again at two to five years and 10–15 years after the injury. All patients had permanent sequelae, with more than 25% being dependent and most receiving a disability pension. Those with a brainstem injury and/or severe anterior lesions suffered the worst outcome. Psychosis occurred often in cases of severe left hemisphere damage and/or anterior lesions, and only when PTA exceeded three months. Absence of social contact created isolation for patients and their families. While the greatest recovery occurred within the first six months, improvement occurred up to three years after the injury. Although a few patients regained some work capacity, it was years after the injury that they did so. (244)

A 30-year follow-up study on 60 patients who suffered a TBI revealed that psychiatric disorders began in 48.3% after the brain injury, including disorders of major depression (26.7% of patients), alcohol abuse (11.7%), panic disorders (8.3%), phobias (8.3%), psychotic disorders (6.7%), and personality disorders (23.3%). The authors felt that due to the high rate of psychiatric disorders after a TBI, psychiatric follow-up is important. TBI can result in decades-long or permanent vulnerability to psychiatric disorders in some individuals. The inclusion criteria for the patients in this study included head trauma sufficient to cause TBI and neurological symptoms (including headache and nausea) lasting at least one week, and at least one other finding (such as loss of consciousness [LOC] for more than one minute, PTA of more than 30 minutes, neurological symptoms during the first three days, and skull fracture or intracerebral hemorrhage). (304)

In a literature search study, Simpson found that patients with a TBI have a 3–4 times greater risk of death by suicide ideation when compared to the general population. Those with a severe TBI have a 1.4 times greater risk of suicide than those with a concussion, and those with high suicide ideation have an increased risk of suicide attempt by a factor of 4.9 when compared to those with low or no suicide ideation. TBI patients with a post-injury psychiatric history or emotional distress had a factor of 7.8 greater risk of suicide attempt when compared with TBI patients who did not have these findings. Those with post-injury moderate-to-high levels of hopelessness had an 8.7-fold greater risk of suicide ideation than those post-injury individuals with minimal or no hopelessness. There is no clear relationship between pre-morbid functioning and post-injury suicide risk. (209)

A study was performed on 1,683 participants who suffered a TBI, of which 14.1–15.5% had moderate to severe major depression and 7.9–9.5% had generalized anxiety disorder at 3–12 months after TBI. It was found that although there were strong concurrent associations between major depression and generalized anxiety disorder after TBI, few received psychological support during rehabilitation, and the authors recommend better monitoring of the psychiatric and psychological status of patients after TBI. Treatment programs including cognitive behavioral therapy or acceptance and commitment therapy may assist with coping. Risk factors that increased the likelihood of developing severe major depression and generalized anxiety disorder were being female, being admitted to an ICU, and having a more severe disability. (205)

In a study of soccer players aged 12–17 years, 47.8% experienced symptoms of concussion during an athletic year, but 4 out of 5 did not realize it. Symptoms lasted at least one day in roughly 24%. The use of football headgear decreased risk of a second concussion. In adolescent football as well as university and professional athletes, the majority of concussions go unrecognized. (43)

A study of 224 fighters including 131 mixed martial arts fighters and 93 boxers was performed, and it was observed on MRI scans that brain volumes were reduced and information processing speed was reduced compared to 22 controls. The greatest reduction in brain volumes were seen in the thalamus and caudate, and this lower volume was associated with lower processing speed. A higher fight exposure score, which combines duration and intensity of a fight career, predicted lower caudate and thalamus volumes and lower processing speed and may be considered for neurological checks or career decisions as to when to retire from the sport. (42)

In athletes suffering boxing concussions, cognitive impairment that was apparent on the day of injury and one to two days post-injury, recovered at three to seven days post-injury. (186)

A study of cognitive function in professional boxers suffering subconcussive sports-related head trauma suggested that a cumulative effect of repeated head trauma was consistent with the development of chronic TBI. (185)

Neuropsychological testing in sports injuries

In a study of 30 amateur athletes who suffered a concussion, computerized neuropsychological testing (verbal and visual memory, reaction time, processing speed, total symptoms) with ImPACT was performed pre-season and one to two days, roughly five days, and roughly 10 days after injury. At day 1 post-injury, 90% of athletes had 2 or more declines in performance, but this decreased to 37% at 10 days. Two athletes did not fully recover within three weeks after injury. (150)

Among athletes who suffered concussions, cognitive testing using the ImPACT computerized test battery was performed within one week of the injury and showed that the symptomatic group performed worse than the asymptomatic concussed group, who themselves performed worse than control subjects. Since the asymptomatic group still performed worse on cognitive testing than controls, there may be lingering impairment to the cognitive process. There may also be underreporting of symptoms by athletes. The authors believe that self-reported symptoms may not be adequate in assessing concussion and evaluating recovery and that neuropsychological testing should be used. (164)

When evaluating high school football players, there were 6 high school students who had suffered a concussion who were compared to their own baseline pre-injury and to 141 nonconcussed high school football players. Even though the concussed students were considered to have suffered mild grade 1 concussions, on their standardized sideline exam, they subsequently scored significantly below the nonconcussed controls as well as their own pre-injury baseline sideline exam score. The sideline examination contained four components: orientation, immediate memory, concentration, and delayed recall. (166)

Conflicting information regarding repeat SRCs and long-term outcome has been reported with a possible explanation given by the author. A study of male college athletes who had suffered self-reported sports-related distant history of concussion found minimal residual neurocognitive deficits. It was felt that the findings of the study suggest that a history of multiple self-reported concussions had little to no impact on long-term cognitive function. The authors mention the possibility of attrition, with those who suffered concussions in high school sports possibly not going on to college. This study did recognize conflicting findings in the literature and suggested future prospective studies. (193)

CHRONIC TRAUMATIC ENCEPHALOPATHY (CTE)

CTE is a progressive neurodegenerative disease that may occur as a result of repetitive injury to the brain. It has been seen in sports in American football players and boxers, but may also occur in participants of ice hockey, professional wrestling, soccer, rugby, and baseball. Patients may experience changes in behavior, irritability, short-term memory loss, mood changes, cognitive decline, dementia, and increased risk of suicide, which typically begin eight to ten years or even decades after the repetitive mild TBI. The disease is a progressive neurodegeneration in which there is deposition of hyperphosphorylated tau (p-tau) and TAR DNA-binding protein 43 (TDP-43). Neuropathological findings include generalized atrophy of the cerebral cortex, medial temporal lobe, and other regions of the brain, and can only be diagnosed post-mortem. Normally, tau is associated with microtubules in axons, and is not toxic, but it can become dissociated from the microtubules as a result of brain trauma. After a mild TBI, subconcussion, and blast injuries, there may be axonal injury, blood-brain barrier breach, injury to the microvasculature, and deposits of p-tau in the perivascular spaces, which may spread to adjacent cortex, and eventually the medial temporal lobe, diencephalon, and brainstem at times, although this mechanism is not clear. The neuropathological progression of CTE has been divided into four stages: (1) stage 1 with perivascular p-tau neurofibrillary tangles in focal epicenters in the deep sulci, associated clinically with headache and decreased concentration; (2) stage 2 with neurofibrillary tangles in superficial cortical layers, associated clinically with depression, mood swings, headache, short-term memory loss; (3) stage 3 with mild cerebral atrophy associated with cognitive impairment, executive dysfunction, depression; and (4) stage 4 with further cerebral atrophy associated clinically with profound short-term memory loss, executive dysfunction, and aggression. Additional neuropathological and clinical findings that have not been mentioned are associated with each of the stages of CTE. There appear to be factors of genetic resistance or susceptibility for developing CTE. Although diagnosis is made based on neuropathological examination of tissue post-mortem, imaging with positron emission tomography (PET), DTI, magnetic resonance spectroscopy and cerebrospinal fluid biomarkers may be useful. (296–299)

CTE has been diagnosed histologically in the brains of donors who had been exposed during life to repeated TBI, typically from soccer, ice hockey, football, boxing, and rugby. A seven-year study awarded by the National Institute of Neurological Disorders and Stroke in December 2015, entitled "Diagnostics, Imaging, and Genetics Network for the Objective Study and Evaluation of Chronic Traumatic Encephalopathy (DIAGNOSE CTE) Research Project" is looking to develop methods in which CTE may be diagnosed while a patient is alive, as opposed to studying their brain after death. In addition to neuropsychological examinations and self-reported measures of cognitive functioning, the testing of potential biomarkers included tau and amyloid PET, MRI and spectroscopy, and collection of blood, saliva, and cerebrospinal fluid. The study is ongoing. (11)

Repetitive TBI, regardless of concussion, may result in early CTE, a progressive tau protein neurodegenerative disease, without relation to the age of the patient (even in teenagers and young adults). These repetitive TBIs may cause increased risk for Alzheimer's disease and other tau protein neurodegenerative diseases. (190)

Zetterberg reported that TBI is frequently seen in contact sports including ice hockey, football, boxing, and horse riding. Although a mild TBI usually resolves within a few weeks, 10–15% of patients will develop a post-concussive syndrome and repetitive head impacts increase the risk of chronic neurological symptoms which may evolve to CTE. (17) In a study of 66 patients with a history of exposure to contact sports, neuropathological examination of the brains showed that 32% had tau pathology consistent with CTE. Of those, 11 played football, 2 boxed, 1 played baseball, 1 basketball, and 5 played multiple sports. One-third of cases had severe CTE pathology, and two-thirds had mild-to-moderate pathology. (300)

In a study of former American football players, the likelihood of finding evidence of CTE pathology at death increased by 30% for every year played, doubled every 2.6 years played, and rose by over 10-fold for every nine years played. Compared to players without CTE, those with CTE were 1/10th as likely to have played less than 4.5 years, and ten times as likely to have played more than 14.5 years. (301)

Among 202 deceased former football players, CTE was neuropathologically diagnosed in 87% of players, who played football a mean of 15 years. Of the 27 players who had mild CTE pathology, 96% had behavioral and, or mood symptoms, 85% had cognitive symptoms, and 33% had signs of dementia. Of 84 players who had severe CTE, 89% had behavioral and, or mood symptoms, 95% had cognitive symptoms, and 85% had signs of dementia. (693)

In rats, there was found to be a seven-day increased window of tissue vulnerability to a second mild TBI when compared to the first with greater volume of tissue damage and increased blood deposition. (434)

VISUAL CHANGES

For the visual system to function, the structure of the globe of the eye must be intact, the optic nerves must function, pupils must dilate and constrict as needed, the cerebral pathways responsible for visual perception must work properly, cranial nerves III, IV, and VI must act in a coordinated manner to move the extraocular muscles of the eye, the brainstem must function to keep both eyes moving in a coordinated manner (any deficit in this would cause diplopia), and the higher executive functioning areas of the brain, including the cortical (visual cortex allows for recognition of objects) and subcortical structures and cerebellum, all must work in perfect harmony with each other. Eye movement dysfunction may be caused by impaired neural connections in the brain which are beyond conscious control. After a TBI, clinical evaluation by a neuro-ophthalmologist may help with the diagnosis and treatment of visual disorders which may exist.

Anatomy of vision

VISUAL SYSTEM

Testing of vision is one of the most sensitive portions of the neurologic examination. Because the anatomy responsible for vision traverses a tremendous portion of the brain, lesions affecting it may produce specific deficits which help with localization of their cause. Vision starts with the reception of light into the eye through the lens and onto the retina, and subsequently the optic nerve exits the eye through an area of the retina known as the optic disc. The optic nerve and retina are outgrowths of the forebrain, and not peripheral nerves. The macula portion of the retina, which is located about two temporal disc diameters to the temporal side of the optic disc, is responsible for visual acuity, with the fovea centralis at its center containing the greatest visual acuity (the central part contains only cone receptors and not rod receptors). The optic nerve, which is more a tract of the brain, contains myelinated axons, and leaves the orbit through the optic canal to join the optic nerve from the other eye and join at the optic chiasm. At the chiasm, fibers from the nasal half of each retina decussate to join with the uncrossed fibers from the temporal side of the opposite retina. The optic tracts then leave the chiasm and travel dorsolaterally to terminate in the lateral geniculate body (LGB) of the thalamus, with other fibers (not terminating in the LGB) which are involved with the pupillary light reflex and eye movements, coursing to end in the superior colliculus and pretectal region of the brainstem. The LGB sends axons in the optic radiation (geniculocalcarine tract) through a portion of the internal capsule, then around the lateral ventricle (this portion of the radiation known as Meyer's loop), to terminate in the primary visual cortex of the occipital lobe (Brodmann area 17). The primary visual sends signals to the surrounding association visual cortex (Brodmann areas 18 and 19), where higher visual function such as processing and recognition of objects and perception of shapes, depth, color, etc., occurs. (694)

This complex anatomy which spans vast and to the critical regions of the brain can be tested and evaluated in many ways. The pupillary light reflex, which describes the constriction of a pupil in response to a bright light shown into the eye, involves that light stimulus causing signals to the pretectal area of the midbrain of the brainstem, with subsequent signals sent to the Edinger-Westphal nucleus of the oculomotor complex, from where parasympathetic preganglionic fibers run on the outside of the oculomotor nerve to stimulate postganglionic neurons in the ciliary ganglion, which cause the sphincter pupillae muscle in the iris to constrict. A direct light reflex represents a response of the eye in which the light was shown, while a consensual light reflex is a response in the other eye. Incidentally, when the brain "herniates," the ipsilateral pupil may dilate because of the temporal lobe pressing on the oculomotor nerve (the fibers for pupillary constriction run on the outside of the nerve, while the motor portion of the nerve is on the inside). The accommodation reflex (pupillary constriction and lens thickening in adapting to near vision) involves visual pathways in the visual association cortex, superior brachium, pretectal area, and superior colliculus. Visual field testing (crudely through bedside testing or formally through a test such as the Goldmann perimeter) is important because a defect may be localized to the optic nerve, optic chiasm, retrochiasmal region, optic radiation or visual cortex. (694)

OCULOMOTOR SYSTEM

The oculomotor system of the eye is also critical as understanding its anatomy and testing helps to localize deficits. Four types of eye movements include saccades, smooth pursuit, vestibulo-optokinetic, and vergence movements. (695)

Saccades are rapid movements of the eye, and allow an object of interest to be placed within the fovea of the eye, and they may be volitional or involuntary (quick phases of vestibular and optokinetic nystagmus). The latency from a stimulus to the onset of eye movement is about 200 msec, with a velocity of approximately 400 degrees per second. The signals for volitional saccades start in the frontal eye fields (Brodmann area 8) which send impulses to the superior colliculi, enabling eye movement in the contralateral direction. (695)

Smooth pursuit is the maintenance of an object near the fovea, and the latency from stimulus to movement is about 125 msec. The neural pathways involved include an image on the retina, with relay of signals to the visual cortex of the occipital lobes, then to the ipsilateral middle temporal visual area, the frontal eye fields, and the pontine nuclei. Following this, there is modification of impulses by the cerebellum and vestibular nuclei, final projection to the ocular motor nuclei to send signals to the muscles of both eyes. This can be evaluated by asking a patient to track objects. (695)

Vestibular-optokinetic eye movements allow the eye to maintain position despite changes in head and body position. The vestibulo-ocular reflex produces compensatory eye movements during high-frequency rotational head movements. Neural inputs come from a combination of the vestibular apparatus in the temporal bone, the visual system, and somatosensors, which are relayed together in the vestibular nuclei to produce a "best estimate" of the head's movement. The latency of signal to eye movement is about 10 msec. Evaluation of this system involves caloric testing in which cold water is irrigated into the external ear, with a normal response being the eyes turning toward the ipsilateral ear, with the quick phase of nystagmus toward the opposite ear. (695)

Vergence eye movements allow both fovea to maintain fixation on an object so that there is perception of one object. Failure of this may result in an individual perceiving an object exists on two separate locations simultaneously (diplopia), or that the two objects are in the same location, causing visual confusion. The latency of movements is about 160 msec, and when there is failure of the two fovea to fixate correctly, it normally occurs for such a short period of time that it does not cause diplopia or confusion. As there are three cranial nerves (cranial nerves III, IV, and VI) that are involved in eye movements, creating in a broad sense horizontal and vertical eye movements, the brain and brainstem must maintain exquisite coordination for both eyes to have a "yoked" movement together in order to maintain binocular gaze. Horizontal eye movement signals originate in the contralateral frontal lobe for saccades, or the ipsilateral occipital lobe for smooth pursuit. Signals course through the internal capsule to the paramedian pontine reticular formation in the pons of the brainstem, then to the ipsilateral sixth nerve nucleus (to send signals to the ipsilateral cranial nerve VI [abducens nerve] causing the lateral rectus muscle to move the eye laterally [abduct]), and also other fibers cross the midline to the contralateral medial longitudinal fasciculus to reach the contralateral oculomotor (cranial nerve III) nucleus, resulting in the medial rectus of the contralateral eye moving that eye medially. This interaction in the brainstem creates "yoked" movements of both eyes. Lesions may produce horizontal eye movement disorders such as internuclear ophthalmoplegia (INO), gaze palsy, and one and a half syndrome. Vertical eye movements involve the pretectal area (vertical gaze center) and brainstem nuclei for cranial nerves III and VI. Disorders of vertical gaze include Parinaud's syndrome and Steele-Richardson-Olszewski's syndrome. (695)

Nystagmus is a biphasic movement with a fast and slow component, with the fast movement defining the direction of the nystagmus. There are many types of nystagmus which may occur, including optokinetic, vestibular, drug-induced, physiologic end-point, gaze-evoked, gaze-paretic, rebound, downbeat, upbeat, periodic alternating, seesaw, spasmus, and convergence retraction. Eye movement disorders may include ocular bobbing, ocular flutter and opsoclonus, ocular dysmetria, square wave jerks, and ocular myoclonus. (695)

Sympathetic innervation of the pupil, responsible for pupillodillator muscles dilating the pupil, starts in the posterior hypothalamus, with projections through the lateral tegmentum of the brainstem to reach the intermediolateral gray matter of the spinal cord (C8 to T2 segments). Fibers then travel through the sympathetic chain to the superior cervical ganglion, and subsequently join the internal carotid artery to enter the cavernous sinus and join the ophthalmic branch of the trigeminal nerve to enter the orbit, ultimately reaching the pupillodilator muscles via the long ciliary nerve. (695)

Parasympathetic innervation of the pupil constricts the pupil. Signals begin in the Edinger-Westphal nucleus of the oculomotor complex in the brainstem, travel with the oculomotor nerve through the subarachnoid space, cavernous sinus, and superior orbital fissure to enter the orbit. Conditions of the pupil include Marcus-Gunn pupil, pharmacologic mydriasis, traumatic mydriasis, Adie's tonic pupil, Hutchinson's pupil, Argyll Robertson pupil, and pinpoint pupils. (695)

Vision and traumatic brain injury

Evaluation of TBI patients for visual changes appears to be reliable in the treatment of concussion. This visual evaluation provides objective measures and is helpful in situations where patients may underreport symptoms or in a pediatric population where patients may not be able to fully report symptoms. (280)

TBI can impact the visual system in a number of ways, including creating defects in the eye structure itself (ocular injury), visual fields (hemianopsia, quadrantanopia, central scotoma) and acuity, pupillary function, accommodation, eye movement including vergence, saccadic and smooth pursuit movements, vestibulo-ocular reflex, visual perception, color vision, visual-spatial functioning, stereopsis, motion vision (akinetopsia), and may cause photophobia, diplopia, blurred vision, nystagmus, loss of vision, and optic nerve abnormalities. Abnormalities of eye movement may be an early sign of TBI. (194, 195)

Direct traumatic causes of visual loss may include ocular injury (trauma to the globe, corneal abrasion, intraocular foreign body, traumatic optic neuropathy, orbital fracture) as well as carotid cavernous fistulas and damage to intracranial visual pathways. Patients who have suffered a TBI may be unaware of or unable to complain of visual loss, and since visual dysfunction may interfere with rehabilitation, formal evaluation of vision should be obtained for TBI patients in rehabilitation. (196)

A proper neuro-ophthalmic exam is important to assess visual dysfunction, as tests of the visual system and eye movements may involve intricate higher cortical pathways. The frontal lobes, which are commonly affected by concussion, play a strong role in eye movement. (197)

A study evaluated patients who sustained a mild TBI and had suffered PCS, and compared them to 36 controls who suffered mild TBI but had a good recovery. The PCS group performed worse on many of the visual tests (including tests of saccades, pursuit, spatial memory and others) and also performed worse on neuropsychological tests. This worsened eye movement function suggested cerebral impairment in motor/visuospatial areas of the brain and subcortical function. The authors felt that oculomotor function testing may be of value in the evaluation of PCS cases. The PCS group had worse performance on several eye-movement functions that are beyond conscious control, indicative of subcortical injury. (198)

A study of 21 mild TBI patients was compared to 26 controls, with evaluation of smooth pursuit eye movements. The findings of increased deficits in pursuit, target prediction, and eye position error in the TBI group were not due to oculomotor impairment or reduced IQ, but were related to deficits in predictive smooth pursuit eye movements and are consistent with possible damage to cerebello-frontal and cortico-cortical connections, indicating that smooth pursuit eye movement impairment may be a sensitive test of executive function and cognitive function deficits. Importantly, oculomotor assessment may be a potential biomarker for detecting changes in patients with PCS. (199, 200)

In a mouse study, it was concluded that TBI-induced traumatic axonal injury (TAI) within the optic nerve provides insight into the pathobiology of TAI, including axonal swelling, disconnection, and proximal and distal dieback changes. (201)

SLEEP DISTURBANCES

One of the most common complaints patients have after suffering a TBI is sleep disturbance, which affects 50% of patients. Of those who have suffered a TBI, 25–29% will have a diagnosed sleep disorder such as insomnia, hypersomnia, apnea and sleep-related movement disorders. Left unrecognized and untreated, sleep problems may interfere with rehabilitation, recovery, and outcomes. (210)

In a study of 98,709 veterans with TBI who were matched with 98,709 veteran controls without having suffered a TBI, a five-year follow-up revealed that 19.6% of the 197,418 veterans developed sleep disorders. At about five years after having suffered a TBI, 23.4% of those with a TBI developed sleep disorders, whereas only 15.8% of those without TBI did. Those who suffered a TBI were 50% more likely to develop a sleep disorder than the non-TBI group after adjusting for age, sex, race, education, and income. Other disorders were more likely to be seen in those who have suffered TBI versus those who did not: psychiatric conditions including mood disorders (22.4% of those who had suffered TBI versus 9.3% of those with no TBI); anxiety (10.5% with TBI patients versus 4.4% in the non-TBI group); PTSD (19.5% versus 4.4%); substance abuse (11.4% versus 5.2%); and smoking or tobacco use (13.5% versus 8.7%). There was a stronger association with sleep disorders among those who suffered a mild TBI than with those who suffered a severe TBI. It was felt that the difference in mechanisms between the two types of injuries may account for the difference in associations with sleep disorders, with mild TBI being associated more with DAI and severe TBI associated more with focal but severe damage. TBI also posed an increased risk of developing a sleep disorder in the future. While the pathophysiology by which TBI may cause sleep disorders is poorly understood, possibilities proposed by DelRosso, Crompton, and Parvizi include "structural brain injuries, including damage to the suprachiasmatic nucleus, optic chasm, hypothalamus, amygdala, and brainstem." (211)

After suffering a TBI, 46% of patients may suffer sleep disorders and 25% may have increased daytime sleepiness. In a study of 40 patients, Castriotta indicated that their finding of no relationship between the presence of sleep disorders and TBI severity or the presence of brain CT scan lesions, confirms literature findings. They felt that sleepy patients had slower reaction times and that their cognitive impairment may be worsened by their sleep disorder. They concluded that "the high prevalence of excessive daytime sleepiness, obstructive sleep apnea, post-traumatic hypersomnia, and narcolepsy after traumatic brain injury leaves us with the conclusion that these subjects should undergo complete sleep evaluations, including NPSG (polysomnography) and MSLT (multiple sleep latency test)." (212)

Half of patients who have suffered a TBI experience sleep disturbance. (210) Dreaming is causally affected by sensations in the body, which serve as a bottom-up source of dreaming and which are related to isomorphisms between the physiology of the sleeping body and phenomenology of the dream. Memories and emotion are top-down processes that shape dream content. Various techniques of dream engineering have been developed in which body stimulation (including haptic, auditory, and olfactory stimulation) has been used to modulate the sleeping body along with concurrent tracking of changes in dream content. Dr. Carr stated, "the dream is understood as in circuit with the body. We then identify past protocols for influencing dream content, many of which have taken advantage of dreaming in circuitry with the body, i.e. linking thirst to dreams of water." (408) As patients who have suffered TBI may experience significant cognitive, neurological, and somatic changes, this technology may potentially have an important role for treatment of these patients in the future.

HEADACHE/PAIN MANAGEMENT

Post-traumatic headaches are very disabling. They often resemble primary headache disorders and, after diagnosis, treatment for a particular headache disorder is implemented. They may be treated with abortive agents as well as prophylactic agents. Post-traumatic headaches often resolve within a few months, but can persist for years.

Post-traumatic headaches are commonly seen after a TBI (secondary headaches) and while acute post-traumatic headaches resolve in three months, they can last longer and become persistent post-traumatic headaches (PPTHs). Symptoms may resemble primary headaches such as tension headaches or migraines. As Labastida-Ramirez in a review article cited Ashina, patients with post-traumatic headaches may experience nausea, vomiting, exacerbation of headache by certain stimuli (light, sound, physical activity and stress), and impaired psychosocial and cognitive function. Also citing Finkel, Baandrup, Kjeldgaard, and Clark, other types of headaches exist, such as cluster-like headache, cervicogenic headache, occipital neuralgia, medication overuse headaches, and others. Labastida-Ramirez cited Larsen in stating that "currently, there is no available data from randomized controlled trials evaluating the therapeutic efficacy of medical interventions specific to persistent PTH (post-traumatic headache), therefore, the therapy mirrors conventional treatment approaches for non-traumatic primary headache disorders." Pharmacological treatment may be aimed at the type of headache that symptoms resemble, whether tension-type headache or migraine headache. Peripheral nerve blocks of the greater and lesser occipital nerves, supraorbital and supratrochlear nerves, and the sphenopalatine ganglion have been performed at times for treatment. Trigger-point injections may also be performed in the occipitalis, frontalis, masseter, temporalis, trapezius, sternocleidomastoid, and other muscles. Physical therapy and massage of the upper cervical spine has been used with success. rTMS has also been used to treat mild TBI-related headache, with further study needed. Surgical decompression of the supraorbital, supratrochlear, and infratrochlear nerves for frontal headaches, transection of the anterior branch of the auriculotemporal nerve or zygomaticotemporal nerve for headaches in the temple region, or occipital nerve decompression or excision (including the greater, lesser or third occipital nerves) have also been performed. Behavior management to address the triggers of headache are also employed. Headaches and cognitive difficulties may be worsened by sleep disorders. (213)

In a study of 212 subjects who were enrolled within one week of suffering a mild TBI, 54% reported having a new or worsened headache as opposed to 18% who had a headache pre-injury. The number increased to 62% at three months, and 69% at six months, but dropped to 58% at one year. Symptoms of migraine were experienced by up to 49%, and tension-type headaches in up to 40% of those experiencing headaches. The most common headache phenotype was migraine or probable migraine. (220)

Of 109 military or veteran patients who suffered moderate and severe TBI, 60% had suffered from headache during the first year after regaining consciousness. During the acute post-traumatic headache period of hospitalization, 38% had acute post-traumatic headaches of any frequency and 28% had headache daily, mostly in a frontal location. The headaches symptoms improved and leveled off by six months, and about 20% had PPTHs. The headaches were not related to the severity of the injury sustained. (221)

Despite the common occurrence of post-traumatic headaches, a literature review showed that evidence-based guidelines for acute or preventive pharmacological treatment are lacking. Commonly used medications for acute post-traumatic headaches include ketorolac, nonsteroidal anti-inflammatory drugs, acetaminophen, and combination medications which may contain caffeine (Cafergot, and Excedrin). (227) Medications used for treatment of migraine headaches include (1) for acute headache, non-steroidal anti-inflammatory drugs, triptans (selective serotonin receptor agonists including sumatriptan, rizatripan, frovatripan, almotripan, zolmitripan, naratripan, and eletripan) (664); (2) for preventive treatment: beta-blockers, anti-epileptics (topiramate) (666), tricyclic antidepressants (amitriptyline) (665) (667), and growing evidence for calcitonin gene-related peptide antibodies (CGRP abs) (erenumab, fremanezumab, eptinezumab, galcanezumab). (668, 213) CGRP receptor antagonists (gepants) such as rimegepant and ubrogepant are also used. (719) Medications used for treatment of tension-type of headache include: (1) for acute headache: non-steroidal anti-inflammatory drugs; (2) for preventative treatment: tricyclic antidepressants. (213, 665, 667)

Excessive use of analgesics in the treatment of post-traumatic headaches may contribute to headaches, and patients should undergo analgesic detoxification. In a group of 104 adolescent concussion patients, 77 had chronic post-traumatic headache, of which 54 met criteria for probable medication overuse headache. Of the 54 patients, 37 patients (68.6%) had improvement or resolution of headaches after discontinuing analgesics. Of the 54 patients with probable medication overuse headache, none had a history of medication overuse prior to concussion and only simple analgesics (such as ibuprofen, acetaminophen, naproxen, etc.) were used. (215)

In a study of 64 active-duty service members who experienced post-traumatic headache of the migraine type, it was concluded that patients with headaches related to concussions may benefit from treatment with onabotulinum toxin A injections. For a population of patients which may have risk of complications from standard treatment (side effects from medications) including cognitive, metabolic, and behavioral side effects, these injections may offer a well-tolerated preventive treatment for PPTH. (216)

In the early 1990s, surgically implanted epidural motor cortex stimulation was found to help neuropathic pain. Subsequently, noninvasive rTMS targeting the primary motor cortex was found to have similar results. Transcranial direct current stimulation (tDCS) has also had some benefit, again targeting the same region in the motor cortex. (494)

RTMS is widely available for the treatment of depression. (495) A literature review, possibly the first to assess rTMS for the treatment of post-concussive symptoms including depression and headache, revealed that this treatment shows promising preliminary results. (218) A study of 29 veterans who were suffering persistent mild TBI headache and were treated with rTMS aimed at the left dorsolateral prefrontal cortex found that this treatment may improve headache symptoms and yield a temporary mood enhancement, but further studies are needed. (217)

Peripheral nerve surgery has been used to address headaches. When headaches are occipitally centered, decompression, or excision of the greater, lesser, and dorsal occipital nerves may be considered for occipital neuralgia related post-concussion headaches. For headaches centered over the temporal regions, endoscopic-assisted surgical transection of the auriculotemporal nerve and the zygomaticotemporal may be used. For headaches located in the frontal region, decompression of the supraorbital, supratrochlear, and infratrochlear nerves can be considered. Nerve excision for frontal headaches for a failed decompression is also a possibility, but the patient will have subsequent forehead numbness and frontal scalp paresthesia. Of 28 patients with post-concussion headaches who underwent occipital nerve surgery, 88% had a successful outcome, with at least a 50% reduction in their headache and 50% were pain free at the time of final follow up. The authors felt that appropriate patient selection, diagnostic nerve blocks, and timely referral to a peripheral nerve surgeon may offer an effective and safe treatment plan for these headaches. (219)

Imaging studies and post-traumatic headache

An imaging study that broke down the post-traumatic headache group and specifically evaluated 58 patients with mild TBI and post-traumatic migraines (PTM), also studied 17 patients with mild TBI but without PTMs and used voxel-based analysis of DTI to compare the two groups. In the mild TBI with PTM group, there was injury to the corpus callosum and fornix/septohippocampal circuit that was not seen in the controls. The authors point out that while other studies of Obermann and Sarmento had looked at gray matter and found neuronal injury and loss in the frontal and parietal regions (based on spectroscopy or volumetric analysis of gray matter), this DTI study evaluated the white matter. They also cited Lee in pointing out "DTI abnormalities in the corpus callosum are commonly seen in non-traumatic migraine" and they cited Bartsch and Moskowitz in stating that "the role of the fornix/septohippocampal circuit in migraines is less clear, but it has been implicated in cortical spreading depression, a propagating, temporary loss of membrane potential in neurons thought to play a part in the pathophysiology of migraines." (228)

In an imaging study that compared 70 patients with a mild TBI to 46 controls, it was found that patients with mild TBI and acute post-traumatic headache showed significant differences in periaqueductal gray functional connectivity. The authors felt that this may reflect the diminished top-down attention regulation of pain perception. The study concluded that this may have value as an early imaging biomarker at three months for those at risk of post-traumatic headache. (222)

Another imaging study of 32 patients with post-traumatic headache, when evaluated with magnetic resonance-based voxel-based morphometry, showed decreases in gray matter in the anterior cingulate and dorsolateral prefrontal cortex after three months, which resolved in one year as the headaches ceased. The structural changes were not present in the acute phase, developed during three months in patients with persistent headaches, and completely reversed in one year, parallel to the cessation of headache and, as the authors state, "confirming their relationship to chronic pain." (223)

In an imaging study comparing 33 patients suffering from PPTH over three months from date of injury with 33 healthy controls, those with PPTH had reduced cerebral cortical thickness in the bilateral frontal regions and right hemisphere parietal regions. In addition, it was found that patients who experienced more frequent headaches had less bilateral superior frontal thickness. (224)

Patients with migraine headaches, PPTH, and controls underwent imaging and differences were found in resting state functional MRI with regard to static functional connectivity and dynamic functional connectivity of pain-processing and visual-processing regions. It was suggested that static and dynamic functional connectivity analysis may be useful for differentiating PPTH from migraine. (225)

A study of 35 patients with chronic post-traumatic headache, 92 patients with migraine headaches, and 49 controls with no headaches was evaluated with regional cerebral blood flow studies using the xenon 133 inhalation technique. The study concluded that since, in comparison to the migraine headache and control groups, there was reduced regional blood flow and regional and hemispheric asymmetries in patients with post-traumatic headaches, there may be an organic basis to chronic post-traumatic headaches. If these findings are confirmed in other studies, the authors indicated that regional blood flow studies may be used as an objective test of organic pathology in minor closed head injury. (226)

EXERCISE

Effect on post-concussion symptoms

Exercise has been found to possibly aggravate post-concussion symptoms. In a study at a university sports medicine clinic, patients who were on average 226 days post-injury but experiencing post-concussion symptoms as a result of sports- or nonsports-related injuries, including falls and motor vehicle collisions, were compared to controls and were found to have limited ability to exercise when compared to controls. They found an increase in severity of post-concussion symptoms as well as the appearance of new symptoms in each of the PCS patients when they exercised and exercise was subsequently stopped. The fact that each of the PCS patients experienced symptoms with exercise led the authors to suggest that the treadmill test may be used to distinguish PCS from other diagnoses, as a lack of symptom exacerbation in a subject may indicate that causes other than PCS may be responsible for prolonged PCS types of symptoms such as headache, dizziness, and stress. (229)

Another way of approaching this is demonstrated in a literature review. It was found that while in the past, the treatment of SRC and PPCS was physical and cognitive rest until symptoms resolved, the current thought may suggest that aerobic exercise may be safe and effective for the treatment of these conditions as long as symptoms are not exacerbated. Further studies will be needed for conclusive guidelines. Exercise intolerance earlier on in the exercise session may be related to autonomic/physiologic dysfunction with respect to cerebral blood flow in SRC and PPCS, but when the intolerance occurs later in the exercise, and is associated with elevated heart rate, the symptoms may be related to vestibulo-ocular or cervical post-traumatic disorders. (230)

Return to play decisions

In the sideline assessment of SRC, evaluation should first begin with assessment for injury to the cervical spine, intracranial bleeding, and other injuries. Assessment of symptoms, a neurological and brief cognitive exam, and balance testing should be performed. It is best to "err on the side of caution when making a return to play decision." (232) Mild TBIs typically have self-limiting cognitive and neurobehavioral sequelae. Athletes usually return to pre-injury functioning within 2–14 days. (143)

The American Medical Society for Sports Medicine in 2013 made recommendations in a position statement regarding concussions in sports. Any athlete who has suffered a concussion should be evaluated by a healthcare provider. Initially, cognitive evaluation, neurological examination, and balance testing should be implemented. Computerized neuropsychological testing can be given as well as paper-and-pencil neuropsychological tests. These tests should not be used in isolation, but rather as part of a larger comprehensive management program. Premature return to play may be associated with decreased reaction time, leading to increased risk of repeat injury and concussion. (169)

POST-TRAUMATIC SEIZURES/ EPILEPSY

Post-traumatic epilepsy is a long-term complication of TBI that, if it develops, usually does so within five years of an injury, but may have a latent period of up to 20 years. As will be discussed next, there are differing opinions as to the importance of EEG in predicting post-traumatic epilepsy. (233)

In a study in mice, it was found that repetitive TBI may cause seizures and this may be related to an atypical response of astrocytes. The injury to the brain was diffuse, as there were no obvious lesions of hemorrhage, pronounced neuroinflammation, or neuronal death. (29)

Post-traumatic seizures have been defined in a variety of ways in the literature. A common method of defining them is as follows: immediate seizures occur less than 24 hours after a TBI; early seizures less than one week after a TBI; and late seizures more than one week after injury. Post-traumatic epilepsy refers to late seizures, which occur more than a week after the injury. Seizures which develop within seven days after a TBI are labeled as provoked seizures, whereas those that occur more than one week post-injury are unprovoked. Patients who develop one unprovoked seizure have a higher risk of another. In patients with a mild TBI, the occurrence of an early seizure did not pose an increased risk for post-traumatic epilepsy. Civilians who experience a severe TBI have up to a 30-fold increased incidence of epilepsy, compared to the general population. These risks are further increased in a soldier population that is exposed to missile and blast injuries. Epilepsy may develop months or years after an injury. Post-traumatic epilepsy accounts for roughly 10–20% of symptomatic epilepsy in the general population. (234, 235)

Researchers studied 2,747 patients with head injury, and the one- and five-year risk of post-traumatic seizures was 7.1% and 11.5% for severe injuries, 0.7% and 1.6% for moderate injuries, and 0.1% and 0.6% for mild injuries (similar to the risk of the general population). (187)

A study was conducted to evaluate seizures in 4,541 patients who suffered a TBI in Olmsted County, MN, from 1935 to 1984. The standardized incidence ratio for all patients was 3.1 (3.1 times what was expected) in the first year post-injury, but decreased to 2.1 for the subsequent four years, with little change thereafter. During the initial five years post-injury, the standardized incidence ratio was slightly higher for patients with a mild injury and LOC versus those with mild injury and PTA but no LOC (2.5 versus 2.1). The study found a strong correlation between the risk of unprovoked seizures and the severity of the TBI; with severe injuries, the increased risk can be present for more than ten years post-injury. Brain contusion and subdural hematoma were the strongest risk factors for late seizures for at least 20 years post-injury. (236)

In a study of patients discharged from hospitals in South Carolina following TBI injuries, the following incidence of post-traumatic epilepsy was found within three years after hospital discharge: 4.4 patients per 100 patients suffering a mild TBI, 7.6 out of 100 for those suffering a moderate TBI, and 13.6 out of 100 for those suffering a severe TBI. The authors point out that this study considered only patients who were hospitalized and that 87.5% of patients with a mild TBI were not admitted to the hospital, suggesting that a "mild TBI" in this study was more severe than in patients not admitted to the hospital. Risk factors for post-traumatic epilepsy included post-traumatic symptoms on hospital discharge, and another association was depression. (94)

A diagnosis of post-traumatic epilepsy is made after a patient experiences two or more seizures one week or more after a TBI. Post-traumatic epilepsy can occur in 10–20% of children following a severe TBI. In a study of 321 children with TBI, 47 children were diagnosed with post-traumatic epilepsy of which 8 children suffered a mild TBI and 39 a severe TBI. An abnormal EEG was present in 79% of those suffering a severe TBI, while those suffering a mild TBI were more likely to have normal EEGs. The authors found that children who suffer post-traumatic epilepsy due to mild TBI are more likely to have a normal head CT and EEG (acute or chronic) and to be on 0–1 anti-epileptic drugs. These children are likely at a higher risk for epilepsy when compared to the general population. (96)

A study of 421 veterans who suffered penetrating brain wounds revealed that 53% had post-traumatic epilepsy. Fifteen years after the injury, 50% of those veterans still had seizures. Compared to the general population, the risk of seizures in the first year was 580-fold higher and still 25-fold higher after ten years. (207)

While early provoked seizures may be controlled with anti-epileptic drug prophylaxis, they are not effective in preventing late unprovoked seizures (post-traumatic epilepsy). Use of antiepileptic drugs may be used in the early period (up to one week after injury) after a TBI and to treat post-traumatic epilepsy. There has not been guidance to use antiepileptic drugs on a long-term basis for the prevention of unprovoked seizures, and these medications may also induce side effects such as cognitive impairment or neurobehavioral difficulties. (233)

There are differing thoughts in the literature as to the usefulness of EEG testing in patients who have not experienced seizures. Chen stated that for the early detection of seizures, patients should ideally receive EEG screening within the first two years after a TBI as this may detect interictal epileptiform discharges before clinical seizures develop. In contrast, literature in the past from Jennett found that after reviewing EEGs from 722 patients with injuries associated with a high risk of late traumatic epilepsy, EEG does not contribute to the prediction of epilepsy after trauma. (233, 237)

In a review, Nuwer felt that in the evaluation of mild TBI, there were felt to be no EEG or quantitative EEG (QEEG) features that were uniquely seen in mild TBI and there is poor correlation with clinical symptoms late after a mild TBI. In the initial months after a mild TBI, EEG abnormalities are more common than clinical symptoms, and while many patients with an abnormal exam have an abnormal EEG, many EEG abnormalities are subclinical. In the later time period after an injury, correlation is poor between EEG and clinical signs and symptoms, imaging, and psychometric tests. EEG does not predict, confirm, or otherwise measure post-concussion symptoms. A normal EEG cannot exclude an acute significant brain injury and a mild EEG abnormality cannot substantiate an objective clinical brain injury. (171)

In a literature review related to TBI and EEG use, it was found that "conventional EEG is important for the evaluation of post-traumatic epilepsy but is not useful as a routine screening measure among individuals with mTBI or post-concussive symptoms." Quantitative EEG may have a role in evaluating post-concussive symptoms and mild TBI. (172)

QEEG refers to the mathematical processing of a digitally recorded EEG. After suffering a mild TBI, although EEG changes may be subtle and difficult to distinguish from EEG changes resulting from other conditions, QEEG may improve the ability to detect electrophysiologic changes. (238) A QEEG-based brain function index (BFI) has been used to evaluate patients with TBI and was shown to scale with severity of impairment in mild TBI patients with the ability for rapid diagnosis. This technology may be a potential future quantitative biomarker for progression or resolution of mild TBI findings. (433)

Patients who experience partial seizures, such as a complex partial seizure, might only exhibit behavioral changes that may be mistaken for mood alterations, catatonia, or apathy. These non-convulsive seizures may be best captured on EEG with video. In treating post-traumatic epilepsy, anti-epileptic drugs should be initiated. In patients whose seizure control is refractory to medications, a neurosurgical procedure may be considered to remove the seizure focus. In those patients for which surgical resection is not feasible, or who have no identifiable epileptic focus or multiple foci or have a focus which is not amenable to surgery, a vagus nerve stimulator may be considered. To prevent abnormal electrical activity in one hemisphere of the brain from generalizing to the other, a neurosurgical procedure of corpus callosotomy may be performed. (233)

In a study of 12 athletes who suffered mild TBI and 12 normal controls, EEG testing performed within five months post-injury revealed a decrease in power in all bandwidths, which was enhanced with standing postures in the mild TBI group as compared to the controls. The authors acknowledge that these findings differ from "currently accepted conventional wisdom" that mild TBI is a transient injury which fully resolves over a matter of days. (173)

BALANCE DIFFICULTIES

Dizziness, vertigo, imbalance, gait disorders, disequilibrium, nausea, and double or blurry vision may be often seen after a patient has suffered a TBI. (677) The etiology of this condition may be peripheral (involving the inner ear including the vestibular labyrinth/semicircular canals within the temporal bone, or the vestibular nerve passing from the temporal bone to the brainstem) or central (involving the central nervous system of the brain and brainstem, including deep nuclei, cortical regions, and interconnecting white matter connections). Initially after a patient suffers a TBI, balance disturbances and dizziness may be unrecognized, as there may appear to be more pressing issues. Clinical evaluation by a neurotologist may help with diagnosis and treatment.

Anatomy of balance

To gain an appreciation as to why the regulation of balance is very sensitive to disruption after a TBI, it is helpful to review the anatomical basis of how intricately balance is regulated. As an overview about the complexity of balance, the canals in the temporal bone sense motion and send signals to the brainstem, which coordinate signals with the spinal cord, the nuclei controlling eye movements, and the cerebellum. The vestibular system has a peripheral and a central component. The peripheral system detects movements and position in space, and has fluid filled spaces. The structure of the vestibular portion includes the utricle and saccule, and the semicircular canals, which detect linear acceleration and position. The peripheral vestibular apparatus sends signals through the vestibular nerves to the brainstem, where a portion of the fibers terminate on the vestibular nuclei, and another portion continue through the inferior cerebellar peduncle to terminate in the cerebellum. Neurons from the vestibular nucleus send descending fibers to the spinal cord (via the vestibulospinal tract), send other fibers up to the oculomotor nuclei (either directly or through the medial longitudinal fasciculus), and send additional fibers to the cerebellum through the inferior cerebellar peduncle. With movement of the head, the semicircular canals create impulses which are sent to the vestibular nuclei, and they subsequently terminate in the nerves to the muscles of the eye (cranial nerves III, IV, and VI). This allows for compensatory eye movements when the head moves, and is known as the vestibulo-occular reflex. (672)

When this system is injured, an individual may experience benign paroxysmal positional vertigo (BPPV), vestibulo-ocular reflex dysfunction, visual motion sensitivity, and balance impairment. (677)

Balance literature

Balance can be evaluated during a physical examination, as well as with formal clinical testing. Assessments may include motor control tests, dynamic visual acuity, audiometry, functional gain assessment, and tests performed during physician examination of the patient. Additional testing may include videonystagmography (VNG), posturography, and electronystagmography (ENG). VNG and ENG are eye movement recording methods, but VNG may be more sensitive than ENG for subtle clinical findings. (670, 671)

After suffering a TBI, Taylor cites Marcus, Davies, Rust, and Arshad noting that up to 57% of patients will suffer from BPPV, which is a transient peripheral dysfunction cause of imbalance, and it can be treated with a maneuver to reposition particles. Marcus and Knoll are cited in recognizing that permanent loss of vestibular function may be related to a fracture or other injury to the inner ear. Vestibular testing may help to assess whether imbalance is due to peripheral or central causes. Taylor cites MacDougall in noting peripheral vestibular function can be evaluated using clinical tests including vestibular-evoked myogenic potentials with oculographic recordings during impulsive head turns (video head impulse testing: vHIT). Testing of balance assesses different sensory organs through the evaluation of caloric testing (placing warm and cool liquids within the external ear canals), oculomotor function testing (turning the patients head), and posturography. When testing caloric and oculomotor function, VNG is used to assess eye movements. Postural stability is evaluated with a sensory organization test. Computerized dynamic posturography is performed, in which there is manipulation of the support surface with eyes open and closed. These methods were used by Taylor to evaluate 99 patients for vestibular dysfunction for a median time of 12 months after having suffered a TBI. After testing, it was found that 33% of the patients had abnormalities in one or more components of the vestibular labyrinth and/or vestibular nerve divisions. (669)

Treatment of imbalance

Vestibular rehabilitation (VR) is utilized to help patients suffering from imbalance in the acute or chronic phase after a TBI. VR is intended to help stabilize gaze, enhance postural stability, and improve vertigo. In a review of randomized controlled trials from 2015 to 2022, which included 33 articles, it was found that the VR group achieved a higher score on the Quality of Life After Brain Injury (QOLIBRI) evaluation, but there were controversial results shown regarding balance and subjective symptoms questionnaire. The study concluded "VR seems useful to reduce symptoms in patients with concussion; however a huge heterogeneity of the studies and of the outcomes used were found." (674) In another literature review looking at the effect of physical therapy on imbalance, there were not felt to be any differences between groups who underwent experimental interventions, virtual reality, VR, control group interventions, and other traditional physical therapy methods. (678) Another study of the effects of VR on imbalance showed that although the treatment sped up recovery for TBI patients with dizziness and balance difficulties, the benefits were lost two months after treatment. (679)

In a group of 207 adults who had suffered a mild-to-moderate TBI and were seen at an outpatient clinic, 66.7% complained of post-traumatic dizziness, which was found to be an independent factor in patients' inability to return to work. Although causes may be related to vestibular, neuronal, or psychiatric pathology, the authors felt that if detected and treated early, patients may resume employment sooner. (242) Persistent vestibular-ocular symptoms may also influence cognitive performance and clinical recovery following SRC. (675) Patients with moderate to severe dizziness report increased post-concussion symptom burden, anxiety, depression, and affected cadence of gain when compared to those with no or mild dizziness. (676)

A canalith repositioning maneuver may have up to an 80% cure rate at 24 hours for peripherally caused BPPV, versus only 10% in controls. A study of 26 nontrauma patients who presented to an emergency department with benign positional vertigo revealed that both the canalith repositioning maneuver and the standard medication treatment regimen had similar and good success and satisfaction by the patients. Canalith repositioning may be considered. It is to be noted that these patients did not suffer a TBI and that before implementing this maneuver in a TBI patient, one must first take precautions to see that no harm will be caused to a potentially injured neck or brain. (240, 241)

Imaging of imbalance

In a study of 30 patients who suffered imbalance or dizziness after an acute TBI and 36 controls, stratification was performed for a comparison of controls versus acute TBI balance impaired versus TBI balance intact patients. These individuals were evaluated with voxel-wise whole-brain MRI. Findings of this report show that balance impairment in acute TBI is vestibular dependent and while much of this disorder may be related to peripheral vestibular function, one-third of cases are related to vestibular agnosia in which the vestibular sensation of self-motion is diminished despite intact peripheral and reflex vestibular function. DTI showed that changes in the right inferior longitudinal fasciculus correlated with vestibular agnosia and patients with agnosia had more balance difficulties than those without it. This may have implications on treatment, because patients who do not report vertigo but have imbalance due to vestibular agnosia, are seven times less likely to have a common inner-ear problem of BPPV evaluated. Objective tests of vestibular function and balance testing are needed to assess vestibular deficit. It was felt that vertigo may only begin to be recognized by a patient after vestibular agnosia recovers. The authors point out that this vestibular cognitive deficit in acute TBI patients may cause imbalance difficulties as a result of disruption of the white-matter microstructure in the inferior longitudinal fasciculus in the right temporal lobe. (243)

NEUROENDOCRINE DYSFUNCTION

In patients who have suffered a moderate to severe TBI, 20–40% will experience pituitary dysfunction and survivors with pituitary hormonal dysfunction may experience an impact on the recovery process and quality of life. As a result of trauma, the primary injury may be direct trauma to the hypothalamus or pituitary gland or stalk. Secondary injuries that may affect other portions of the brain, such as elevated levels of neurotransmitters, ischemia, and inflammation, can affect pituitary function as well. The most commonly affected will be growth hormone and FSH/LH, with ACTH and TSH less affected and, therefore, the greatest effects will be of diminished growth hormone and, to a lesser extent, hypogonadism, hypothyroidism, hypocortisolism, diabetes insipidus, and decreased bone density. While some findings may be transient in the acute phase, others may be long term. In the chronic phase, which begins at three months after the injury and depending upon what the endocrine dysfunction is, a patient may experience fatigue, reduced attention, poor judgment, impaired memory, irritability, anxiety, depression, lethargy, insomnia, and a decrease in libido. Endocrine testing may be considered and hormone replacement given when indicated. (308–310)

DISABILITY AND RETURN TO WORK

TBI, depending upon the severity, can have a strong adverse impact on a patient's ability to return to independent living and work. Different studies have shown different return-to-work rates. The following discussion looks at different methods of analysis regarding a patient's ability to return to work and independent living after suffering a TBI.

In the United States, roughly 3.2–5.3 million people live with disability related to TBI, and about 43% of those hospitalized for TBI have residual disability a year after discharge from the hospital. (256, 260) In 2005, roughly 1.1% of the US population, or 3.17 million people, were suffering from long-term disability from TBI, resulting in possible limitations in their ability to work and perform daily activities. There may also be an increased need for ongoing medical care, rehabilitation, and support. (188) After suffering a TBI, the ability to be employed contributes to a patient's sense of well-being, social integration, and pursuit of leisure and home activities. (583)

Mild TBI: Return to work

In a TRACK-TBI pilot study, 152 subjects who had suffered a mild TBI were evaluated regarding their return-to-work status. Three-month post-concussion symptoms (irritability, sadness, nervousness, or being "more emotional") predicted delayed return to work at six months. In addition, having difficulties in the certain domains (physical, cognitive, emotional, sleep) was associated with a significantly reduced likelihood of return to work at six months post-injury (56% unable to return to work). In conclusion, the study felt that return to work after a mild TBI is associated with significant psychosocial and financial impacts, which may exacerbate the mild TBI symptoms and impede recovery. The three-month post-injury point is an important time at which post-concussion symptoms and return-to-work status should be addressed, and they are predictive for six-month return to work status. (582)

At six months post-injury, 1,566 individuals who had suffered a mild TBI were evaluated for return to work. In that group, 26.1% of individuals experienced post-concussion symptoms and 9.8% experienced PTSD symptoms, of which 81% also had post-concussion symptoms. Patients experiencing both post-concussion symptoms and PTSD reported the lowest health-related quality of life (HRQoL). In total, at six months post-injury, 74.3% returned to work at their pre-injury level. Roughly half of the patients with post-concussion symptoms and/or PTSD symptoms had not returned to work at their pre-injury level. (584)

A group of 47 patients in Finland who suffered mild TBI were divided into two groups, uncomplicated, which had no findings, and complicated who had positive findings of an intracranial abnormality on the day of injury brain CT or a three- to four-week post-injury MRI scan. Uncomplicated mild TBI patients returned to work about six days after injury, while the complicated group did so about 36 days after injury, but there were no differences in their neurocognitive tests or self-report measures at three to four weeks post-injury. The authors point out that one reason the complicated mild TBI patients were off from work for a longer period of time is that their doctors are likely to grant longer periods of sick leave when there is objective scan evidence of a brain injury. (157)

A literature review looked at how cognition affects return to work for mild and moderate TBI patients and concluded that cognition predicts and facilitates return to work post-TBI. It was felt that cognitive assessment and rehabilitation deserve more attention across the continuum of TBI treatment. Greater focus on executive functioning, attention, memory, information processing, and verbal skills are important, as proficiency increases the likelihood of successful return to work. (580)

In 109 patients who suffered a mild TBI, return to work was significantly adversely impacted with increased headaches. It was felt that headaches possibly may be a confounding variable for other injury characteristics such as cognitive functioning. (585) When 245 patients who suffered a mild TBI were evaluated, 17.3% had exited the workforce four years later in addition to 15.5% who had limitations at work because of their injury. It appeared that the symptom of taking longer to think even one month post-injury, predicted work loss. (586)

Moderate/Severe TBI: Return to work

In a study of TBI patients in the United States who completed inpatient rehabilitation between 2001 and 2010, 60.4% were unemployed at two years post-injury. Of those who were employed, 35% were employed part time. Contributing factors to being unemployed were older age at the time of injury, nonemployed pre-injury status, nonprivate insurance payment sources, lower levels of education, and longer length of stay in the hospital. (311)

In a study of 288,009 TBI survivors in the United States who were hospitalized, using a logistic regression model based upon TBI injuries in the South Carolina Traumatic Brain Injury Follow-up Registry, and applying it to the 288,009 hospitalized TBI survivors, it was estimated that 124,626 (roughly 43%) had developed long-term disability and likely need support and rehabilitative care. (182)

Five-year outcomes showed significant mortality and morbidity in those patients who had suffered a TBI requiring acute inpatient rehabilitation. In a review of TBI patients who required and were treated with acute inpatient rehabilitation in the United States from 2001 to 2007, there were an average of 13,700 patients age 16 and older who were treated annually. It was noted that by five years after the injury, 1 in 5 patients had died. Of those who survived, 12% were institutionalized, one-third were not independent in daily activities, 57% were moderately or severely disabled, 29% were dissatisfied with life, and 55% of those who were previously employed were no longer employed. Poorer outcomes were associated with older age. Interestingly, the authors point out that while those aged 30–59 years at the time of injury showed the greatest life dissatisfaction and depression, persons who were older at the time of injury suffered the worst health status outcomes and functional independence. (189)

Of 195 TBI patients studied, it was found that one to two years after injury, older patients were more likely to become physically and financially dependent upon others and less likely to return to work. Increasing age was found to negatively affect neurological outcome. (291)

In a study that looked at 108 patients with TBI and separated them into two groups, one which followed commands upon discharge from inpatient rehabilitation (early recovery group) and one group which did not (late recovery), outcomes were assessed five years later. In the early group, 8–21% (depending upon which functional item was tested) functioned independently at discharge, and at five years, 56–85% did so, whereas in the late group, 19–36% were independent at five years. Those within the early group have seen more improvement in mobility and self-care than in memory and problem solving. While the number of those who achieved independence increased in the first two years, it did not during years 2–5, indicating that recovery was not statistically significant after 5 years. At five years, depending upon the functional domain, 30-70% of patients in the late recovery group remained completely dependent. (295)

Of 466 hospitalized head injured patients, a higher severity of head injuries was associated with greater dependence on others, worse GOS ratings, dependent living, and unemployment. (177)

Among 113 patients who were hospitalized with moderate-to-severe TBI, the employment rate pre-injury was 80%, 15% at three months postinjury, and 55% after three years. Those with psychiatric symptoms and impaired cognitive function were less likely to have gained employment. As depression and anxiety are common psychiatric problems in post-TBI patients, the authors suggest that cognitive rehabilitation and treatment of psychiatric symptoms are important for vocational rehabilitation programs. (312)

History of previous TBI was found to have an adverse impact on the outcome of a subsequent TBI (even a mild TBI), resulting in an increase of post-concussive symptoms, increased mood issues, worsened verbal learning and slower processing speed, as well as a lower satisfaction with life. At six months post-injury, most patients with no previous TBI had returned to work, whereas many of those with a previous TBI remained unemployed (patients who were unemployed at the time of injury were excluded from this study). (28)

A study of 86 patients who suffered a severe TBI with a median initial GCS score of 6, were evaluated eight years after the injury. After eight years, only 15% did not experience neurological disability, while most had several complaints, and balance and motor difficulties, along with headaches, were the most common complaints. Ten percent of patients developed epilepsy and 25% had significant anxiety or depression. Patients who had a lower initial GCS score, longer ICU stay, lower GOSE at ICU discharge and at one year after injury, had a lower GOSE at eight years. Academic achievement boded for better ability to work after TBI. Almost half of the subjects were working eight years after the injury (average return to work was more than two years after injury) of which 25% reduced their working hours, and more than one-third had reduced income. Unemployment prior to the injury was associated with a similar status post-injury. Those who returned to work had difficulties at work, with possible job instability. The authors point out that other studies show differing return-to-work rates. (245)

In contrast regarding rates of return to work, a study of 637 patients in Denmark who suffered severe TBI found that return to work occurred mainly within two years, and while 30% attempted to return to work, only 16% achieved long-term employment with no public assistance, and this dropped to 11% at 2.5–5 years after the injury. (246)

IMPACT ON CAREGIVERS

Caring for an individual who has suffered a TBI, whether mild, moderate or severe, involves significant care at different levels. An individual who has suffered a severe TBI may require around the clock-skilled attendant care. There cognitive abilities may be severely impaired, and they may require significant help with many daily activities pertaining to personal hygiene, eating, dressing, etc. An individual who has suffered a mild TBI may also require care of a different nature and magnitude. They may have a small or large number of symptoms which have resulted from injury to the cortical regions of the brain as well as the white matter connections. They may have significant changes in personality and behavior, with impulsivity, mood swings, anger, and anxiety potentially interfering with the care which is being given to them. They may feel a loss of self, how they became as they are, and what they can and cannot do. They may react when they compare their present status to the life they had prior to the injury. (673)

Those providing long-term care for a relative who has suffered a TBI, whether they be spouses or parents, were more likely to have anxiety and depression if the TBI patients were suffering from cognitive, behavioral, and emotional changes. Direct caregivers may experience a significant emotional burden. (292)

MOVEMENT DISORDERS: PARKINSON'S DISEASE

When 325,870 military veterans were studied, half with TBI and the remainder controls without a TBI, with an average follow-up of 4.6 years, it was found that a mild TBI is associated with a 56% increased risk of developing Parkinson's disease when compared with non-TBI patients. The increased risk was 83% after a moderate-to-severe TBI. This is taken in the context of the fact that most patients in the study did not develop Parkinson's disease. (18)

In those over the age of 55 who have suffered a TBI, the risk over the next five to seven years of developing Parkinson's disease was increased by 44% (1.7% of TBI patients versus 1.1% of control non-TBI trauma patients developed Parkinson's disease). The risk increases significantly with more severe or more frequent TBIs. (19)

SPASTICITY

Spasticity, beginning as early as one week following TBI, is one of the barriers preventing re-entry for a patient into the community. Medical treatments include oral medications (baclofen, tizanidine, diazepam, dantrolene sodium), intrathecal baclofen, orthopedic surgical procedures (tendon transfers and lengthening, etc.), neurosurgical procedures (dorsal rhizotomies, etc.), injections (botulinum toxin, phenol nerve blocks), and rehabilitation (casting, splinting, movement). (30)

SWALLOWING DIFFICULTIES

Swallowing disorders are commonly seen after severe TBI and may be more prevalent in patients with worsened cognitive status and poor oral-motor musculature. Factors that increase likelihood of dysphagia include lower initial GCS score, presence of a tracheostomy, and longer time on a ventilator (more than two weeks). Aspiration commonly occurs in these patients. (287)

REHABILITATION AND THERAPY

Much has been written in Chapter 10 as well as in this chapter regarding short- and long-term care and treatment of TBI and the comorbidities which may be anticipated. This section will discuss rehabilitation and therapy in additional details.

Rehabilitation of TBI patients should make efforts to assess patients and optimize their function, while at the same time reduce their disability. It requires a multi-disciplinary approach, focusing on the vast and varying needs and deficits of patients. Therapy and other interventions must address all aspects of a patients' needs, whether they be physical, neurological, medical, cognitive, psychological, emotional, language related, social, family related, and vocational. Other complications of severe TBI which might interfere with treatment include heterotopic ossification, agitation, dysautonomia, motivation, and spasticity. (700) Oftentimes problematic areas are unrecognized or underrecognized, and not addressed. Varying problematic issues can create a compounding effect upon each other, if not addressed. Persistent issues may include sleep disturbance, headaches, visuospatial deficits, cognitive dysfunction, and behavioral issues. (700) In cases of severe TBI, there may be lifelong needs for rehabilitation.

Important aspects of rehabilitation after TBI include education, physical therapy, physical rehabilitation, computer-based management, practicing tasks of activities of daily living, cognitive therapy, cognitive/behavioral feedback, speech therapy and rehabilitation, occupational therapy, vocational rehabilitation, compensatory memory and visual strategies, focus on swallowing, attention to communicating, and psychological evaluation and treatment. (687) Other aspects can also be included. Areas of interest for the future include further research on neuroplasticity, stem cells, neural stimulation (rTMS), nutrition, and medications which may have early and late protective effects on the brain. (701)

Neuroplasticity may be enhanced by physiotherapy, speech and language therapy, neuropsychology, cognitive rehabilitation therapy, and other treatments. (701)

Sixty-six members of the Neurocritical Care Society and the American Congress of Rehabilitation Medicine who cared for ICU patients were surveyed to obtain guidance regarding the incorporation of rehabilitation into the care of patients who suffered a moderate or severe TBI. Those responding to the survey included 27 physicians, 8 advanced practice providers (nurse practitioners and physician assistants), 16 therapists (physical, speech and occupational), 6 nurses, 5 neurocritical care fellowship physicians, 3 residents, and 1 additional respondent. Ninety-eight percent recommended initiating rehabilitation in the ICU. Despite differences on timing guidance, physical and occupational therapy can start after ICP and vital signs are stabilized, and speech therapy is started after extubation. The health providers that contributed to the decision to initiate treatment included the specialties of neurosurgery, trauma surgery, physical therapy, occupational therapy, speech therapy, physiatry, and neurology in addition to family members at times. It was noted that this guidance was given by practitioners who cared for patients in the ICU and may have bias. (697)

Physical therapy

Physical therapy is important to help patients who have suffered TBI with maximization of their physical potential and to decrease risk of complications. Injured patients may suffer from paresis, paralysis, immobility, apraxia, and other disorders. They may develop complications from immobility including pressure sores, decubitus ulcers, pneumonia, deep venous thrombosis, contractures, weakness.

Physical therapy, when initiated early after an injury, is associated with reduced hospital and ICU stays for patients who have suffered trauma with or without TBI. Those who have experienced trauma without TBI had reduced risk of suffering a deep venous thrombosis, pulmonary embolus, pneumonia, and pressure ulcers when therapy was started earlier as compared to later in their care. (702)

Cognitive rehabilitation therapy

Cognitive rehabilitation is based on the principles of brain neuroplasticity and restoration. A literature review of 11 studies was performed, analyzing the effects that cognitive rehabilitation had on functional and structural neural modifications. Due to the range of severity of TBI in different studies, as well as the varying methods to cerebral patterns of post-treatment activation, only general trends emerged. It was felt that cognitive training promotes neural reorganization following TBI, which decreases the risk of creating a spiral of negative neuroplastic changes, and might otherwise lead to the disuse of previously healthy neural tissue, permitting it to undergo accelerated aging, atrophy, and other white matter changes often seen in chronic stages of moderate and severe TBI. (684)

Patients with cognitive impairments may benefit from compensatory interventions including the use of paper or a smart phone for reminders of tasks and contacts, as well as other phone apps to help with goal management training. Emerging technologies of neuromodulation including transcranial direct cortical stimulation and rTMS may be possibilities in the future. Marklund cited McDonald regarding clinical trials of the medication methylphenidate to treat attention disturbance after moderate-to-severe TBI. (701) Medications such as modafinil may act as a central nervous stimulant, which may be useful as an adjunctive therapy for patients with TBI who are experiencing fatigue. Borghol felt that modafinil "appears to be relatively safe compared to most other CNS stimulants and might be a valuable asset to patients to patients with TBI who are experiencing fatigue/excessive daytime sleepiness." It also appears to be a good option when other psychostimulants have failed. (706)

One hundred fifteen allied health professionals, including neuropsychologists and occupational therapists from 29 countries were surveyed, and it was observed that both cognitive training and functional compensation approaches were commonly utilized in caring for patients with a TBI. Factors considered in treating patients were their social support network, motivation in rehabilitation, multidisciplinary team collaboration, and goal setting. (685) Virtual reality may potentially provide an effective assessment and rehabilitation tool for treating cognitive and behavioral impairments in TBI patients. (686)

Speech language pathology rehabilitation

Speech language pathologists are important in the treatment of patients experiencing communication problems after a head injury. (698) They also have an important role in addressing voice and swallowing difficulties. (699)

Music therapy

In a randomized controlled trial of 40 patients who had suffered a moderate-to-severe TBI, evaluations were done using neuropsychological testing and MRI structural and functional imaging, and patients underwent a 10-week music-based neurological rehabilitation (MBNR). It was found that MBNR can ameliorate cognitive and behavioral symptoms after TBI. In addition, MBNR may induce neuroplasticity. Their analysis showed that there was an increase in functional connectivity between the fronto-parietal network and nodes of the sensorimotor network, in addition to connectivity between the dorsal attention network and the visual network. (680)

Hyperbaric oxygen therapy

A study was conducted on 44 patients who suffered a moderate or severe TBI and 40 controls to look at the effect of hyperbaric oxygen (HBO) treatment on brain dysfunction after a TBI. The authors concluded "HBO improves consciousness, cognitive function, and prognosis in patients with severe or moderate TBI through decreasing TBI-induced hematoma volumes, promoting the recovery of EEG rhythms, and modulating the expression of serum neuron-specific enolase, S100B, glial fibrillary acidic protein, brain-derived neurotrophic factor, nerve growth factor, and vascular endothelial growth factor." (681) Another randomized controlled trial of 158 patients who suffered a moderate to severe TBI, and who underwent HBO therapy, concluded that early intensified rehabilitation combined with HBO is helpful for the recovery of cognitive as well as activities of daily life and movement abilities of patients. (682)

Mindfulness meditation training

A study was performed to evaluate the impact of mindfulness meditation training (MMT) on health, cognition, and large-scale networks in the brain. Forty-six healthy adults underwent resting state functional MRI before and after completing 31 days of MMT, and they were compared to control subjects who underwent an active control intervention. In the MMT group, it was found an increase in interconnectivity between the DMN, the salience network (SN), and the CEN. The authors suggest that the MMT changes the interaction between the SN and the DMN and CEN networks, more in favor of the CEN. (683)

CLINICAL TRIALS IN TRAUMATIC BRAIN INJURY

A search of the website clinicaltrials.com (accessed on January 28, 2023) revealed 1,531 search results (including recruiting, completed, and withdrawn) when searching for "TBI (Traumatic Brain Injury)." (688)

Several of the areas being studied include the following:

- *Behavioral:* High-intensity stepping training and conventional therapy
- *Diagnostic test:* CT perfusion
- Light therapy for moderate TBI
- Deep brain stimulation
- *Behavioral:* Self-advocacy for independent life (SAIL) after TBI

- Depth electrode detection of cortical spreading depolarization after TBI
- Near-infrared phototherapy in veterans with TBI
- Fast MR for young children with TBI
- Group lifestyle balance for individuals with TBI
- Study of modified stem cells in TBI
- Imaging of TBI metabolism using hyperpolarized carbon-13 pyruvate
- TBI and yoga
- S100B as pre-head CT scan screening after mild TBI
- Etc.

12

Life care planning and socioeconomic consequences

LIFE CARE PLANNING

Life care planning for a person with traumatic brain injury (TBI) must take into account all of the bodily functions because injury to the brain can result in complications to most organ systems in the body. Problems a TBI patient may experience in the future include but are not limited to:

- Cranial complications (vision, hearing, smell, taste, facial paralysis, etc.)
- Neurological complications (seizures, headache, fatigue, weakness, sensory loss, spasticity, impaired mobility, hypertonia, apraxia, ataxia, aphasia, agnosia, post-traumatic hydrocephalus, etc.)
- Cognitive impairment (difficulty with memory, attention, arousal, language, and communications)
- Behavioral and emotional disorders (personality changes, psychiatric complications, depression, anxiety, PTSD, aggression, agitation, problems with alcohol and drugs, etc.)
- Social issues (difficulty communicating, family difficulties with impact on relationships, loss of relationships, dependence upon others)
- Difficulty performing activities of daily living
- Sleep disorders
- Employment concerns (inability to return to work, decrease in previous level of functioning)
- Balance difficulties (dizziness, difficulty with gait, falls)
- Pulmonary complications (pneumonia, pulmonary embolism, etc.)
- Endocrine disorders
- Metabolic abnormalities
- Cardiovascular complications (deep venous thrombosis [DVT], pulmonary embolism, etc.)
- Musculoskeletal complications (spasticity, weakness, muscle atrophy, contractures, heterotopic ossification, osteoporosis, fractures)
- Gastrointestinal complications (dysphagia requiring a feeding tube, etc.)
- Genitourinary complications (incontinence, urinary retention, urinary tract infections)
- Renal and bladder stones, sexual dysfunction, etc.
- Skin issues (decubitus ulcers, skin breakdown, etc.)
- Accelerated aging process (faster physical and mental/cognitive decline [increased risk of Alzheimer's and Parkinson's disease] and increased likelihood of additional injuries due to reduced physical and neurological skills and judgment) (214, 703)

Additional detailed information about short- and long-term problems, complications, and comorbidities which may arise following a TBI is provided in Chapters 10 (Recovery and Rehabilitation) and 11 (Long-Term Outcome: Prognosis).

A life care plan should, based upon collaboration with treating providers, anticipate likely future care needs of the TBI patient and their associated costs.

DOI: 10.1201/9781003354154-12

Types of services which should be addressed in a life care plan will depend upon the nature and severity of deficits. Future medical care with physicians, psychologists, therapists, and other rehabilitative providers will likely be needed. Future surgery may be anticipated. Individuals may need help with skilled or unskilled care providers, depending upon their needs. They might require assistance from homemakers, yard maintenance support personnel, and life skill trainers. Collaboration with the patient's treating providers will help to determine current and anticipated future needs. If the services are very intensive (possibly after a moderate or severe TBI), home care or long-term residential care may be required. Adaptive architectural changes may be required in the home to assure safety. Items like grab bars, shower chairs, raised toilet seats, ramps, and modifications to a vehicle may be needed. General safety features such as smoke and carbon monoxide detectors should be considered. Patients may lose their support at home as they get older or their life situation changes, and their needs for additional assistance should be anticipated and accounted for by a life care planner. Future medication needs should be anticipated. Durable medical equipment and their anticipated replacements may be needed. Discussions and evaluations may be helpful. (712)

Life expectancy (LE) was evaluated in 279 patients who suffered a TBI, and had a follow-up period of 22–27 years. LE was found to be shortened by −0.51 years in patients who have suffered a mild TBI (similar to the general population), 4.11 years in those who have suffered moderate TBI, and 13.77 years in those with a severe TBI. Those patients who died within the first two years post-injury were excluded from this study. (27)

SOCIOECONOMIC CONSEQUENCES

In a review of literature of a decade, Dismuke found that the utilization and cost of healthcare varied depending on the population studies, severity of TBI, and presence of other mental health comorbidities. (709)

According to Eibner in *Invisible Wounds of War*, the 2005 annual first year post-TBI costs for U.S. military service members on a per-case basis (in 2007 dollars) were estimated to be $27,259–$32,759 for mild TBI cases and $268,903–$408,519 for moderate-to-severe TBI cases. The authors point out that some cases of mild TBI go undiagnosed and untreated and, therefore, the mild TBI group likely represents the more severe-mild TBI cases. For mild TBI cases, productivity losses accounted for 47–57% of total costs. The authors point out that the estimated costs were drawn from costs related to civilian patients, and that the estimates of prevalence, treatment, and costs they used to compute overall cost estimates are likely conservative. The authors also indicate that the estimates are not comprehensive because they were unable to include important cost categories, including caretaker burden, substance abuse comorbidity, other TBI-related health problems, violence, and difficulty with family functioning. They also do not take into account future costs arising from substance abuse, domestic violence, homelessness, family strain, and other concerns. In addition, while the estimates are for the first year post-TBI, many of the sequelae and associated costs, especially for the moderate-to-severe TBI cases, will continue in the long term. Taking this into account, the authors felt that even their "high" estimate is likely conservative, but does demonstrate that the costs of TBI are substantial and are primarily driven by loss of productivity and life associated with TBI, rather than treatment costs. (231)

In a study of veterans, those who suffered blast-related mild TBI had the highest annual utilization of healthcare, with 26.31 visits (annual cost of $6,480) versus 20.43 visits (annual cost $4,901) in those with non-blast-related mild TBI, versus 16.62 (annual cost $4,061) visits in those without a mild TBI. Those with blast-related mild TBI were found to be more likely to suffer from headache, post-traumatic stress disorder, anxiety, and nicotine dependence. It is to be noted that the cost figures were converted to 2018 dollar values. (248)

In a 1995 study, mean initial hospitalization charges for acute care and rehabilitation was $17,015 for mild TBI and $133,467 for severe TBI, with mean follow-up charges (rehospitalizations, physician visits, medications, outpatient treatment, equipment/supplies, attendant care) for four years at $2,323 and $54,701 for the two groups, respectively. (704)

Humphreys concluded that a successful TBI rehabilitation program may provide cost savings to an individual patient as well as society. Ashley's 1991 study of cost savings of post-acute TBI rehabilitation, indicating that in 1991 dollars, the cost of care and treatment for different options of TBI care was as follows: (1) annual life care without rehabilitation: $226,000; (2) estimated post-acute rehabilitation program cost: $450,000; (3) annual life care cost with attended home placement: $49,688; and (4) annual life care cost in behavioral group home placement: $84,082. (705) In the United Kingdom, specialist rehabilitation for severe TBI saved four billion pounds for an eight years national cohort of patients. (710) In 2016, the annual incremental healthcare costs for the US population of non-fatal TBI patients covered by a private health insurance, Medicaid or Medicare, was $40.6 billion. (711)

A 2019 literature review of in-hospital costs (from various countries) after a severe TBI revealed a range of $2,130 to $401,808 per patient. Factors increasing cost included length of stay, surgical intervention, and higher TBI severity. Of note, there were variations between studies due to methodological heterogeneity and different patient treatments. Costs differed in different countries. (707) A 2006 retrospective analysis of 25,783 cases of pediatric TBI found an annual cost of over $1 billion for total hospital charges. (708)

It must be remembered that although there are costs which can be associated with various treatments and life care planning accommodations, no economic value can be placed on the sometimes devastating and life-altering impact which TBI places on patients and those around them.

References

1. Park SQ, Bae HG, Yoon SM, Shim JJ, Yun IG, Choi SK. Morphological characteristics of the thalamoperforating arteries. *J Korean Neurosurg Soc*. 2010;47(1):36–41. https://doi.org/10.3340/jkns.2010.47.1.36
2. von Bartheld CS, Bahney J, Herculano-Houzel S. The search for true numbers of neurons and glial cells in the human brain: A review of 150 years of cell counting. *J Comp Neurol*. 2016;524(18):3865–3895. https://doi.org/10.1002/cne.24040
3. Javaid S, Farooq T, Rehman Z, et al. Dynamics of choline-containing phospholipids in traumatic brain injury and associated comorbidities. *Int J Mol Sci*. 2021;22(21):11313. https://doi.org/10.3390/ijms222111313
4. Armstrong RA. Risk factors for Alzheimer's disease. *Folia Neuropathol*. 2019;57(2):87–105. https://doi.org/10.5114/fn.2019.85929
5. Gardner RC, Yaffe K. Epidemiology of mild traumatic brain injury and neurodegenerative disease. *Mol Cell Neurosci*. 2015; 66(Pt B):75–80. https://doi.org/10.1016/j.mcn.2015.03.001
6. Frieden TR, Houry D, Baldwin G. Report to congress: Traumatic brain injury in the United States: Epidemiology and rehabilitation. Centers of disease control and prevention. National Center for Injury Prevention and Control: Division of Unintentional Injury Prevention. Atlanta, GA. 2015.
7. Hulkower MB, Poliak DB, Rosenbaum SB, Zimmerman ME, Lipton ML. A decade of DTI in traumatic brain injury: 10 years and 100 articles later. *AJNR Am J Neuroradiol*. 2013;34(11):2064–2074. https://doi.org/10.3174/ajnr.A3395
8. Dewan MC, Rattani A, Gupta S, et al. Estimating the global incidence of traumatic brain injury. *J Neurosurg*. 2018:1–18. Advance online publication. https://doi.org/10.3171/2017.10.JNS17352
9. Meaney DF, Morrison B, Dale Bass C. The mechanics of traumatic brain injury: A review of what we know and what we need to know for reducing its societal burden. *J Biomech Sci Eng*. 2014;136(2):021008. https://doi.org/10.1115/1.4026364
10. McKee AC. The neuropathology of chronic traumatic encephalopathy: The status of the literature. *Semin Neurol*. 2020;40(4):359–369. https://doi.org/10.1055/s-0040-1713632
11. Alosco ML, Mariani ML, Adler CH, et al. Developing methods to detect and diagnose chronic traumatic encephalopathy during life: Rationale, design, and methodology for the DIAGNOSE CTE Research Project. *Alzheimers Res Ther*. 2021;13(1):136. https://doi.org/10.1186/s13195-021-00872-x
12. Peterson AB, Zhou H, Thomas KE, Daugherty J. Surveillance report: Traumatic brain injury-related hospitalizations and death by age group, sex, and mechanism of injury- United States, 2016 and 2017. Centers for disease control and prevention, U.S. Department of the Health and Human Services. 2021. https://www.cdc.gov/traumaticbraininjury/pdf/TBI-surveillance-report-2016-2017-508.pdf
13. Dewan MC, Mummareddy N, Wellons JC 3rd, Bonfield CM. Epidemiology of global pediatric traumatic brain injury: Qualitative review. *World Neurosurg*. 2016;91:497–509. https://doi.org/10.1016/j.wneu.2016.03.045

14. Tagliaferri F, Compagnone C, Korsic M, Servadei F, Kraus J. A systematic review of brain injury epidemiology in Europe. *Acta Neurochir.* 2006;148(3):255–268. https://doi.org/10.1007/s00701-005-0651-y
15. Faul M, Coronado V. Epidemiology of traumatic brain injury. *Handb Clin Neurol.* 2015;127:3–13. https://doi.org/10.1016/B978-0-444-52892-6.00001-5
16. Thompson HJ, McCormick WC, Kagan SH. Traumatic brain injury in older adults: Epidemiology, outcomes, and future implications. *J Am Geriatr Soc.* 2006;54(10):1590–1595. https://doi.org/10.1111/j.1532-5415.2006.00894.x
17. Zetterberg H, Winblad B, Bernick C, et al. Head trauma in sports - clinical characteristics, epidemiology and biomarkers. *J Intern Med.* 2019;285(6):624–634. https://doi.org/10.1111/joim.12863
18. Gardner RC, Byers AL, Barnes DE, Li Y, Boscardin J, Yaffe K. Mild TBI and risk of Parkinson disease: A chronic effects of neurotrauma consortium study. *Neurology.* 2018;90(20):e1771–e1779. https://doi.org/10.1212/WNL.0000000000005522
19. Gardner RC, Burke JF, Nettiksimmons J, Goldman S, Tanner CM, Yaffe K. Traumatic brain injury in later life increases risk for Parkinson disease. *Ann Neurol.* 2015;77(6):987–995. https://doi.org/10.1002/ana.24396
20. Ponsford J, Alway Y, Gould KR. Epidemiology and natural history of psychiatric disorders after TBI. *J Neuropsychiatry Clin Neurosci.* 2018;30(4):262–270. https://doi.org/10.1176/appi.neuropsych.18040093
21. Barnes DE, Byers AL, Gardner RC, Seal KH, Boscardin WJ, Yaffe K. Association of mild traumatic brain injury with and without loss of consciousness with dementia in US military veterans. *JAMA Neurol.* 2018;75(9):1055–1061. https://doi.org/10.1001/jamaneurol.2018.0815
22. Schwenkreis P, Gonschorek A, Berg F, et al. Prospective observational cohort study on epidemiology, treatment and outcome of patients with traumatic brain injury (TBI) in German BG hospitals. *BMJ Open.* 2021;11(6):e045771. https://doi.org/10.1136/bmjopen-2020-045771
23. Rickels E, von Wild K, Wenzlaff P. Head injury in Germany: A population-based prospective study on epidemiology, causes, treatment and outcome of all degrees of head-injury severity in two distinct areas. *Brain Inj.* 2010;24(12):1491–1504. https://doi.org/10.3109/02699052.2010.498006
24. Leo P, McCrea M. Epidemiology. In: Laskowitz D, et al., editors. *Translational research in traumatic brain injury.* Boca Raton, FL; London; New York: CRC Press/Taylor and Francis Group, 2016, p. 1–16.
25. Tverdal C, Aarhus M, Rønning P, et al. Incidence of emergency neurosurgical TBI procedures: A population-based study. *BMC Emerg Med.* 2022;22(1):1. https://doi.org/10.1186/s12873-021-00561-w
26. Emami P, Czorlich P, Fritzsche FS, et al. Impact of Glasgow Coma Scale score and pupil parameters on mortality rate and outcome in pediatric and adult severe traumatic brain injury: A retrospective, multicenter cohort study. *J Neurosurg.* 2017;126(3):760–767. https://doi.org/10.3171/2016.1.JNS152385
27. Groswasser Z, Peled I. Survival and mortality following TBI. *Brain Inj.* 2018;32(2):149–157. https://doi.org/10.1080/02699052.2017.1379614
28. Dams-O'Connor K, Spielman L, Singh A, et al. The impact of previous traumatic brain injury on health and functioning: A TRACK-TBI study. *J Neurotrauma.* 2013;30(24):2014–2020. https://doi.org/10.1089/neu.2013.3049
29. Shandra O, Winemiller AR, Heithoff BP, et al. Repetitive diffuse mild traumatic brain injury causes an atypical astrocyte response and spontaneous recurrent seizures. *J Neurosci.* 2019;39(10):1944–1963. https://doi.org/10.1523/JNEUROSCI.1067-18.2018
30. Bose P, Hou J, Thompson FJ. Traumatic brain injury (TBI)-induced spasticity: Neurobiology, treatment, and rehabilitation. In: Kobeissy FH, editor. *Brain neurotrauma: Molecular, neuropsychological, and rehabilitation aspects.* Boca Raton, FL; London; New York: CRC Press/Taylor & Francis, 2015, p. 155–168.
31. Khairat A, Waseem M. Epidural hematoma. In: *StatPearls.* Treasure Island, FL: StatPearls Publishing, 2021.

32. Wilberger JE Jr, Harris M, Diamond DL. Acute subdural hematoma: Morbidity, mortality, and operative timing. *J Neurosurg.* 1991;74(2):212–218. https://doi.org/10.3171/jns.1991.74.2.0212
33. Elsayed NM. Toxicology of blast overpressure. *Toxicology.* 1997;121(1):1–15. https://doi.org/10.1016/s0300-483x(97)03651-2
34. Elder GA, Cristian A. Blast-related mild traumatic brain injury: Mechanisms of injury and impact on clinical care. *Mt Sinai J Med.* 2009, 76(2):111–118. https://doi.org/10.1002/msj.20098
35. Kennedy JE, Leal FO, Lewis JD, Cullen MA, Amador RR. Posttraumatic stress symptoms in OIF/OEF service members with blast-related and non-blast-related mild TBI. *Neuro Rehabil.* 2010;26(3):223–231. https://doi.org/10.3233/NRE-2010-0558
36. Mathews ZR, Koyfman A. Blast injuries. *J Emerg Med.* 2015;49(4):573–587. https://doi.org/10.1016/j.jemermed.2015.03.013
37. Kocsis JD, Tessler A. Pathology of blast-related brain injury. *J Rehabil Res Dev.* 2009;46(6):667–672. https://doi.org/10.1682/jrrd.2008.08.0100
38. Belanger HG, Proctor-Weber Z, Kretzmer T, Kim M, French LM, Vanderploeg RD. Symptom complaints following reports of blast versus non-blast mild TBI: Does mechanism of injury matter? *Clin Neuropsychol.* 2011;25(5):702–715. https://doi.org/10.1080/13854046.2011.566892
39. Bochicchio GV, Lumpkins K, O'Connor J, et al. Blast injury in a civilian trauma setting is associated with a delay in diagnosis of traumatic brain injury. *Am Surg.* 2008;74(3), 267–270.
40. Rosenfeld JV, McFarlane AC, Bragge P, Armonda RA, Grimes JB, Ling GS. Blast-related traumatic brain injury. *Lancet Neurol.* 2013;12(9):882–893. https://doi.org/10.1016/S1474-4422(13)70161-3
41. Kovacs SK, Leonessa F, Ling GS. Blast TBI models, neuropathology, and implications for seizure risk. *Front Neurol.* 2014;5:47. https://doi.org/10.3389/fneur.2014.00047
42. Bernick C, Banks SJ, Shin W, et al. Repeated head trauma is associated with smaller thalamic volumes and slower processing speed: The professional Fighters' brain health study. *Br J Sports Med.* 2015;49(15):1007–1011. https://doi.org/10.1136/bjsports-2014-093877
43. Delaney JS, Al-Kashmiri A, Drummond R, Correa JA. The effect of protective headgear on head injuries and concussions in adolescent football (soccer) players. *Br J Sports Med.* 2008;42(2):110–115. https://doi.org/10.1136/bjsm.2007.037689
44. https://health.mil/Military-Health-Topics/Centers-of-Excellence/Traumatic-Brain-Injury-Center-of-Excellence/DOD-TBI-Worldwide-Numbers, (Accessed on February 8, 2023).
45. Honeybul S, Janzen C, Kruger K, Ho KM. Decompressive craniectomy for severe traumatic brain injury: Is life worth living? *J Neurosurg.* 2013;119(6):1566–1575. https://doi.org/10.3171/2013.8.JNS13857
46. Marion DW, Curley KC, Schwab K, Hicks RR, mTBI Diagnostics Workgroup. Proceedings of the military mTBI diagnostics workshop, St. Pete Beach, August 2010. *J Neurotrauma.* 2011;28(4):517–526. https://doi.org/10.1089/neu.2010.1638
47. Masel BE, DeWitt DS. Traumatic brain injury: A disease process, not an event. *J Neurotrauma.* 2010;27(8):1529–1540. https://doi.org/10.1089/neu.2010.1358
48. Menon DK, Schwab K, Wright DW, Maas AI, Demographics and Clinical Assessment Working Group of the International and Interagency Initiative toward Common Data Elements for Research on Traumatic Brain Injury and Psychological Health. Position statement: Definition of traumatic brain injury. *Arch Phys Med Rehabil.* 2010;91(11):1637–1640. https://doi.org/10.1016/j.apmr.2010.05.017
49. Ryan LM, Warden DL. Post concussion syndrome. *Int Rev Psychiatry (Abingdon, England).* 2003;15(4):310–316. https://doi.org/10.1080/09540260310001606692
50. Toth A. Magnetic resonance imaging application in the area of mild and acute traumatic brain injury: Implications for diagnostic markers? In: Kobeissy FH, editor. *Brain neurotrauma: Molecular, neuropsychological, and rehabilitation aspects.* Boca Raton, FL; London; New York: CRC Press/Taylor & Francis, 2015, p. 329–340.

51. Chong CD, Schwedt TJ. Research imaging of brain structure and function after concussion. *Headache*. 2018;58(6):827–835. https://doi.org/10.1111/head.13269
52. Hasan KM, Keser Z, Schulz PE, Wilde EA. Multimodal advanced imaging for concussion. *Neuroimaging Clin N Am*. 2018;28(1):31–42. https://doi.org/10.1016/j.nic.2017.09.001
53. Centers for Disease Control and Prevention. about Chronic Diseases. https://www.cdc.gov/chronicdisease/about/index.htm. (Accessed February, 2022.)
54. Teasdale G, Jennett B. Assessment of coma and impaired consciousness. A practical scale. *Lancet (London, England)*. 1974;2(7872):81–84. https://doi.org/10.1016/s0140-6736(74)91639-0
55. Laskowski RA, Creed JA, Raghupathi R. Pathophysiology of mild TBI: Implications for altered signaling pathways. In: Kobeissy FH, editor. *Brain neurotrauma: Molecular, neuropsychological, and rehabilitation aspects*. Boca Raton, FL; London; New York: CRC Press/Taylor & Francis, 2015, p. 35–42.
56. Jennett B, Bond M. Assessment of outcome after severe brain damage. *Lancet (London, England)*. 1975;1(7905):480–484. https://doi.org/10.1016/s0140-6736(75)92830-5
57. Wilson L, Boase K, Nelson LD, et al. A manual for the Glasgow outcome scale-extended interview. *J Neurotrauma*. 2021;38(17):2435–2446. https://doi.org/10.1089/neu.2020.7527
58. Lin K, Wroten M. Ranchos Los Amigos. In: *StatPearls*. Treasure Island, FL: StatPearls Publishing, 2021.
59. Gill-Thwaites H, Munday R. The sensory modality assessment and rehabilitation technique (SMART): A valid and reliable assessment for vegetative state and minimally conscious state patients. *Brain Inj*. 2004;18(12):1255–1269. https://doi.org/10.1080/02699050410001719952
60. Böhmer AE, Oses JP, Schmidt AP, et al. Neuron-specific enolase, S100B, and glial fibrillary acidic protein levels as outcome predictors in patients with severe traumatic brain injury. *Neurosurgery*. 2011;68(6):1624–1631. https://doi.org/10.1227/NEU.0b013e318214a81f
61. Perel P, Arango M, Clayton T, et al. Predicting outcome after traumatic brain injury: Practical prognostic models based on large cohort of international patients. *BMJ*. 2008;336(7641):425–429. https://doi.org/10.1136/bmj.39461.643438.25
62. Bir SC, Maiti TK, Ambekar S, Nanda A. Incidence, hospital costs and in-hospital mortality rates of epidural hematoma in the US. *Clin Neurol Neurosurg*. 2015;138:99–103. https://doi.org/10.1016/j.clineuro.2015.07.021
63. Aromatario M, Torsello A, D'Errico S, et al. Traumatic epidural and subdural hematoma: Epidemiology, outcome, and dating. *Medicina (Kaunas, Lithuania)*. 2021;57(2):125. https://doi.org/10.3390/medicina57020125
64. Goodman JC. Neuropathology of traumatic brain injury. In: Winn HR, editor. *Youmans and Winn neurological surgery*. 7th ed. Philadelphia, PA: Elsevier, 2017; p. 2765–2777.
65. Bigler ED. Neuropathology of mild traumatic brain injury: Correlation to neurocognitive and neurobehavioral findings. In: Kobeissy FH, editor. *Brain neurotrauma: Molecular, neuropsychological, and rehabilitation aspects*. Boca Raton, FL; London; New York: CRC Press/Taylor & Francis, 2015, p. 433–450.
66. Reeves TM, Phillips LL, Povlishock JT. Myelinated and unmyelinated axons of the corpus callosum differ in vulnerability and functional recovery following traumatic brain injury. *Exp Neurol*. 2005;196(1):126–137. https://doi.org/10.1016/j.expneurol.2005.07.014
67. Castellani RJ, Perry G. Dementia pugilistica revisited. *J Alzheimers Dis*. 2017;60(4):1209–1221. https://doi.org/10.3233/JAD-170669
68. Mckee AC, Abdolmohammadi B, Stein TD. The neuropathology of chronic traumatic encephalopathy. *Handb Clin Neurol*. 2018;158:297–307. https://doi.org/10.1016/B978-0-444-63954-7.00028-8
69. Vanltallie TB. Traumatic brain injury (TBI) in collision sports: Possible mechanisms of transformation into chronic traumatic encephalopathy (CTE). *Metab Clin Exp*. 2019;100S:153943. https://doi.org/10.1016/j.metabol.2019.07.007

70. Mira RG, Lira M, Cerpa W. Traumatic brain injury: Mechanisms of glial response. *Front Physiol.* 2021;12:740939. https://doi.org/10.3389/fphys.2021.740939
71. Dickerson MR, Murphy SF, Urban MJ, White Z, VandeVord PJ. Chronic anxiety- and depression-like behaviors are associated with glial-driven pathology following repeated blast induced neurotrauma. *Front Behav Neurosci.* 2021; 15:787475. https://doi.org/10.3389/fnbeh.2021.787475
72. Lewis LM, Schloemann DT, Papa L, et al. Utility of serum biomarkers in the diagnosis and stratification of mild traumatic brain injury. *Acad Emerg Med.* 2017;24(6):710–720. https://doi.org/10.1111/acem.13174
73. Khellaf A, Khan DZ, Helmy A. Recent advances in traumatic brain injury. *J Neurol.* 2019;266(11):2878–2889. https://doi.org/10.1007/s00415-019-09541-4
74. Huibregtse ME, Bazarian JJ, Shultz SR, Kawata K. The biological significance and clinical utility of emerging blood biomarkers for traumatic brain injury. *Neurosci Biobehav Rev.* 2021;130:433–447. https://doi.org/10.1016/j.neubiorev.2021.08.029
75. Unterberg AW, Stover J, Kress B, Kiening KL. Edema and brain trauma. *Neuroscience.* 2004;129(4):1021–1029. https://doi.org/10.1016/j.neuroscience.2004.06.046
76. Blixt J, Svensson M, Gunnarson E, Wanecek M. Aquaporins and blood-brain barrier permeability in early edema development after traumatic brain injury. *Brain Res.* 2015; 1611:18–28. https://doi.org/10.1016/j.brainres.2015.03.004
77. Barzó P, Marmarou A, Fatouros P, Hayasaki K, Corwin F. Contribution of vasogenic and cellular edema to traumatic brain swelling measured by diffusion-weighted imaging. *J Neurosurg.* 1997;87(6):900–907. https://doi.org/10.3171/jns.1997.87.6.0900
78. Marmarou A, Signoretti S, Fatouros PP, Portella G, Aygok GA, Bullock MR. Predominance of cellular edema in traumatic brain swelling in patients with severe head injuries. *J. Neurosurg.* 2006;104(5):720–730. https://doi.org/10.3171/jns.2006.104.5.720
79. Steiner J, Bernstein HG, Bielau H, et al. Evidence for a wide extra-astrocytic distribution of S100B in human brain. *BMC Neurosci.* 2007;8:2. https://doi.org/10.1186/1471-2202-8-2
80. Zetterberg H, Hietala MA, Jonsson M, et al. Neurochemical aftermath of amateur boxing. *Arch Neurol.* 2006; 63(9):1277–1280. https://doi.org/10.1001/archneur.63.9.1277
81. Rubenstein R, Chang B, Yue JK, et al. Comparing plasma phospho tau, total tau, and phospho tau-total tau ratio as acute and chronic traumatic brain injury biomarkers. *JAMA Neurol.* 2017; 74(9):1063–1072. https://doi.org/10.1001/jamaneurol.2017.0655
82. Papa L, Brophy GM, Welch RD, et al. Time course and diagnostic accuracy of glial and neuronal blood biomarkers GFAP and UCH-L1 in a large cohort of trauma patients with and without mild traumatic brain injury. *JAMA Neurol.* 2016;73(5):551–560. https://doi.org/10.1001/jamaneurol.2016.0039
83. Sapin V, Gaulmin R, Aubin R, Walrand S, Coste A, Abbot M. Blood biomarkers of mild traumatic brain injury: State of art. *Neuro-Chirurgie.* 2021;67(3):249–254. https://doi.org/10.1016/j.neuchi.2021.01.001
84. Amoo M, Henry J, O'Halloran PJ, et al. S100B, GFAP, UCH-L1 and NSE as predictors of abnormalities on CT imaging following mild traumatic brain injury: A systematic review and meta-analysis of diagnostic test accuracy. *Neurosurg Rev.* 2022;45(2):1171–1193. https://doi.org/10.1007/s10143-021-01678-z
85. Seidenfaden SC, Kjerulff JL, Juul N, et al. Diagnostic accuracy of prehospital serum S100B and GFAP in patients with mild traumatic brain injury: A prospective observational multicenter cohort study - "the PreTBI I study". *Scand J Trauma Resusc Emerg Med.* 2021;29(1):75. https://doi.org/10.1186/s13049-021-00891-5
86. Kraus GE, Bucholz RD, Smith KR Jr, Awwad EE. Open depressed skull fracture missed on computed tomography: A case report. *Am J Emerg Med.* 1991;9(1):34–36. https://doi.org/10.1016/0735-6757(91)90010-h

87. Carney N, Totten AM, O'Reilly C, et al. *Guidelines for the management of severe traumatic brain injury*. 4th ed. Brain Trauma Foundation, 2016 September. https://braintrauma.org/uploads/03/12/Guidelines_for_Manage-ment_of_Severe_TBI_4th_Edition.pdf
88. Chen SH, Chen Y, Fang WK, Huang DW, Huang KC, Tseng SH. Comparison of craniotomy and decompressive craniectomy in severely head-injured patients with acute subdural hematoma. *J Trauma*. 2011;71(6):1632–1636. https://doi.org/10.1097/TA.0b013e3182367b3c
89. Edwards P, Arango M, Balica L, et al. Final results of MRC CRASH, a randomised placebo-controlled trial of intravenous corticosteroid in adults with head injury-outcomes at 6 months. *Lancet (London, England)*. 2005;365(9475):1957–1959. https://doi.org/10.1016/S0140-6736(05)66552-X
90. Härtl R, Gerber LM, Ni Q, Ghajar J. Effect of early nutrition on deaths due to severe traumatic brain injury. *J Neurosurg*. 2008;109(1):50–56. https://doi.org/10.3171/JNS/2008/109/7/0050
91. Denson K, Morgan D, Cunningham R, et al. Incidence of venous thromboembolism in patients with traumatic brain injury. *Am J Surg*. 2007;193(3):380–384. https://doi.org/10.1016/j.amjsurg.2006.12.004
92. Geerts WH, Code KI, Jay RM, Chen E, Szalai JP. A prospective study of venous thromboembolism after major trauma. *N Engl J Med*. 1994;331(24):1601–1606. https://doi.org/10.1056/NEJM199412153312401
93. Torbic H, Forni AA, Anger KE, Degrado JR, Greenwood BC. Use of antiepileptics for seizure prophylaxis after traumatic brain injury. *Am J Health Syst Pharm*. 2013;70(9):759–766. https://doi.org/10.2146/ajhp120203
94. Ferguson PL, Smith GM, Wannamaker BB, Thurman DJ, Pickelsimer EE, Selassie AW. A population-based study of risk of epilepsy after hospitalization for traumatic brain injury. *Epilepsia*. 2010;51(5):891–898. https://doi.org/10.1111/j.1528-1167.2009.02384.x
95. Zimmermann LL, Diaz-Arrastia R, Vespa PM. Seizures and the role of anticonvulsants after traumatic brain injury. *Neurosurg Clin N Am*. 2016;27(4):499–508. https://doi.org/10.1016/j.nec.2016.06.001
96. Park JT, DeLozier SJ, Chugani HT. Epilepsy due to mild TBI in children: An experience at a tertiary referral center. *J Clin Med*. 2021;10(23):5695. https://doi.org/10.3390/jcm10235695
97. Sahuquillo J, Dennis JA. Decompressive craniectomy for the treatment of high intracranial pressure in closed traumatic brain injury. *Cochrane Database Syst Rev*. 2019;12(12):CD003983. https://doi.org/10.1002/14651858.CD003983.pub3
98. Zusman BE, Kochanek PM, Jha RM. Cerebral edema in traumatic brain injury: A historical framework for current therapy. *Curr Treat Options Neurol*. 2020;22(3):9. https://doi.org/10.1007/s11940-020-0614-x
99. Huang SJ, Hong WC, Han YY, et al. Clinical outcome of severe head injury using three different ICP and CPP protocol-driven therapies. *J Clin Neurosci*. 2006;13(8):818–822. https://doi.org/10.1016/j.jocn.2005.11.034
100. Maloney-Wilensky E, Le Roux P. The physiology behind direct brain oxygen monitors and practical aspects of their use. *Childs Nerv Syst*. 2010;26(4):419–430. https://doi.org/10.1007/s00381-009-1037-x
101. Green JA, Pellegrini DC, Vanderkolk WE, Figueroa BE, Eriksson EA. Goal directed brain tissue oxygen monitoring versus conventional management in traumatic brain injury: An Analysis of in Hospital recovery. *Neurocrit Care*. 2013;18(1):20–25. https://doi.org/10.1007/s12028-012-9797-7
102. Fatima N, Shuaib A, Chughtai TS, Ayyad A, Saqqur M. The role of transcranial Doppler in traumatic brain injury: A systemic review and meta-analysis. *Asian J Neurosurg*. 2019;14(3):626–633. https://doi.org/10.4103/ajns.AJNS_42_19
103. Ziegler D, Cravens G, Poche G, Gandhi R, Tellez M. Use of transcranial Doppler in patients with severe traumatic brain injuries. *J Neurotrauma*. 2017;34(1):121–127. https://doi.org/10.1089/neu.2015.3967
104. Soustiel JF, Mahamid E, Chistyakov A, Shik V, Benenson R, Zaaroor M. Comparison of moderate hyperventilation and mannitol for control of intracranial pressure control in patients with severe traumatic brain injury–a study of cerebral blood flow and metabolism. *Acta Neurochir*. 2006;148(8):845–851. https://doi.org/10.1007/s00701-006-0792-7

105. Bullock MR, Chesnut R, Ghajar J, et al., & Surgical Management of Traumatic Brain Injury Author Group. Surgical management of acute epidural hematomas. *Neurosurgery*. 2006;58(3 Suppl):S7–S15; discussion Si-iv. PMID: 16710967.
106. Bullock MR, Chesnut R, Ghajar J, et al., & Surgical Management of Traumatic Brain Injury Author Group. Surgical management of traumatic parenchymal lesions. *Neurosurgery*. 2006;58(3 Suppl):S25–S46; discussion Si-iv. https://doi.org/10.1227/01.NEU.0000210365.36914.E3
107. Bullock MR, Chesnut R, Ghajar J, et al., & Surgical Management of Traumatic Brain Injury Author Group. Surgical management of acute subdural hematomas. *Neurosurgery*. 2006;58(3 Suppl):S16–S24; discussion Si–iv. PMID: 16710968.
108. Cooper DJ, Rosenfeld JV, Murray L, et al. Decompressive craniectomy in diffuse traumatic brain injury. *N Engl J Med*. 2011;364(16):1493–1502. https://doi.org/10.1056/NEJMoa1102077
109. Haydel MJ, Preston CA, Mills TJ, Luber S, Blaudeau E, DeBlieux PM. Indications for computed tomography in patients with minor head injury. *N Engl J Med*. 2000;343(2):100–105. https://doi.org/10.1056/NEJM200007133430204
110. Noguchi K, Ogawa T, Seto H, et al. Subacute and chronic subarachnoid hemorrhage: Diagnosis with fluid-attenuated inversion-recovery MR imaging. *Radiology*. 1997;203(1):257–262. https://doi.org/10.1148/radiology.203.1.9122404
111. Schweitzer AD, Niogi SN, Whitlow CT, Tsiouris AJ. Traumatic brain injury: Imaging patterns and complications. *RadioGraphics*. 2019;39(6):1571–1595. https://doi.org/10.1148/rg.2019190076
112. Haacke EM, Xu Y, Cheng YC, Reichenbach JR. Susceptibility weighted imaging (SWI). *Magn Reson Med*. 2004;52(3):612–618. https://doi.org/10.1002/mrm.20198
113. Babikian T, Freier MC, Tong KA, et al. Susceptibility weighted imaging: Neuropsychologic outcome and pediatric head injury. *Pediatr Neurol*. 2005;33(3):184–194. https://doi.org/10.1016/j.pediatrneurol.2005.03.015
114. Liu AY, Maldjian JA, Bagley LJ, Sinson GP, Grossman RI. Traumatic brain injury: Diffusion-weighted MR imaging findings. *AJNR Am J Neuroradiol*. 1999;20(9):1636–1641.
115. Mac Donald CL, Johnson AM, Cooper D, et al. Detection of blast-related traumatic brain injury in US Military personnel. *N Engl J Med*. 2011;364(22):2091–2100. https://doi.org/10.1056/NEJMoa1008069
116. Tator CH, Davis HS, Dufort PA, et al. Postconcussion syndrome: Demographics and predictors in 221 patients. *J Neurosurg*. 2016;125(5):1206–1216. https://doi.org/10.3171/2015.6.JNS15664
117. Eierud C, Craddock RC, Fletcher S, et al. Neuroimaging after mild traumatic brain injury: Review and meta-analysis. *NeuroImage Clin*. 2014;4:283–294. https://doi.org/10.1016/j.nicl.2013.12.009
118. Croall I, Smith FE, Blamire AM. Magnetic resonance spectroscopy for traumatic brain injury. *Top Magn Reson Imaging*. 2015;24(5):267–274. https://doi.org/10.1097/RMR.0000000000000063
119. Huang MX, Theilmann RJ, Robb A, et al. Integrated imaging approach with MEG and DTI to detect mild traumatic brain injury in military and civilian patients. *J. Neurotrauma*. 2009;26(8):1213–1226. https://doi.org/10.1089/neu.2008.0672
120. Huang MX, Nichols S, Robb A, et al. An automatic MEG low-frequency source imaging approach for detecting injuries in mild and moderate TBI patients with blast and non-blast causes. *NeuroImage*. 2012;61(4):1067–1082. https://doi.org/10.1016/j.neuroimage.2012.04.029
121. Byrnes KR, Wilson CM, Brabazon F, et al. FDG-PET imaging in mild traumatic brain injury: A critical review. *Front Neuroenergetics*. 2014;5:13. https://doi.org/10.3389/fnene.2013.00013
122. Kraus GE, Bernstein TW, Satter M, Ezzeddine B, Hwang DR, Mantil J. A technique utilizing positron emission tomography and magnetic resonance/computed tomography image fusion to aid in surgical navigation and tumor volume determination. *J Image Guid Surg*. 1995;1(6):300–307. https://doi.org/10.1002/(SICI)1522-712X(1995)1:6<300::AID-IGS2>3.0.CO;2-E

123. Padma MV, Jacobs M, Sequeira P, et al. Functional imaging in Lhermitte-Duclose disease. *Mol Imaging Biol*. 2004;6(5): 319–323. https://doi.org/10.1016/j.mibio.2004.06.005
124. Padma MV, Jacobs M, Kraus G, et al. Radiation-induced medulloblastoma in an adult: A functional imaging study. *Neurol India*. 2004;52(1):91–93.
125. Padma MV, Said S, Jacobs M, et al. Prediction of pathology and survival by FDG PET in gliomas. *J Neurooncol*. 2003;64(3):227–237. https://doi.org/10.1023/a:1025665820001
126. Raji CA, Tarzwell R, Pavel D, et al. Clinical utility of SPECT neuroimaging in the diagnosis and treatment of traumatic brain injury: A systematic review. *PLoS One*. 2014;9(3):e91088. https://doi.org/10.1371/journal.pone.0091088
127. Irimia A, Wang B, Aylward SR, et al. Neuroimaging of structural pathology and connectomics in traumatic brain injury: Toward personalized outcome prediction. *NeuroImage Clin*. 2012;1(1):1–17. https://doi.org/10.1016/j.nicl.2012.08.002
128. Ranzenberger LR, Snyder T. Diffusion tensor imaging. In: *StatPearls*. Treasure Island, FL: StatPearls Publishing, 2021.
129. Kraus MF, Susmaras T, Caughlin BP, Walker CJ, Sweeney JA, Little DM. White matter integrity and cognition in chronic traumatic brain injury: A diffusion tensor imaging study. *Brain*. 2007;130(Pt 10):2508–2519. https://doi.org/10.1093/brain/awm216
130. Kraus JF, Nourjah P. The epidemiology of mild, uncomplicated brain injury. *J Trauma*. 1988;28(12):1637–1643. https://doi.org/10.1097/00005373-198812000-00004
131. Ledig C, Heckemann RA, Hammers A, et al. Robust whole-brain segmentation: Application to traumatic brain injury. *Med Image Anal*. 2015;21(1):40–58. https://doi.org/10.1016/j.media.2014.12.003
132. Calvillo M, Fan D, Irimia A. Multimodal imaging of cerebral microhemorrhages and white matter degradation in geriatric patients with mild traumatic brain injury. *Methods Mol Biol (Clifton, N.J.)*. 2020;2144:223–236. https://doi.org/10.1007/978-1-0716-0592-9_20
133. Rostowsky KA, Maher AS, Irimia A. Macroscale white matter alterations due to traumatic cerebral microhemorrhages are revealed by diffusion tensor imaging. *Front Neuro*. 2018;9:948. https://doi.org/10.3389/fneur.2018.00948
134. Wilde EA, McCauley SR, Hunter JV, et al. Diffusion tensor imaging of acute mild traumatic brain injury in adolescents. *Neurology*. 2008;70(12):948–955. https://doi.org/10.1212/01.wnl.0000305961.68029.54
135. Vijayakumari AA, Parker D, Osmanlioglu Y, et al. Free water volume fraction: An imaging biomarker to characterize moderate-to-severe traumatic brain injury. *J Neurotrauma*. 2021;38(19):2698–2705. https://doi.org/10.1089/neu.2021.0057
136. Moen KG, Brezova V, Skandsen T, Håberg AK, Folvik M, Vik A. Traumatic axonal injury: The prognostic value of lesion load in corpus callosum, brain stem, and thalamus in different magnetic resonance imaging sequences. *J Neurotrauma*. 2014;31(17):1486–1496. https://doi.org/10.1089/neu.2013.3258
137. Venkatasubramanian PN, Keni P, Gastfield R, et al. Diffusion tensor imaging detects acute and subacute changes in corpus callosum in blast-induced traumatic brain injury. *ASN Neuro*. 2020;12:1759091420922929. https://doi.org/10.1177/1759091420922929
138. Gardner A, Iverson GL, Stanwell P. A systematic review of proton magnetic resonance spectroscopy findings in sport-related concussion. *J Neurotrauma*. 2014;31(1):1–18. https://doi.org/10.1089/neu.2013.3079
139. Gardner A, Kay-Lambkin F, Stanwell P, et al. A systematic review of diffusion tensor imaging findings in sports-related concussion. *J Neurotrauma*. 2012;29(16):2521–2538. https://doi.org/10.1089/neu.2012.2628
140. Voormolen DC, Cnossen MC, Polinder S, von Steinbuechel N, Vos PE, Haagsma JA. Divergent classification methods of post-concussion syndrome after mild traumatic brain injury: Prevalence rates, risk factors, and functional outcome. *J Neurotrauma*. 2018;35(11):1233–1241. https://doi.org/10.1089/neu.2017.5257

141. Heskestad B, Waterloo K, Baardsen R, Helseth E, Romner B, Ingebrigtsen T. No impact of early intervention on late outcome after minimal, mild and moderate head injury. *Scand J Trauma Resusc Emerg Med.* 2010;18:10. https://doi.org/10.1186/1757-7241-18-10
142. Ponsford J, Willmott C, Rothwell A, et al. Impact of early intervention on outcome following mild head injury in adults. *J Neurol Neurosurg Psychiatry.* 2002; 73(3):330–332. https://doi.org/10.1136/jnnp.73.3.330
143. Iverson GL. Outcome from mild traumatic brain injury. *Curr Opin Psychiatry.* 2005;18(3):301–317. https://doi.org/10.1097/01.yco.0000165601.29047.ae
144. Randolph C, McCrea M, Barr WB. Is neuropsychological testing useful in the management of sport-related concussion? *J Athl Train.* 2005;40(3):139–152.
145. Jones C, Harasym J, Miguel-Cruz A, Chisholm S, Smith-MacDonald L, Brémault-Phillips S. Neurocognitive assessment tools for military personnel with mild traumatic brain injury: Scoping literature review. *JMIR Mental Health.* 2021;8(2):e26360. https://doi.org/10.2196/26360
146. Arrieux JP, Cole WR, Ahrens AP. A review of the validity of computerized neurocognitive assessment tools in mild traumatic brain injury assessment. *Concussion (London, England).* 2017;2(1):CNC31. https://doi.org/10.2217/cnc-2016-0021
147. Broglio SP, Macciocchi SN, Ferrara MS. Neurocognitive performance of concussed athletes when symptom free. *J Athl. Train.* 2007;42(4):504–508.
148. Schatz P, Pardini JE, Lovell MR, Collins MW, Podell K. Sensitivity and specificity of the Impact test battery for concussion in athletes. *Arch Clin Neuropsychol.* 2006;21(1):91–99. https://doi.org/10.1016/j.acn.2005.08.001
149. Erlanger D, Feldman D, Kutner K, et al. Development and validation of a web-based neuropsychological test protocol for sports-related return-to-play decision-making. *Arch Clin Neuropsychol.* 2003;18(3):293–316.
150. Iverson GL, Brooks BL, Collins MW, Lovell MR. Tracking neuropsychological recovery following concussion in sport. *Brain Inj.* 2006;20(3):245–252. https://doi.org/10.1080/02699050500487910
151. Blanchfield Army Community Hospital Public Affairs. Pre-deployment screening establishes baseline to fight TBI. (2018, March 22). https://www.army.mil/arti-cle/202517/pre_deployment_screening_establishes_baseline_to_fight_tbi
152. Meyers JE, Vincent AS. Automated neuropsychological assessment metrics (v4) military battery: Military normative data. *Mil Med.* 2020;185(9–10):e1706–e1721. https://doi.org/10.1093/milmed/usaa066
153. Hoge CW, McGurk D, Thomas JL, Cox AL, Engel CC, Castro CA. Mild traumatic brain injury in US Soldiers returning from Iraq. *N Engl J Med.* 2008;358(5):453–463. https://doi.org/10.1056/NEJMoa072972
154. Mac Donald CL, Johnson AM, Wierzechowski L, et al. Prospectively assessed clinical outcomes in concussive blast vs nonblast traumatic brain injury among evacuated US military personnel. *JAMA Neurol.* 2014;71(8): 994–1002. https://doi.org/10.1001/jamaneurol.2014.1114
155. Karr JE, Areshenkoff CN, Duggan EC, Garcia-Barrera MA. Blast-related mild traumatic brain injury: A bayesian random-effects meta-analysis on the cognitive outcomes of concussion among military personnel. *Neuropsychol Rev.* 2014;24(4):428–444. https://doi.org/10.1007/s11065-014-9271-8
156. Echemendia RJ, Thelen J, Meeuwisse W, et al. Neuropsychological assessment of professional ice hockey players: A cross-cultural examination of baseline data across language groups. *Arch Clin Neuropsychol.* 2020;35(3):240–256. https://doi.org/10.1093/arclin/acz077
157. Iverson GL, Lange RT, Wäljas M, et al. Outcome from complicated versus uncomplicated mild traumatic brain injury. *Rehabil Res Pract.* 2012;2012:415740. https://doi.org/10.1155/2012/415740
158. Polinder S, Cnossen MC, Real R, et al. A multidimensional approach to post-concussion symptoms in mild traumatic brain injury. *Front Neurol.* 2018;9:1113. https://doi.org/10.3389/fneur.2018.01113

159. Hiploylee C, Dufort PA, Davis HS, et al. Longitudinal study of postconcussion syndrome: Not everyone recovers. *J Neurotrauma*. 2017;34(8):1511–1523. https://doi.org/10.1089/neu.2016.4677
160. Guskiewicz KM, McCrea M, Marshall SW, et al. Cumulative effects associated with recurrent concussion in collegiate football players: The NCAA concussion study. *JAMA*. 2003;290(19):2549–2555. https://doi.org/10.1001/jama.290.19.2549
161. Spencer RJ, Drag LL, Walker SJ, Bieliauskas LA. Self-reported cognitive symptoms following mild traumatic brain injury are poorly associated with neuropsychological performance in OIF/OEF veterans. *J Rehabil Res Dev*. 2010; 47(6):521–530. https://doi.org/10.1682/jrrd.2009.11.0181
162. Silverberg ND, Crane PK, Dams-O'Connor K, et al. Developing a cognition endpoint for traumatic brain injury clinical trials. *J Neurotrauma*. 2017;34(2):363–371. https://doi.org/10.1089/neu.2016.4443
163. Schretlen DJ, Shapiro AM. A quantitative review of the effects of traumatic brain injury on cognitive functioning. *Int Rev Psychiatry (Abingdon, England)*. 2003;15(4):341–349. https://doi.org/10.1080/09540260310001606728
164. Fazio VC, Lovell MR, Pardini JE, Collins MW. The relation between post concussion symptoms and neurocognitive performance in concussed athletes. *NeuroRehabilitation*. 2007;22(3):207–216.
165. McCrory P, Meeuwisse W, Dvořák J, et al. Consensus statement on concussion in sport-the 5th international conference on concussion in sport held in Berlin, October 2016. *Br J Sports Med*. 2017;51(11):838–847. https://doi.org/10.1136/bjsports-2017-097699
166. McCrea M, Kelly JP, Kluge J, Ackley B, Randolph C. Standardized assessment of concussion in football players. *Neurology*. 1997;48(3):586–588. https://doi.org/10.1212/wnl.48.3.586
167. Guskiewicz KM, Ross SE, Marshall SW. Postural stability and neuropsychological deficits after concussion in collegiate athletes. *J Athl Train*. 2001;36(3):263–273.
168. Cavanaugh JT, Guskiewicz KM, Giuliani C, Marshall S, Mercer V, Stergiou N. Detecting altered postural control after cerebral concussion in athletes with normal postural stability. *Br J Sports Med*. 2005;39(11):805–811. https://doi.org/10.1136/bjsm.2004.015909
169. Harmon KG, Drezner JA, Gammons M, et al. American Medical society for sports medicine position statement: Concussion in sport. *Br J Sports Med*. 2013;47(1):15–26. https://doi.org/10.1136/bjsports-2012-091941
170. Guskiewicz KM, Riemann BL, Perrin DH, Nashner LM. Alternative approaches to the assessment of mild head injury in athletes. *Med Sci Sports Exerc*. 1997;29(7 Suppl):S213–S221. https://doi.org/10.1097/00005768-199707001-00003
171. Nuwer MR, Hovda DA, Schrader LM, Vespa PM. Routine and quantitative EEG in mild traumatic brain injury. *Clin Neurophysiol*. 2005;116(9):2001–2025. https://doi.org/10.1016/j.clinph.2005.05.008
172. Ianof JN, Anghinah R. Traumatic brain injury: An EEG point of view. *Dement Neuropsychol*. 2017;11(1):3–5. https://doi.org/10.1590/1980-57642016dn11-010002
173. Thompson J, Sebastianelli W, Slobounov S. EEG and postural correlates of mild traumatic brain injury in athletes. *Neurosci Lett*. 2005;377(3):158–163. https://doi.org/10.1016/j.neulet.2004.11.090
174. Mittenberg W, Canyock EM, Condit D, Patton C. Treatment of post-concussion syndrome following mild head injury. *J Clin Exp Neuropsychol*. 2001;23(6):829–836. https://doi.org/10.1076/jcen.23.6.829.1022
175. Mittenberg W, Tremont G, Zielinski RE, Fichera S, Rayls KR. Cognitive-behavioral prevention of postconcussion syndrome. *Arch Clin Neuropsychol*. 1996;11(2):139–145.
176. Tiersky LA, Anselmi V, Johnston MV, et al. A trial of neuropsychologic rehabilitation in mild-spectrum traumatic brain injury. *Arch Phys Med Rehabil*. 2005;86(8):1565–1574. https://doi.org/10.1016/j.apmr.2005.03.013
177. Dikmen SS, Ross BL, Machamer JE, Temkin NR. One year psychosocial outcome in head injury. *J Int Neuropsychol Soc*. 1995;1(1):67–77. https://doi.org/10.1017/s1355617700000126

178. Fay TB, Yeates KO, Taylor HG, et al. Cognitive reserve as a moderator of postconcussive symptoms in children with complicated and uncomplicated mild traumatic brain injury. *J Int Neuropsychol Soc*. 2010;16(1):94–105. https://doi.org/10.1017/S1355617709991007
179. Riggio S, Wong M. Neurobehavioral sequelae of traumatic brain injury. *Mt Sinai J Med*. 2009;76(2):163–172. https://doi.org/10.1002/msj.20097
180. Lundin A, de Boussard C, Edman G, Borg J. Symptoms and disability until 3 months after mild TBI. *Brain Inj*. 2006;20(8):799–806. https://doi.org/10.1080/02699050600744327
181. McCrea M, Guskiewicz KM, Marshall SW, et al. Acute effects and recovery time following concussion in collegiate football players: The NCAA concussion study. *JAMA*. 2003;290(19):2556–2563. https://doi.org/10.1001/jama.290.19.2556
182. Selassie AW, Zaloshnja E, Langlois JA, Miller T, Jones P, Steiner C. Incidence of long-term disability following traumatic brain injury hospitalization, United States, 2003. *J. Head Trauma Rehabil*. 2008;23(2): 123–131. https://doi.org/10.1097/01.HTR.0000314531.30401.39
183. Levin HS, Gary HE Jr, Eisenberg HM, et al. Neurobehavioral outcome 1 year after severe head injury. Experience of the traumatic coma data bank. *J. Neurosurg*. 1990;73(5):699–709. https://doi.org/10.3171/jns.1990.73.5.0699
184. Lange RT, Brickell TA, French LM, et al. Neuropsychological outcome from uncomplicated mild, complicated mild, and moderate traumatic brain injury in US military personnel. *Arch Clin Neuropsychol*. 2012;27(5): 480–494. https://doi.org/10.1093/arclin/acs059
185. Ravdin LD, Barr WB, Jordan B, Lathan WE, Relkin NR. Assessment of cognitive recovery following sports related head trauma in boxers. *Clin J Sport Med*. 2003; 13(1):21–27. https://doi.org/10.1097/00042752-200301000-00005
186. Bleiberg J, Cernich AN, Cameron K, et al. Duration of cognitive impairment after sports concussion. *Neurosurgery*. 2004;54(5):1073–1080. https://doi.org/10.1227/01.neu.0000118820.33396.6a
187. Annegers JF, Grabow JD, Groover RV, Laws ER Jr, Elveback LR, Kurland LT. Seizures after head trauma: A population study. *Neurology*. 1980;30(7 Pt 1):683–689. https://doi.org/10.1212/wnl.30.7.683
188. Zaloshnja E, Miller T, Langlois JA, Selassie AW. Prevalence of long-term disability from traumatic brain injury in the civilian population of the United States, 2005. *J Head Trauma Rehabil*. 2008;23(6):394–400. https://doi.org/10.1097/01.HTR.0000341435.52004.ac
189. Corrigan JD, Cuthbert JP, Harrison-Felix C, et al. US population estimates of health and social outcomes 5 years after rehabilitation for traumatic brain injury. *J Head Trauma Rehabil*. 2014;29(6):E1–E9. https://doi.org/10.1097/HTR.0000000000000020
190. Tagge CA, Fisher AM, Minaeva OV, et al. Concussion, microvascular injury, and early tauopathy in young athletes after impact head injury and an impact concussion mouse model. *Brain*. 2018;141(2):422–458. https://doi.org/10.1093/brain/awx350
191. Gronwall D, Wrightson P. Cumulative effect of concussion. *Lancet (London, England)*. 1975;2(7943):995–997. https://doi.org/10.1016/s0140-6736(75)90288-3
192. Königs M, de Kieviet JF, Oosterlaan J. Post-traumatic amnesia predicts intelligence impairment following traumatic brain injury: A meta-analysis. *J. Neurol. Neurosurg. Psychiatry*. 2012;83(11):1048–1055. https://doi.org/10.1136/jnnp-2012-302635
193. Bruce JM, Echemendia RJ. History of multiple self-reported concussions is not associated with reduced cognitive abilities. *Neurosurgery*. 2009;64(1):100–106. https://doi.org/10.1227/01.NEU.0000336310.47513.C8
194. Armstrong RA. Visual problems associated with traumatic brain injury. *Clin Exp Optom*. 2018;101(6):716–726. https://doi.org/10.1111/cxo.12670
195. Sen N. An insight into the vision impairment following traumatic brain injury. *Neurochem Int*. 2017;111:103–107. https://doi.org/10.1016/j.neuint.2017.01.019
196. Atkins EJ, Newman NJ, Biousse V. Post-traumatic visual loss. *Rev Neurosci*. 2008;5(2):73–81.

197. Ventura RE, Balcer LJ, Galetta SL, Rucker JC. Ocular motor assessment in concussion: Current status and future directions. *J Neurol Sci.* 2016;361:79–86. https://doi.org/10.1016/j.jns.2015.12.010
198. Heitger MH, Jones RD, Macleod AD, Snell DL, Frampton CM, Anderson TJ. Impaired eye movements in post-concussion syndrome indicate suboptimal brain function beyond the influence of depression, malingering or intellectual ability. *Brain.* 2009;132(Pt 10):2850–2870. https://doi.org/10.1093/brain/awp181
199. Suh M, Kolster R, Sarkar R, McCandliss B, Ghajar J, & Cognitive and Neurobiological Research Consortium. Deficits in predictive smooth pursuit after mild traumatic brain injury. *Neurosci Lett.* 2006;401(1–2):108–113. https://doi.org/10.1016/j.neulet.2006.02.074
200. Taghdiri F, Varriano B, Tartaglia MC. Assessment of oculomotor function in patients with postconcussion syndrome: A systematic review. *J Head Trauma Rehabil.* 2017;32(5):E55–E67. https://doi.org/10.1097/HTR.0000000000000286
201. Wang J, Hamm RJ, Povlishock JT. Traumatic axonal injury in the optic nerve: Evidence for axonal swelling, disconnection, dieback, and reorganization. *J Neurotrauma.* 2011;28(7):1185–1198. https://doi.org/10.1089/neu.2011.1756
202. Jorge R, Robinson RG. Mood disorders following traumatic brain injury. *Int Rev Psychiatry (Abingdon, England).* 2003;15(4):317–327. https://doi.org/10.1080/09540260310001606700
203. Stein MB, Jain S, Giacino JT, et al. Risk of posttraumatic stress disorder and major depression in civilian patients after mild traumatic brain injury: A TRACK-TBI study. *JAMA Psychiatry.* 2019;76(3):249–258. https://doi.org/10.1001/jamapsychiatry.2018.4288
204. Tateno A, Jorge RE, Robinson RG. Clinical correlates of aggressive behavior after traumatic brain injury. *J Neuropsychiatry Clin Neurosci.* 2003;15(2):155–160. https://doi.org/10.1176/jnp.15.2.155
205. Wang B, Zeldovich M, Rauen K, et al., & Center-TBI Participants And Investigators. Longitudinal analyses of the reciprocity of depression and anxiety after traumatic brain injury and its clinical implications. *J Clin Med.* 2021;10(23):5597. https://doi.org/10.3390/jcm10235597
206. Gilbert KS, Kark SM, Gehrman P, Bogdanova Y. Sleep disturbances, TBI and PTSD: Implications for treatment and recovery. *Clin Psychol Rev.* 2015;40:195–212. https://doi.org/10.1016/j.cpr.2015.05.008
207. Salazar AM, Jabbari B, Vance SC, Grafman J, Amin D, Dillon JD. Epilepsy after penetrating head injury. I. Clinical correlates: A report of the Vietnam head injury study. *Neurology.* 1985;35(10):1406–1414. https://doi.org/10.1212/wnl.35.10.1406
208. Rochat L, Beni C, Annoni JM, Vuadens P, Van der Linden M. How inhibition relates to impulsivity after moderate to severe traumatic brain injury. *J Int Neuropsychol Soc.* 2013;19(8):890–898. https://doi.org/10.1017/S1355617713000672
209. Simpson G, Tate R. Suicidality in people surviving a traumatic brain injury: Prevalence, risk factors and implications for clinical management. *Brain Inj.* 2007;21(13–14):1335–1351. https://doi.org/10.1080/02699050701785542
210. Mathias JL, Alvaro PK. Prevalence of sleep disturbances, disorders, and problems following traumatic brain injury: A meta-analysis. *Sleep Med.* 2012;13(7):898–905. https://doi.org/10.1016/j.sleep.2012.04.006
211. Leng Y, Byers AL, Barnes DE, Peltz CB, Li Y, Yaffe K. Traumatic brain injury and incidence risk of sleep disorders in nearly 200,000 US veterans. *Neurology.* 2021;96(13):e1792–e1799. https://doi.org/10.1212/WNL.0000000000011656
212. Castriotta RJ, Wilde MC, Lai JM, Atanasov S, Masel BE, Kuna ST. Prevalence and consequences of sleep disorders in traumatic brain injury. *J Clin Sleep Med.* 2007; 3(4):349–356.
213. Labastida-Ramírez A, Benemei S, Albanese M, et al, & European Headache Federation School of Advanced Studies (EHF-SAS). Persistent post-traumatic headache: A migrainous loop or not? The clinical evidence. *J. Headache Pain.* 2020;21(1):55. https://doi.org/10.1186/s10194-020-01122-5

214. Ripley DL, Weed RO. Life care planning for acquired brain injury. In: Weed RO, Berens DE, editors. *Life care planning and case management*. 4th ed. New York; Abingdon; Oxon: Routledge, 2019; p. 367–399.
215. Heyer GL, Idris SA. Does analgesic overuse contribute to chronic post-traumatic headaches in adolescent concussion patients? *Pediatr Neurol*. 2014;50(5):464–468. https://doi.org/10.1016/j.pediatrneurol.2014.01.040
216. Yerry JA, Kuehn D, Finkel AG. Onabotulinum toxin A for the treatment of headache in service members with A history of mild traumatic brain injury: A cohort study. *Headache*. 2015;55(3):395–406. https://doi.org/10.1111/head.12495
217. Leung A, Metzger-Smith V, He Y, et al. Left dorsolateral prefrontal cortex rTMS in alleviating MTBI related headaches and depressive symptoms. *Neuromodulation*. 2018;21(4):390–401. https://doi.org/10.1111/ner.12615
218. Mollica A, Safavifar F, Fralick M, Giacobbe P, Lipsman N, Burke MJ. Transcranial magnetic stimulation for the treatment of concussion: A systematic review. *Neuromodulation*. 2021;24(5):803–812. https://doi.org/10.1111/ner.13319
219. Ducic I, Sinkin JC, Crutchfield KE. Interdisciplinary treatment of post-concussion and post-traumatic headaches. *Microsurgery*. 2015;35(8):603–607. https://doi.org/10.1002/micr.22503
220. Lucas S, Hoffman JM, Bell KR, Dikmen S. A prospective study of prevalence and characterization of headache following mild traumatic brain injury. *Cephalalgia*. 2014;34(2):93–102. https://doi.org/10.1177/0333102413499645
221. Walker WC, Seel RT, Curtiss G, Warden DL. Headache after moderate and severe traumatic brain injury: A longitudinal analysis. *Arch Phys Med Rehabil*. 2005;86(9):1793–1800. https://doi.org/10.1016/j.apmr.2004.12.042
222. Niu X, Bai L, Sun Y, et al. Disruption of periaqueductal grey-default mode network functional connectivity predicts persistent post-traumatic headache in mild traumatic brain injury. *J Neurol Neurosurg Psychiatry*. 2019;90(3):326–332. https://doi.org/10.1136/jnnp-2018-318886
223. Obermann M, Nebel K, Schumann C, et al. Gray matter changes related to chronic posttraumatic headache. *Neurology*. 2009;73(12):978–983. https://doi.org/10.1212/WNL.0b013e3181b8791a
224. Chong CD, Berisha V, Chiang CC, Ross K, Schwedt TJ. Less cortical thickness in patients with persistent post-traumatic headache compared with healthy controls: An MRI study. *Headache*. 2018;58(1):53–61. https://doi.org/10.1111/head.13223
225. Dumkrieger G, Chong CD, Ross K, Berisha V, Schwedt TJ. Static and dynamic functional connectivity differences between migraine and persistent post-traumatic headache: A resting-state magnetic resonance imaging study. *Cephalalgia*. 2019;39(11):1366–1381. https://doi.org/10.1177/0333102419847728
226. Gilkey SJ, Ramadan NM, Aurora TK, Welch KM. Cerebral blood flow in chronic posttraumatic headache. *Headache*. 1997;37(9):583–587. https://doi.org/10.1046/j.1526-4610.1997.3709583.x
227. Larsen EL, Ashina H, Iljazi A, et al. Acute and preventive pharmacological treatment of post-traumatic headache: A systematic review. *J Headache Pain*. 2019;20(1):98. https://doi.org/10.1186/s10194-019-1051-7
228. Alhilali LM, Delic J, Fakhran S. Differences in callosal and forniceal diffusion between patients with and without postconcussive migraine. *AJNR Am J Neuroradiol*. 2017;38(4):691–695. https://doi.org/10.3174/ajnr.A5073
229. Kozlowski KF, Graham J, Leddy JJ, Devinney-Boymel L, Willer BS. Exercise intolerance in individuals with postconcussion syndrome. *J Athl Train*. 2013;48(5):627–635. https://doi.org/10.4085/1062-6050-48.5.02
230. Haider MN, Bezherano I, Wertheimer A, et al. Exercise for sport-related concussion and persistent post-concussive symptoms. *Sports Health*. 2021;13(2):154–160. https://doi.org/10.1177/1941738120946015
231. Eibner C, Ringel JS, Kilmer B, Pacula L, Diaz C. The cost of post-deployment mental health and cognitive conditions. In: Tanielian T, Jaycox LH, editors. *Invisible wounds of war: Psychological and cognitive injuries, their consequences, and services to assist recovery*. Santa Monica, CA; Arlington, VA; Pittsburgh, PA: Rand Corporation, 2008; p. 169–241.

232. Putukian M. Clinical evaluation of the concussed athlete: A view from the sideline. *J Athl Train*. 2017;52(3):236–244. https://doi.org/10.4085/1062-6050-52.1.08
233. Chen JW, Ruff RL, Eavey R, Wasterlain CG. Posttraumatic epilepsy and treatment. *J Rehabil Res Dev*. 2009;46(6):685–696. https://doi.org/10.1682/jrrd.2008.09.0130
234. Lowenstein DH. Epilepsy after head injury: An overview. *Epilepsia*. 2009;50(Suppl 2):4–9. https://doi.org/10.1111/j.1528-1167.2008.02004.x
235. Lucke-Wold BP, Nguyen L, Turner RC, et al. Traumatic brain injury and epilepsy: Underlying mechanisms leading to seizure. *Seizure*. 2015;33:13–23. https://doi.org/10.1016/j.seizure.2015.10.002
236. Annegers JF, Hauser WA, Coan SP, Rocca WA. A population-based study of seizures after traumatic brain injuries. *N Engl J Med*. 1998;338(1):20–24. https://doi.org/10.1056/NEJM199801013380104
237. Jennett B, Van De Sande J. EEG prediction of post-traumatic epilepsy. *Epilepsia*. 1975;16(2):251–256. https://doi.org/10.1111/j.1528-1157.1975.tb06055.x
238. Schmitt S, Dichter MA. Electrophysiologic recordings in traumatic brain injury. *Handb Clin Neurol*. 2015;127:319–339. https://doi.org/10.1016/B978-0-444-52892-6.00021-0
239. Roberts RM, Mathias JL, Rose SE. Relationship between diffusion tensor imaging (DTI) findings and cognition following pediatric TBI: A meta-analytic review. *Dev Neuropsychol*. 2016;41(3):176–200. https://doi.org/10.1080/87565641.2016.1186167
240. Sacco RR, Burmeister DB, Rupp VA, Greenberg MR. Management of benign paroxysmal positional vertigo: A randomized controlled trial. *J Emerg Med*. 2014;46(4):575–581. https://doi.org/10.1016/j.jemermed.2013.08.116
241. Kerber KA. Benign paroxysmal positional vertigo: Opportunities squandered. *Ann NY Acad Sci*. 2015;1343:106–112. https://doi.org/10.1111/nyas.12721
242. Chamelian L, Feinstein A. Outcome after mild to moderate traumatic brain injury: The role of dizziness. *Arch Phys Med Rehabil*. 2004;85(10):1662–1666. https://doi.org/10.1016/j.apmr.2004.02.012
243. Calzolari E, Chepisheva M, Smith RM, et al. Vestibular agnosia in traumatic brain injury and its link to imbalance. *Brain*. 2021;144(1):128–143. https://doi.org/10.1093/brain/awaa386
244. Thomsen IV. Late outcome of very severe blunt head trauma: A 10–15 year second follow-up. *J Neurol Neurosurg Psychiatry*. 1984;47(3):260–268. https://doi.org/10.1136/jnnp.47.3.260
245. Ruet A, Bayen E, Jourdan C, et al. A detailed overview of long-term outcomes in severe traumatic brain injury eight years post-injury. *Front Neurol*. 2019;10:120. https://doi.org/10.3389/fneur.2019.00120
246. Odgaard L, Johnsen SP, Pedersen AR, Nielsen JF. Return to work after severe traumatic brain injury: A nationwide follow-up study. *J Head Trauma Rehabil*. 2017;32(3):E57–E64. https://doi.org/10.1097/HTR.0000000000000239
247. Tang Y, Nyengaard JR, De Groot DM, Gundersen HJ. Total regional and global number of synapses in the human brain neocortex. *Synapse*. 2001;41(3):258–273. https://doi.org/10.1002/syn.1083
248. Dismuke-Greer C, Hirsch S, Carlson K, et al. Health services utilization, health care costs, and diagnoses by mild traumatic brain injury exposure: A chronic effects of neurotrauma consortium study. *Arch Phys Med Rehabil*. 2020;101(10):1720–1730. https://doi.org/10.1016/j.apmr.2020.06.008
249. Marion DW, Firlik A, McLaughlin MR. Hyperventilation therapy for severe traumatic brain injury. *New Horizons (Baltimore, Md.)*. 1995;3(3):439–447.
250. Kraus G, Popp P. *Unexpected: Body trade 2*. Jonesboro, AR: TouchPoint Press, 2016.
251. Kraus G, Popp P. *Body trade*. Kosciusko, MS: TouchPoint Press, 2014.
252. Zimmer C. 100 trillion connections. *Sci Am*. 2011;304(1):58–63. https://doi.org/10.1038/scientificamerican0111-58
253. Fields RD. The brain learns in unexpected ways: Neuroscientists have discovered a set of unfamiliar cellular mechanisms for making fresh memories. *Sci Am*. 2020;322(3):74–79.

254. LoBue C, Munro C, Schaffert J, et al. Traumatic brain injury and risk of long-term brain changes, accumulation of pathological markers, and developing dementia: A review. *J Alzheimer's Dis*. 2019;70(3): 629–654. https://doi.org/10.3233/JAD-190028
255. Dikmen S, Machamer J, Temkin N. Mild traumatic brain injury: Longitudinal study of cognition, functional status, and post-traumatic symptoms. *J Neurotrauma*. 2017;34(8):1524–1530. https://doi.org/10.1089/neu.2016.4618
256. Corrigan JD, Selassie AW, Orman JA. The epidemiology of traumatic brain injury. *J Head Trauma Rehabil*. 2010;25(2):72–80. https://doi.org/10.1097/HTR.0b013e3181ccc8b4
257. Thurman DJ, Alverson C, Dunn KA, Guerrero J, Sniezek JE. Traumatic brain injury in the United States: A public health perspective. *J Head Trauma Rehabil*. 1999;14(6):602–615. https://doi.org/10.1097/00001199-199912000-00009
258. Iaccarino C, Carretta A, Nicolosi F, Morselli C. Epidemiology of severe traumatic brain injury. *J Neurosurg Sci*. 2018;62(5):535–541. https://doi.org/10.23736/S0390-5616.18.04532-0
259. Cook AM, Morgan Jones G, Hawryluk GWJ, et al. Guidelines for the acute treatment of cerebral edema in neurocritical care patients. *Neurocrit Care*. 2020;32(3): 647–666. https://doi.org/10.1007/s12028-020-00959-7. PMID: 32227294; PMCID: PMC7272487.
260. Langlois JA, Rutland-Brown W, Wald MM. The epidemiology and impact of traumatic brain injury: A brief overview. *J Head Trauma Rehabil*. 2006;21(5):375–378. https://doi.org/10.1097/00001199-200609000-00001
261. Coronado VG, Haileyesus T, Cheng TA, et al. Trends in sports- and recreation-related traumatic brain injuries treated in US emergency departments: The national electronic injury surveillance system-all injury program (NEISS-AIP) 2001–2012. *J Head Trauma Rehabil*. 2015;30(3):185–197. https://doi.org/10.1097/HTR.0000000000000156
262. Phipps H, Mondello S, Wilson A, et al. Characteristics and impact of US Military blast-related mild traumatic brain injury: A systematic review. *Front Neurol*. 2020; 11:559318. https://doi.org/10.3389/fneur.2020.559318
263. McCrea M, Hammeke T, Olsen G, Leo P, Guskiewicz K. Unreported concussion in high school football players: Implications for prevention. *Clin J Sport Med*. 2004; 14(1):13–17. https://doi.org/10.1097/00042752-200401000-00003
264. Campbell WW. The examination in coma. In: *DeJong's the neurologic examination*. 7th ed. Philadelphia, PA; Baltimore, MD; New York; London; Buenos Aires, Hong Kong, Sydney, Tokyo: Wolters Kluwer and Lippincott Williams & Wilkins, 2013; p. 745–762.
265. Silva MA. Review of the neurobehavioral symptom inventory. *Rehabil Psychol*. 2021;66(2): 170–182. https://doi.org/10.1037/rep0000367
266. Bagiella E, Novack TA, Ansel B, et al. Measuring outcome in traumatic brain injury treatment trials: Recommendations from the traumatic brain injury clinical trials network. *J Head Trauma Rehabil*. 2010;25(5):375–382. https://doi.org/10.1097/HTR.0b013e3181d27fe3
267. Ansell BJ, Keenan JE. The Western neuro sensory stimulation profile: A tool for assessing slow-to-recover head-injured patients. *Arch Phys Med Rehabil*. 1989;70(2):104–108.
268. Rappaport M, Hall KM, Hopkins K, Belleza T, Cope DN. Disability rating scale for severe head trauma: Coma to community. *Arch Phys Med Rehabil*. 1982;63(3):118–123.
269. Campbell WW. Gross and microscopic anatomy of the cerebral hemishperes. In: *DeJong's the neurologic examination*. 7th ed. Philadelphia, PA; Baltimore, MD; New York; London; Buenos Aires, Hong Kong, Sydney, Tokyo: Wolters Kluwer and Lippincott Williams and Wilkins, 2013; p. 47–64.
270. Campbell WW. Functions of the cerebral cortex and regional cerebral diagnosis. In: *DeJong's the neurologic examination*. 7th ed. Philadelphia, PA; Baltimore, MD; New York; London; Buenos Aires, Hong Kong, Sydney, Tokyo: Wolters Kluwer and Lippincott Williams and Wilkins, 2013; p. 65–74.

271. Campbell WW. An overview of brainstem and cranial nerve anatomy. In: *DeJong's the neurologic examination*. 7th ed. Philadelphia, PA; Baltimore, MD; New York; London; Buenos Aires, Hong Kong, Sydney, Tokyo: Wolters Kluwer and Lippincott Williams and Wilkins, 2013; p. 123–136.
272. Campbell WW. Cerebellar function. In: *DeJong's the neurologic examination*. 7th ed. Philadelphia, PA; Baltimore, MD; New York; London; Buenos Aires, Hong Kong, Sydney, Tokyo: Wolters Kluwer and Lippincott Williams and Wilkins, 2013; p. 611–632.
273. Shahlaie K, Zwienenberg-Lee M, Muizelaar JP. Neuropathology of traumatic brain injury. In: Winn HR, editor. *Youmans and Winn neurological surgery*. 7th ed. Philadelphia, PA: Elsevier, 2017; p. 2843–2859.
274. Aisiku IP, Silvestri DM, Robertson CS. Critical care management of traumatic brain injury. In: Winn HR, editor. *Youmans and Winn neurological surgery*. 7th ed. Philadelphia, PA: Elsevier, 2017; p. 2876–2897.
275. Haitsma IK, Maas AI. Advanced monitoring in the intensive care unit: Brain tissue oxygen tension. *Curr Opin Crit Care*. 2002;8(2):115–120. https://doi.org/10.1097/00075198-200204000-00005
276. Glenn MB, Shih SL. Rehabilitation following TBI. In: Tsao JW, editor. *Traumatic brain injury: A Clinician's guide to diagnosis, management, and rehabilitation*. 2nd ed. Switzerland: Springer, 2020; p. 293–328.
277. American Psychiatric Association. *Diagnostic and statistical manual of mental disorders*. 5th ed. Washington, DC; London, England: American Psychiatric Publishing, 2013, p. 602–605, 624.
278. American Psychiatric Association. *Diagnostic and statistical manual of mental disorders*. 4th ed. Washington, DC: American Psychiatric Association, 1994, p. 703–706.
279. Gardner AJ, Tonks J, Potter S, et al. Neuropsychological assessment of mTBI in adults. In: Tsao JW, editor. *Traumatic brain injury: A Clinician's guide to diagnosis, management, and rehabilitation*. 2nd ed. Switzerland: Springer, 2020; p. 57–74.
280. Ditta LC, Weber NK, Robinson-Freeman KE, et al. Visual disturbances and mild traumatic brain injury (mTBI). In: Tsao JW, editor. *Traumatic brain injury: A Clinician's guide to diagnosis, management, and rehabilitation*. 2nd ed. Switzerland: Springer, 2020; p. 215–224.
281. Nichol AD, Higgins AM, Gabbe BJ, Murray LJ, Cooper DJ, Cameron PA. Measuring functional and quality of life outcomes following major head injury: Common scales and checklists. *Injury*. 2011;42(3):281–287. https://doi.org/10.1016/j.injury.2010.11.047
282. Shukla D, Devi BI, Agrawal A. Outcome measures for traumatic brain injury. *Clin Neurol Neurosurg*. 2011;113(6):435–441. https://doi.org/10.1016/j.clineuro.2011.02.013
283. Hall KM, Bushnik T, Lakisic-Kazazic B, Wright J, Cantagallo A. Assessing traumatic brain injury outcome measures for long-term follow-up of community-based individuals. *Arch Phys Med Rehabil*. 2001;82(3):367–374. https://doi.org/10.1053/apmr.2001.21525
284. Olson CR, Colby CL. The organization of cognition. In: Kandel ER, Schwartz JH, Jessell TM, Siegelbaum SA, Hudspeth AJ, editors. *Principles of neural science*. 5th ed. New York; Chicago, IL; San Francisco, CA; Lisbon; Madrid; Mexico City; Milan; New Delhi; San Juan; Seoul; Singapore; Sydney; Toronto: McGraw Medical, 2013; p. 392–411.
285. Lutkenhoff ES, Wright MJ, Shrestha V, et al. The subcortical basis of outcome and cognitive impairment in TBI: A longitudinal cohort study. *Neurology*. 2020;95(17):e2398–e2408. https://doi.org/10.1212/WNL.0000000000010825
286. Martin RM, Wright MJ, Lutkenhoff ES, et al. Traumatic hemorrhagic brain injury: Impact of location and resorption on cognitive outcome. *J Neurosurg*. 2017;126(3):796–804. https://doi.org/10.3171/2016.3.JNS151781
287. Mackay LE, Morgan AS, Bernstein BA. Swallowing disorders in severe brain injury: Risk factors affecting return to Oral intake. *Arch Phys Med Rehabil*. 1999;80(4):365–371. https://doi.org/10.1016/s0003-9993(99)90271-x

288. Casaletto KB, Heaton RK. Neuropsychological assessment: Past and future. *J Int Neuropsychol Soc.* 2017;23(9–10):778–790. https://doi.org/10.1017/S1355617717001060
289. Martins NRB, Erlhagen W, Freitas RA. Non-destructive whole-brain monitoring using nanorobots: Neural electrical data rate requirements. *Int J Mach Conscious.* 2012 June;04(01). https://doi.org/10.1142/S1793843012400069
290. Vallat-Azouvi C, Swaenepoël M, Ruet A, et al. Relationships between neuropsychological impairments and functional outcome eight years after severe traumatic brain injury: Results from the Paris-TBI study. *Brain Inj.* 2021;35(9):1001–1010. https://doi.org/10.1080/02699052.2021.1933180
291. Testa JA, Malec JF, Moessner AM, Brown AW. Outcome after traumatic brain injury: Effects of aging on recovery. *Arch Phys Med Rehabil.* 2005;86(9):1815–1823. https://doi.org/10.1016/j.apmr.2005.03.010
292. Ponsford J, Olver J, Ponsford M, Nelms R. Long-term adjustment of families following traumatic brain injury where comprehensive rehabilitation has been provided. *Brain Inj.* 2003;17(6):453–468. https://doi.org/10.1080/0269905031000070143
293. Mostert C, Singh RD, Gerritsen M, et al. Long-term outcome after severe traumatic brain injury: A systematic literature review. *Acta Neurochir.* 2022;164(3):599–613. https://doi.org/10.1007/s00701-021-05086-6
294. Ahmadi SA, Meier U, Lemcke J. Detailed long-term outcome analysis after decompressive craniectomy for severe traumatic brain injury. *Brain Inj.* 2010;24(13–14):1539–1549. https://doi.org/10.3109/02699052.2010.523049
295. Whyte J, Nakase-Richardson R, Hammond FM, et al. Functional out- comes in traumatic disorders of consciousness: 5-year outcomes from the national institute on disability and rehabilitation research traumatic brain injury model systems. *Arch Phys Med Rehabil.* 2013;94(10):1855–1860. https://doi.org/10.1016/j.apmr.2012.10.041
296. Baugh CM, Stamm JM, Riley DO, et al. Chronic traumatic encephalopathy: Neurodegeneration following repetitive concussive and subconcussive brain trauma. *Brain Imaging Behav.* 2012;6(2):244–254. https://doi.org/10.1007/s11682-012-9164-5
297. McKee AC, Stein TD, Kiernan PT, Alvarez VE. The neuropathology of chronic traumatic encephalopathy. *Brain Pathol (Zurich, Switzerland).* 2015;25(3):350–364. https://doi.org/10.1111/bpa.12248
298. McKee AC, Stern RA, Nowinski CJ, et al. The spectrum of disease in chronic traumatic encephalopathy. *Brain.* 2013; 136(Pt 1):43–64. https://doi.org/10.1093/brain/aws307
299. McKee AC, Daneshvar DH, Alvarez VE, Stein TD. The neuropathology of sport. *Acta Neuropathol.* 2014;127(1):29–51. https://doi.org/10.1007/s00401-013-1230-6
300. Bieniek KF, Ross OA, Cormier KA, et al. Chronic traumatic encephalopathy pathology in a neurodegenerative disorders brain bank. *Acta Neuropathol.* 2015;130(6):877–889. https://doi.org/10.1007/s00401-015-1502-4
301. Mez J, Daneshvar DH, Abdolmohammadi B, et al. Duration of American football play and chronic traumatic encephalopathy. *Ann Neurol.* 2020;87(1):116–131. https://doi.org/10.1002/ana.25611
302. Deb S, Lyons I, Koutzoukis C. Neurobehavioural symptoms one year after a head injury. *Br J Psychiatry.* 1999;174:360–365. https://doi.org/10.1192/bjp.174.4.360
303. Deb S, Lyons I, Koutzoukis C, Ali I, McCarthy G. Rate of psychiatric illness 1 year after traumatic brain injury. *Am J Psychiatry.* 1999;156(3):374–378. https://doi.org/10.1176/ajp.156.3.374
304. Koponen S, Taiminen T, Portin R, et al. Axis I and II psychiatric disorders after traumatic brain injury: A 30-year follow-up study. *Am J Psychiatry.* 2002;159(8):1315–1321. https://doi.org/10.1176/appi.ajp.159.8.1315
305. Fleminger S, Ponsford J. Long term outcome after traumatic brain injury. *BMJ.* 2005;331(7530):1419–1420. https://doi.org/10.1136/bmj.331.7530.1419
306. French LM, Lange RT, Brickell T. Subjective cognitive complaints and neuropsychological test performance following military-related traumatic brain injury. *J Rehabil Res Dev.* 2014;51(6):933–950. https://doi.org/10.1682/JRRD.2013.10.0226

307. Morton N, Barker L. The contribution of injury severity, executive and implicit functions to awareness of deficits after traumatic brain injury (TBI). *J Int Neuropsychol Soc*. 2010;16(6):1089–1098. https://doi.org/10.1017/S1355617710000925
308. Sav A, Rotondo F, Syro LV, Serna CA, Kovacs K. Pituitary pathology in traumatic brain injury: A review. *Pituitary*. 2019;22(3):201–211. https://doi.org/10.1007/s11102-019-00958-8
309. Gasco V, Cambria V, Bioletto F, Ghigo E, Grottoli S. Traumatic brain injury as frequent cause of hypopituitarism and growth hormone deficiency: Epidemiology, diagnosis, and treatment. *Front Endocrinol*. 2021;12:634415. https://doi.org/10.3389/fendo.2021.634415
310. Gray S, Bilski T, Dieudonne B, Saeed S. Hypopituitarism after traumatic brain injury. *Cureus*. 2019;11(3):e4163. https://doi.org/10.7759/cureus.4163
311. Cuthbert JP, Harrison-Felix C, Corrigan JD, Bell JM, Haarbauer-Krupa JK, Miller AC. Unemployment in the United States after traumatic brain injury for working-age individuals: Prevalence and associated factors 2 years postinjury. *J Head Trauma Rehabil*. 2015;30(3):160–174. https://doi.org/10.1097/HTR.0000000000000090
312. Grauwmeijer E, Heijenbrok-Kal MH, Haitsma IK, Ribbers GM. A prospective study on employment outcome 3 years after moderate to severe traumatic brain injury. *Arch Phys Med Rehabil*. 2012;93(6):993–999. https://doi.org/10.1016/j.apmr.2012.01.018
313. Martins N, Angelica A, Chakravarthy K, et al. Human Brain/Cloud interface. *Front Neurol*. 2019;13:112. https://doi.org/10.3389/fnins.2019.00112
314. Kraus GE, Bailey GJ. *Microsurgical anatomy of the brain: A stereo atlas*. Baltimore: Williams & Wilkins, 1994, p. 24, 131.
315. Selwyn R, Hockenbury N, Jaiswal S, Mathur S, Armstrong RC, Byrnes KR. Mild traumatic brain injury results in depressed cerebral glucose uptake: An (18)FDG PET study. *J Neurotrauma*. 2013;30(23):1943–1953. https://doi.org/10.1089/neu.2013.2928
316. Nakayama N, Okumura A, Shinoda J, Nakashima T, Iwama T. Relationship between regional cerebral metabolism and consciousness disturbance in traumatic diffuse brain injury without large focal lesions: An FDG-PET study with statistical parametric mapping analysis. *J Neurol Neurosurg Psychiatry*. 2006;77(7):856–862. https://doi.org/10.1136/jnnp.2005.080523
317. Koerte IK, Muehlmann M. Diffusion tensor imaging. In: Mulert C, Shenton ME, editors. *MRI in psychiatry*. Berlin; Heidelberg: Springer, 2014; p. 77–86.
318. Emsell L, Hecke WV, Tournier JD. Introduction to diffusion tensor imaging. In: Hecke WV, Emsell L, Sunaert S, editors. *Diffusion tensor imaging*. New York; Heidelberg: Springer, 2016; p. 7–22.
319. Kay T, Harrington DE, Adams R, et al. Definition of mild traumatic brain injury. *J Head Trauma Rahabil*. 1993;8(3):86–87.
320. Centers for Disease Control and Prevention. Symptoms of Mild TBI and Concussion. (2021, May 12). https://www.cdc.gov/traumaticbraininjury/concussion/symp-toms.html
321. Wycoco V, Shroff M, Sudhakar S, Lee W. White matter anatomy: What the radiologist needs to know. *Neuroimaging Clin N Am*. 2013;23(2):197–216. https://doi.org/10.1016/j.nic.2012.12.002
322. Mori S, Oishi K, Jiang H, et al. Stereotaxic white matter atlas based on diffusion tensor imaging in an ICBM template. *NeuroImage*. 2008;40(2):570–582. https://doi.org/10.1016/j.neuroimage.2007.12.035
323. Aggarwal M, Zhang J, Pletnikova O, Crain B, Troncoso J, Mori S. Feasibility of creating A high-resolution 3D diffusion tensor imaging based atlas of the human brainstem: A case study at 11.7 T. *NeuroImage*. 2013;74:117–127. https://doi.org/10.1016/j.neuroimage.2013.01.061
324. McMahon P, Hricik A, Yue JK, et al., & TRACK-TBI Investigators. Symptomatology and functional outcome in mild traumatic brain injury: Results from the prospective TRACK-TBI study. *J Neurotrauma*. 2014;31(1):26–33. https://doi.org/10.1089/neu.2013.2984
325. Hoffman M. *Cognitive, conative and behavioral neurology: An evolutional perspective*. Switzerland: Springer, 2016, p. 83–98; 145–156; 131–220.

326. Das JM, Naqvi IA. *Anton syndrome*. Treasure Island, FL: Stat Pearls Publishing, 2022.
327. Weiller C, Reisert M, Peto I, Hennig J, Makris N, Petrides M, Rijntjes M, Egger K. The ventral pathway of the human brain: A continuous association tract system. *NeuroImage*. 2021;234:117977. https://doi.org/10.1016/j.neuroimage.2021.117977
328. Hubbard EM, Ramachandran VS. Neurocognitive mechanisms of synesthesia. *Neuron*. 2005;48(3):509–520. https://doi.org/10.1016/j.neuron.2005.10.012
329. Freud E, Plaut DC, Behrmann M. 'What' is happening in the dorsal visual pathway. *Trends Cogn Sci*. 2016;20(10):773–784. https://doi.org/10.1016/j.tics.2016.08.003
330. Hu AM, Ma YL, Li YX, Han ZZ, Yan N, Zhang YM. Association between changes in white matter microstructure and cognitive impairment in white matter lesions. *Brain Sci*. 2022;12(4):482. https://doi.org/10.3390/brainsci12040482
331. Johnson CP, Juranek J, Kramer LA, Prasad MR, Swank PR, Ewing-Cobbs L. Predicting behavioral deficits in pediatric traumatic brain injury through uncinate fasciculus integrity. *J Int Neuropsychol Soc*. 2011;17(4):663–673. https://doi.org/10.1017/S1355617711000464
332. Dennis EL, Caeyenberghs K, Hoskinson KR, et al. White matter disruption in pediatric traumatic brain injury: Results from ENIGMA pediatric moderate to severe traumatic brain injury. *Neurology*. 2021;97(3):e298–e309. Advance online publication. https://doi.org/10.1212/WNL.0000000000012222
333. Willis MA, Haines DE. The limbic system. In: Haines DE, Mahailoff GA, editors. *Fundamental neuroscience for basic and clinical applications*. 5th ed. Elsevier, 2018; p. 457–467
334. Irimia A, Chambers MC, Torgerson CM, et al. Patient-tailored connectomics visualization for the assessment of white matter atrophy in traumatic brain injury. *Front Neurol*. 2012;3:10. https://doi.org/10.3389/fneur.2012.00010
335. Yeh FC, Irimia A, Bastos D, Golby AJ. Tractography methods and findings in brain tumors and traumatic brain injury. *NeuroImage*. 2021;245:118651. https://doi.org/10.1016/j.neuroimage.2021.118651
336. Radwan AM, Sunaert S, Schilling K, et al. An atlas of white matter anatomy, its variability, and reproducibility based on constrained spherical deconvolution of diffusion MRI. *NeuroImage*. 2022;254:119029. https://doi.org/10.1016/j.neuroimage.2022.119029
337. Baker CM, Burks JD, Briggs RG, et al. A connectomic atlas of the human cerebrum-chapter 1: Introduction, methods, and significance. *Oper Neurosurg (Hagerstown, Md.)*. 2018;15(suppl_1):S1–S9. https://doi.org/10.1093/ons/opy253
338. Salas CE, Castro O, Yuen KS, Radovic D, d'Avossa G, Turnbull OH. Just can't hide it': A behavioral and lesion study on emotional response modulation after right prefrontal damage. *Soc Cogn Affect Neurosci*. 2016;11(10):1528–1540. https://doi.org/10.1093/scan/nsw075
339. Poologaindran A, Lowe SR, Sughrue ME. The cortical organization of language: Distilling human connectome insights for supratentorial neurosurgery. *J Neurosurg*. 2020;134(6):1959–1966. https://doi.org/10.3171/2020.5.JNS191281
340. Glasser MF, Coalson TS, Robinson EC, et al. A multi-modal parcellation of human cerebral cortex. *Nature*. 2016; 536(7615):171–178. https://doi.org/10.1038/nature18933
341. Brodmann K. Vergleichende lokalisationslehre der grosshirnrinde in ihren prinzipien dargestellt auf grund des zellenbaues. In: Garey LJ, translator. (2006). *Brodmann's localisation in the cerebral cortex*. Lausanne, Switzerland: Springer, 1909.
342. Zilles K. Brodmann: A Pioneer of human brain mapping—his impact on concepts of cortical organization. *Brain*. 2018;141(11):3262–3278. https://doi.org/10.1093/brain/awy273
343. Nieuwenhuys R. The myeloarchitectonic studies on the human cerebral cortex of the Vogt-Vogt school, and their significance for the interpretation of functional neuroimaging data. *Brain Struct Funct*. 2013;218(2):303–352. https://doi.org/10.1007/s00429-012-0460-z
344. Bassett DS, Sporns O. Network neuroscience. *Nat Neurosci*. 2017;20(3):353–364. https://doi.org/10.1038/nn.4502

345. Herbet G, Duffau H. Revisiting the functional anatomy of the human brain: Toward a meta-networking theory of cerebral functions. *Physiol Rev.* 2020;100(3): 1181–1228. https://doi.org/10.1152/physrev.00033.2019
346. Stam CJ. Modern network science of neurological disorders. Nature reviews. *Neuroscience.* 2014;15(10):683–695. https://doi.org/10.1038/nrn3801
347. Lefaucheur JP. Transcranial magnetic stimulation. *Handb Clin Neurol.* 2019;160:559–580. https://doi.org/10.1016/B978-0-444-64032-1.00037-0
348. Gazzaniga MS, Doron KW, Funk CM. Looking toward the future: Perspectives on examining the architecture and function of the human brain as a complex system. In: Gazzaniga MS, Bizzi E, Caramazza A, Chalupa LM, et al., editors. *The cognitive neuro-sciences.* 4th ed. Cambridge, MA; London, England: A Bradford Book, The MIT Press, 2009, p. 1247–1254.
349. Sporns O. *Networks of the brain.* Cambridge: The MIT Press, 2011.
350. Spetzler RF, Martin NA. A proposed grading system for arteriovenous malformations. *J Neurosurg.* 1986;65(4):476–483. https://doi.org/10.3171/jns.1986.65.4.0476. PMID: 3760956.
351. Spetzler RF, Ponce FA. A 3-tier classification of cerebral arteriovenous malformations. Clinical article. *J Neurosurg.* 2011; 114(3):842–849. https://doi.org/10.3171/2010.8.JNS10663. Epub 2010 Oct 8. PMID: 20932095.
352. Geschwind N. Disconnexion syndromes in animals and man. I. *Brain.* 1965;88(2):237–294. https://doi.org/10.1093/brain/88.2.237. PMID: 5318481.
353. Russin JJ, Spetzler RF. Microsurgical management of aneurysms of the posterior cerebral, superior cerebellar, and anterior inferior cerebellar arteries. In: Spetzler RF, Kalani MYS, Nakaji P, editors. *Neurovascular surgery.* 2nd ed. New York: Thieme Medical Publishers, Inc, 2015. Chapter 57, p. 661–678.
354. Berker EA, Berker AH, Smith A. Translation of Broca's 1865 report. Localization of speech in the third left frontal convolution. *Arch Neurol.* 1986;43(10):1065–1072. https://doi.org/10.1001/archneur.1986.00520100069017. PMID: 3530216.
355. Stephan KE, Fink GR, Marshall JC. Mechanisms of hemispheric specialization: Insights from analyses of connectivity. *Neuropsychologia.* 2007 January 28;45(2):209–228. https://doi.org/10.1016/j.neuropsychologia.2006.07.002. Epub 2006 Sep 1. PMID: 16949111; PMCID: PMC2638113.
356. Sperry R. Consciousness, personal identity and the divided brain. *Neuropsychologia.* 1984;22(6):661–673. https://doi.org/10.1016/0028-3932(84)90093-9. PMID: 6084824.
357. Spetzler RF, Zabramski JM, McDougall CG, et al. Analysis of saccular aneurysms in the barrow ruptured aneurysm trial. *J Neurosurg.* 2018;128(1):120–125. https://doi.org/10.3171/2016.9.JNS161301. Epub 2017 Feb 24. PMID: 28298031.
358. de Haan EHF, Corballis PM, Hillyard SA, et al. Split-Brain: What we know now and why this is important for understanding consciousness. *Neuropsychol Rev.* 2020; 30(2):224–233. https://doi.org/10.1007/s11065-020-09439-3. Epub 2020 May 12. PMID: 32399946; PMCID: PMC7305066.
359. Gazzaniga MS. The split-brain: Rooting consciousness in biology. *Proc Natl Acad Sci U S A.* 2014 December 23;111(51): 18093–18094. https://doi.org/10.1073/pnas.1417892111. PMID: 25538285; PMCID: PMC4280607.
360. Thiel A, Habedank B, Herholz K, et al. From the left to the right: How the brain compensates progressive loss of language function. *Brain Lang.* 2006;98(1):57–65. https://doi.org/10.1016/j.bandl.2006.01.007. Epub 2006 Mar 7. PMID: 16519926.
361. Amunts K, Schleicher A, Bürgel U, Mohlberg H, Uylings HB, Zilles K. Broca's region revisited: Cytoarchitecture and intersubject variability. *J Comp Neurol.* 1999 September 20;412(2):319–341. https://doi.org/10.1002/(sici)1096-9861(19990920)412:2<319::aid-cne10>3.0.co;2-7. PMID: 10441759.

362. Benson RR, Meda SA, Vasudevan S, et al. Global white matter analysis of diffusion tensor images is predictive of injury severity in traumatic brain injury. *J Neurotrauma.* 2007;24(3):446–459. https://doi.org/10.1089/neu.2006.0153. PMID: 17402851.
363. Wada T, Asano Y, Shinoda J. Decreased fractional anisotropy evaluated using tract-based spatial statistics and correlated with cognitive dysfunction in patients with mild traumatic brain injury in the chronic stage. *AJNR Am J Neuroradiol.* 2012;33(11):2117–2122. https://doi.org/10.3174/ajnr.A3141. Epub 2012 Jun 21. PMID: 22723057; PMCID: PMC7965599.
364. Croall ID, Cowie CJ, He J, et al. White matter correlates of cognitive dysfunction after mild traumatic brain injury. *Neurology.* 2014;83(6):494–501. https://doi.org/10.1212/WNL.0000000000000666. Epub 2014 Jul 16. PMID: 25031282; PMCID: PMC4142001.
365. Veeramuthu V, Narayanan V, Kuo TL, et al. Diffusion tensor imaging parameters in mild traumatic brain injury and its correlation with early neuropsychological impairment: A longitudinal study. *J Neurotrauma.* 2015;32(19):1497–1509. https://doi.org/10.1089/neu.2014.3750. Epub 2015 Jun 11. PMID: 25952562; PMCID: PMC4589266.
366. Palacios EM, Sala-Llonch R, Junque C, et al. Long-term declarative memory deficits in diffuse TBI: Correlations with cortical thickness, white matter integrity and hippocampal volume. *Cortex.* 2013;49(3):646–657. https://doi.org/10.1016/j.cortex.2012.02.011. Epub 2012 Mar 8. PMID: 22482692.
367. Mayer AR, Ling J, Mannell MV, et al. A prospective diffusion tensor imaging study in mild traumatic brain injury. *Neurology.* 2010 February 23;74(8):643–650. https://doi.org/10.1212/WNL.0b013e3181d0ccdd. Epub 2010 Jan 20. PMID: 20089939; PMCID: PMC2830922.
368. Inglese M, Raz E. Functional neuroradiology of traumatic brain injury. In: Faro SH, Mohamed FB, Law M, Ulmer JL, editors. *Functional neuroradiology principles and clinical applications.* New York: Springer, 2011; p. 229–246.
369. Sharp DJ, Ham TE. Investigating white matter injury after mild traumatic brain injury. *Curr Opin Neurol.* 2011;24(6):558–563. https://doi.org/10.1097/WCO.0b013e32834cd523. PMID: 21986682.
370. Tsougos I. *Advanced MR imaging from theory to clinical practice.* Boca Raton: CRC Press, 2018. Chapter 7, Functional magnetic resonance imaging (fMRI); p. 141–160.
371. Gordon EM, May GJ, Nelson SM. MRI-based measures of intracortical myelin are sensitive to a history of TBI and are associated with functional connectivity. *Neuroimage.* 2019 October 15;200:199–209. https://doi.org/10.1016/j.neuroimage.2019.06.026. Epub 2019 Jun 13. PMID: 31203023; PMCID: PMC6703948.
372. Wilde EA, Ramos MA, Yallampalli R, et al. Diffusion tensor imaging of the cingulum bundle in children after traumatic brain injury. *Dev Neuropsychol.* 2010;35(3):333–351. https://doi.org/10.1080/87565641003696940. PMID: 20446136; PMCID: PMC3229222.
373. Kumar R, Gupta RK, Husain M, et al. Comparative evaluation of corpus callosum DTI metrics in acute mild and moderate traumatic brain injury: Its correlation with neuropsychometric tests. *Brain Inj.* 2009;23(7):675–685. https://doi.org/10.1080/02699050903014915. PMID: 19557571.
374. Cohen AL, Soussand L, Corrow SL, Martinaud O, Barton JJS, Fox MD. Looking beyond the face area: Lesion network mapping of prosopagnosia. *Brain.* 2019;142(12):3975–3990. https://doi.org/10.1093/brain/awz332. PMID: 31740940; PMCID: PMC6906597.
375. Margulies DS, Böttger J, Watanabe A, Gorgolewski KJ. Visualizing the human connectome. *Neuroimage.* 2013 October 15; 80:445–461. https://doi.org/10.1016/j.neuroimage.2013.04.111. Epub 2013 May 6. PMID: 23660027.
376. Cazalis F, Feydy A, Valabrègue R, Pélégrini-Issac M, Pierot L, Azouvi P. fMRI study of problem-solving after severe traumatic brain injury. *Brain Inj.* 2006;20(10):1019–1028. https://doi.org/10.1080/02699050600664384. PMID: 17060134.

377. Tang CY, Eaves E, Dams-O'Connor K, et al. Diffuse disconnectivity in tBi: A resting state fMRI and Dti study. *Transl Neurosci.* 2012;3(1):9–14. https://doi.org/10.2478/s13380-012-0003-3. PMID: 23459252; PMCID: PMC3583347.
378. Thompson WH, Thelin EP, Lilja A, Bellander BM, Fransson P. Functional resting- state fMRI connectivity correlates with serum levels of the S100B protein in the acute phase of traumatic brain injury. *Neuroimage Clin.* 2016;12:1004–1012. https://doi.org/10.1016/j.nicl.2016.05.005. PMID: 27995066; PMCID: PMC5153599.
379. Lawrence TP, Steel A, Ezra M, et al. MRS and DTI evidence of progressive posterior cingulate cortex and corpus callosum injury in the hyper-acute phase after traumatic brain injury. *Brain Inj.* 2019;33(7):854–868. https://doi.org/10.1080/02699052.2019.1584332. Epub 2019 Mar 8. PMID: 30848964; PMCID: PMC6619394.
380. Tang-Schomer MD, Johnson VE, Baas PW, Stewart W, Smith DH. Partial interruption of axonal transport due to microtubule breakage accounts for the formation of periodic varicosities after traumatic axonal injury. *Exp Neurol.* 2012;233(1):364–372. https://doi.org/10.1016/j.expneurol.2011.10.030. Epub 2011 Nov 4. PMID: 22079153; PMCID: PMC3979336.
381. Gasparovic C, Yeo R, Mannell M, et al. Neurometabolite concentrations in gray and white matter in mild traumatic brain injury: An 1H-magnetic resonance spectroscopy study. *J Neurotrauma.* 2009;26(10): 1635–1643. https://doi.org/10.1089/neu.2009.0896. PMID: 19355814; PMCID: PMC2822798.
382. Lindsey HM, Hodges CB, Greer KM, Wilde EA, Merkley TL. Diffusion-weighted imaging in mild traumatic brain injury: A systematic review of the literature. *Neuro-Psychol Rev.* 2021 March 15. https://doi.org/10.1007/s11065-021-09485-5. Epub ahead of print. PMID: 33721207.
383. Koch C, Hepp K. Quantum mechanics in the brain. *Nature.* 2006 March 30;440(7084):611. https://doi.org/10.1038/440611a. PMID: 16572152.
384. Rudolf R, Khan MM, Witzemann V. Motor endplate-anatomical, functional, and molecular concepts in the historical perspective. *Cells.* 2019 April 27;8(5):387. https://doi.org/10.3390/cells8050387. PMID: 31035624; PMCID: PMC6562597.
385. Hawkins J, Ahmad S. Why neurons have thousands of synapses, a theory of sequence memory in neocortex. *Front Neural Circuits.* 2016 March 30;10:23. https://doi.org/10.3389/fncir.2016.00023. PMID: 27065813; PMCID: PMC4811948.
386. Miri A, Azim E, Jessell TM. Edging toward entelechy in motor control. *Neuron.* 2013 Oct 30;80(3):827–834. https://doi.org/10.1016/j.neuron.2013.10.049. PMID: 24183031.
387. Barach JH. Entelechy and scientific determinism in medicine. *Ann Med Hist.* 1932 Sep;4(5):474–486. PMID: 33944184; PMCID: PMC7945271.
388. Spetzler RF, Rhoton AL, Nakaji P, Kawashima M. *Color atlas of cerebral revascularization: Anatomy, techniques, clinical cases.* New York: Thieme, 2013.
389. Koch C. What is consciousness? *Nature.* 2018; 557(7704):S8–S12. https://doi.org/10.1038/d41586-018-05097-x. PMID: 29743705.
390. Newton SI. *Newton's principia: The mathematical principles of natural philosophy.* New York: Daniel Adee, 1846.
391. Abbott EA. *Flatland a romance of many dimensions.* 2nd ed. Oxford: Oxford University Press, 1884.
392. Fan L, Li H, Zhuo J, et al. The human brainnetome atlas: A new brain atlas based on connectional architecture. *Cereb Cortex.* 2016;26(8):3508–3526. https://doi.org/10.1093/cercor/bhw157. Epub 2016 May 26. PMID: 27230218; PMCID: PMC4961028.
393. Zador A. The connectome as a DNA sequencing problem. In: Marcus G, Freeman J, editors. *The future of the brain: Essays by the world's leading scientists.* Princeton, NJ: Princeton University Press, 2015; p. 40–49.
394. Church G, Marblestone A, Kalhor R. Rosetta Brain. In: Marcus G, Freeman J, editors. *The future of the brain: Essays by the world's leading scientists.* Princeton, NJ: Princeton University Press, 2015; p. 50–66.

395. Zador AM, Dubnau J, Oyibo HK, Zhan H, Cao G, Peikon ID. Sequencing the connectome. *PLoS Biol.* 2012;10(10):e1001411. https://doi.org/10.1371/journal.pbio.1001411. Epub 2012 Oct 23. PMID: 23109909; PMCID: PMC3479097.
396. Sporns O. Network neuroscience. In: Marcus G, Freeman J, editors. *The future of the brain: Essays by the world's leading scientists.* Princeton, NJ: Princeton University Press, 2015; p. 90–99.
397. The Nobel Prize in Physiology or Medicine 1981 [Internet]. Nobelprize.org. [cited 2022 August 28]. Available from: https://www.nobelprize.org/prizes/medicine/1981/summary/
398. Hubel DH, Wiesel TN. *Brain and visual perception: The story of a 25-year collaboration.* New York, NY: Oxford University Press, 2004, p. 104–140.
399. Randall L. *Warped passages: Unravelling the universe's hidden dimensions.* Harlow, England: Penguin Books, 2006.
400. Poeppel D. The neurobiology of language. In: Marcus G, Freeman J, editors. *The future of the brain: Essays by the world's leading scientists.* Princeton, NJ: Princeton University Press, 2015; p. 139–148.
401. Block N. Consciousness, big science, and conceptual clarity. In: Marcus G, Freeman J, editors. *The future of the brain: Essays by the world's leading scientists.* Princeton, NJ: Princeton University Press, 2015; p. 161–176.
402. Marcus G. The computational brain. In: Marcus G, Freeman J, editors. *The future of the brain: Essays by the world's leading scientists.* Princeton, NJ: Princeton University Press, 2015; p. 205–218.
403. Donoghue J. Neurotechnology. In: Marcus G, Freeman J, editors. *The future of the brain: Essays by the world's leading scientists.* Princeton, NJ: Princeton University Press, 2015; p. 219–233.
404. Sampaio-Baptista C, Johansen-Berg H. White matter plasticity in the adult brain. *Neuron.* 2017 December 20;96(6):1239–1251. https://doi.org/10.1016/j.neuron.2017.11.026. PMID: 29268094; PMCID: PMC5766826.
405. Fields RD. A new mechanism of nervous system plasticity: Activity-dependent myelination. *Nat Rev Neurosci.* 2015; 16(12): 756–767. https://doi.org/10.1038/nrn4023. PMID: 26585800; PMCID: PMC6310485.
406. Marner L, Nyengaard JR, Tang Y, Pakkenberg B. Marked loss of myelinated nerve fibers in the human brain with age. *J Comp Neurol.* 2003 July 21;462(2):144–152. https://doi.org/10.1002/cne.10714. PMID: 12794739.
407. Ekerdt CEM, Kühn C, Anwander A, Brauer J, Friederici AD. Word learning reveals white matter plasticity in preschool children. *Brain Struct Funct.* 2020;225(2):607–619. https://doi.org/10.1007/s00429-020-02024-7. Epub 2020 Feb 18. PMID: 32072249; PMCID: PMC7046568.
408. Carr M, Haar A, Amores J, et al. Dream engineering: Simulating worlds through sensory stimulation. *Conscious Cogn.* 2020;83:102955. https://doi.org/10.1016/j.concog.2020.102955. Epub 2020 Jul 8. PMID: 32652511; PMCID: PMC7415562.
409. Kumar A, Wroten M. Agnosia. 2022 February 2. In: *StatPearls [Internet].* Treasure Island, FL: StatPearls Publishing, 2022. PMID: 29630208.
410. Marotta JJ, Behrmann M. Agnosia. In: Ramachandran VS, editor. *Encyclopedia of the human brain: Volume 1.* Amsterdam: Elsevier, 2002; p. 59–70.
411. Rapcsak SZ, Beeson PM. Agraphia. In: Ramachandran VS, editor. *Encyclopedia of the human brain: Volume 1.* Amsterdam: Elsevier, 2002; p. 71–86.
412. Friedman RB. Alexia. In: Ramachandran VS, editor. *Encyclopedia of the human brain: Volume 1.* Amsterdam: Elsevier, 2002; p. 111–117.
413. Connor LT, Obler LK. Anomia. In: Ramachandran VS, editor. *Encyclopedia of the human brain: Volume 1.* Amsterdam: Elsevier, 2002; p. 137–143.
414. Heilman KM, Gonzalez-Rothi LJ. Apraxia. In: Ramachandran VS, editor. *Encyclopedia of the human brain: Volume 1.* Amsterdam: Elsevier, 2002; p. 193–197.

415. Vaid J. Bilingualism. In: Ramachandran VS, editor. *Encyclopedia of the human brain: Volume 1*. Amsterdam: Elsevier, 2002; p. 417–434.
416. Goldenberg G. Body perception disorders. In: Ramachandran VS, editor. *Encyclopedia of the human brain: Volume 1*. Amsterdam: Elsevier, 2002; p. 443–458.
417. Crank M, Fox PT. Broca's area. In: Ramachandran VS, editor. *Encyclopedia of the human brain: Volume 1*. Amsterdam: Elsevier, 2002; p. 569–586.
418. Knowlton BJ. Categorization. In: Ramachandran VS, editor. *Encyclopedia of the human brain: Volume 1*. Amsterdam: Elsevier, 2002; p. 603–609.
419. Coslett HB. Dyslexia. In: Ramachandran VS, editor. *Encyclopedia of the human brain: Volume 2*. Amsterdam: Elsevier, 2002; p. 135–146.
420. Kemenoff LA, Miller BL, Kramer JH. Frontal lobe. In: Ramachandran VS, editor. *Encyclopedia of the human brain: Volume 2*. Amsterdam: Elsevier, 2002; p. 317–325.
421. Doty RL. Olfaction. In: Ramachandran VS, editor. *Encyclopedia of the human brain: Volume 3*. Amsterdam: Elsevier, 2002; p. 717–727.
422. De Haan EHF. Prosopagnosia. In: Ramachandran VS, editor. *Encyclopedia of the human brain: Volume 4*. Amsterdam: Elsevier, 2002; p. 67–74.
423. Saffran EM. Wernicke's area. In: Ramachandran VS, editor. *Encyclopedia of the human brain: Volume 4*. Amsterdam: Elsevier, 2002; p. 805–828.
424. Wickens AP. *A history of the brain: From stone age surgery to modern neuroscience*. Hove, East Sussex: Psychology Press, 2015.
425. Das M J, Saadabadi A. Abulia. 2022 May 2. In: *StatPearls [Internet]*. Treasure Island, FL: StatPearls Publishing, 2022 Jan–. PMID: 30725778.
426. Teles RV. Phineas Gage's great legacy. *Dement Neuropsychol*. 2020;14(4):419–421. https://doi.org/10.1590/1980-57642020dn14-040013. PMID: 33354296; PMCID: PMC7735047.
427. Stapp HP. Quantum theory and the role of mind in nature. *Found Phys*. 2001 October;31(10):1465–1499.
428. Ward BK. Is there a link between quantum mechanics and consciousness? In: Smith CUM, Whitaker H, editors. *Brain, mind and consciousness in the history of neuroscience*. New York: Springer, 2014; p. 273–302.
429. Phillips KG, Beretta A, Whitaker HA. Mind and brain: Toward an understanding of dualism. In: Smith CUM, Whitaker H, editors. *Brain, mind and consciousness in the history of neuroscience*. New York: Springer, 2014; p. 355–369.
430. Ascoli GA. The mind-brain relationship as a mathematical problem. *ISRN Neurosci*. 2013 April 14;2013:261364. https://doi.org/10.1155/2013/261364. PMID: 24967307; PMCID: PMC4045549.
431. Lee AL. Advanced imaging of traumatic brain injury. *Korean J Neurotrauma*. 2020 April 27;16(1):3–17. https://doi.org/10.13004/kjnt.2020.16.e12. PMID: 32395447; PMCID: PMC7192808.
432. Smith LGF, Milliron E, Ho ML, et al. Advanced neuroimaging in traumatic brain injury: An overview. *Neurosurg Focus*. 2019;47(6):E17. https://doi.org/10.3171/2019.9.FOCUS19652 Erratum in: Neurosurg Focus. 2021 Jan;50(1):E22. PMID: 32364704.
433. Hanley D, Prichep LS, Badjatia N, et al. A brain electrical activity electroencephalographic-based biomarker of functional impairment in traumatic brain injury: A multi-site validation trial. *J Neurotrauma*. 2018;35(1):41–47. https://doi.org/10.1089/neu.2017.5004. Epub 2017 Sep 21. PMID: 28599608.
434. Donovan V, Bianchi A, Hartman R, Bhanu B, Carson MJ, Obenaus A. Computational analysis reveals increased blood deposition following repeated mild traumatic brain injury. *Neuroimage Clin*. 2012 August 23;1(1):18–28. https://doi.org/10.1016/j.nicl.2012.08.001. PMID: 24179733; PMCID: PMC3757717.
435. Rutgers DR, Toulgoat F, Cazejust J, Fillard P, Lasjaunias P, Ducreux D. White matter abnormalities in mild traumatic brain injury: A diffusion tensor imaging study. *AJNR Am J Neuroradiol*. 2008;29(3):514–519. https://doi.org/10.3174/ajnr.A0856. Epub 2007 Nov 26. PMID: 18039754; PMCID: PMC8118864.

436. Hutchinson EB, Schwerin SC, Radomski KL, et al. Detection and distinction of mild brain injury effects in a ferret model using diffusion tensor MRI (DTI) and DTI-driven tensor-based morphometry (D-TBM). *Front Neurosci.* 2018 August 17;12:573. https://doi.org/10.3389/fnins.2018.00573. PMID: 30174584; PMCID: PMC6107703.
437. Boes AD, Prasad S, Liu H, et al. Network localization of neurological symptoms from focal brain lesions. *Brain.* 2015;138(Pt 10): 3061–3075. https://doi.org/10.1093/brain/awv228. Epub 2015 Aug 10. PMID: 26264514; PMCID: PMC4671478.
438. Paydar A, Fieremans E, Nwankwo JI, et al. Diffusional kurtosis imaging of the developing brain. *AJNR Am J Neuroradiol.* 2014;35(4):808–814. https://doi.org/10.3174/ajnr.A3764. Epub 2013 Nov 14. PMID: 24231848; PMCID: PMC7965814.
439. Kotian RP, Prakashini K, Nair S, Babu MS. Consistency of fractional anisotropy values using different combinations of b-value and time of echo (TE) in diffusion tensor imaging of normal brain white matter. *J Clin Diagn Res.* 2018 December;12(12):1–4
440. Schimrigk SK, Bellenberg B, Schlüter M, et al. Diffusion tensor imaging-based fractional anisotropy quantification in the corticospinal tract of patients with amyotrophic lateral sclerosis using a probabilistic mixture model. *AJNR Am J Neuroradiol.* 2007 April;28(4):724–730. PMID: 17416829; PMCID: PMC7977339.
441. Veraart J, Poot DH, Van Hecke W, et al. More accurate estimation of diffusion tensor parameters using diffusion kurtosis imaging. *Magn Reson Med.* 2011;65(1):138–145. https://doi.org/10.1002/mrm.22603. PMID: 20878760.
442. Tournier JD, Yeh CH, Calamante F, Cho KH, Connelly A, Lin CP. Resolving crossing fibres using constrained spherical deconvolution: Validation using diffusion-weighted imaging phantom data. *Neuroimage.* 2008 August 15;42(2):617–625. https://doi.org/10.1016/j.neuroimage.2008.05.002. Epub 2008 May 9. PMID: 18583153.
443. Lazar M, Jensen JH, Xuan L, Helpern JA. Estimation of the orientation distribution function from diffusional kurtosis imaging. *Magn Reson Med.* 2008;60(4):774–781. https://doi.org/10.1002/mrm.21725. PMID: 18816827; PMCID: PMC2562250.
444. Jang SH, Seo JP. Delayed degeneration of the left fornical crus with verbal memory impairment in a patient with mild traumatic brain injury: A case report. *Medicine (Baltimore).* 2017;96(51):e9219. https://doi.org/10.1097/MD.0000000000009219. PMID: 29390470; PMCID: PMC5758172.
445. Kenney K, Iacono D, Edlow BL, et al. Dementia after moderate-severe traumatic brain injury: Coexistence of multiple proteinopathies. *J Neuropathol Exp Neurol.* 2018;77(1):50–63. https://doi.org/10.1093/jnen/nlx101. PMID: 29155947; PMCID: PMC5939622.
446. Harrington DL, Hsu PY, Theilmann RJ, et al. Detection of chronic blast-related mild traumatic brain injury with diffusion tensor imaging and support vector machines. *Diagnostics (Basel).* 2022 April 14;12(4):987. https://doi.org/10.3390/diagnostics12040987. PMID: 35454035; PMCID: PMC9030428.
447. Yeh PH, Guan Koay C, Wang B, et al. Compromised neurocircuitry in chronic blast-related mild traumatic brain injury. *Hum Brain Mapp.* 2017;38(1):352–369. https://doi.org/10.1002/hbm.23365. Epub 2016 Sep 15. PMID: 27629984; PMCID: PMC6867097.
448. Michel BF, Sambuchi N, Vogt BA. Impact of mild traumatic brain injury on cingulate functions. *Handb Clin Neurol.* 2019;166: 151–162. https://doi.org/10.1016/B978-0-444-64196-0.00010-8. PMID: 31731910.
449. Ivanov I, Fernandez C, Mitsis EM, et al. Blast exposure, white matter integrity, and cognitive function in Iraq and Afghanistan combat veterans. *Front Neurol.* 2017 April 21;8:127. https://doi.org/10.3389/fneur.2017.00127. PMID: 28484418; PMCID: PMC5399028.
450. Levin HS, Wilde E, Troyanskaya M, et al. Diffusion tensor imaging of mild to moderate blast-related traumatic brain injury and its sequelae. *J Neurotrauma.* 2010;27(4):683–694. https://doi.org/10.1089/neu.2009.1073. PMID: 20088647.

451. Guenette JP, Stern RA, Tripodis Y, et al. Automated versus manual segmentation of brain region volumes in former football players. *Neuroimage Clin.* 2018 March 21;18:888–896. https://doi.org/10.1016/j.nicl.2018.03.026. PMID: 29876273; PMCID: PMC5988230.
452. Ross DE, Ochs AL, Seabaugh JM, Shrader CR. Alzheimer's disease neuroimaging initiative. Man versus machine: Comparison of radiologists' interpretations and NeuroQuant® volumetric analyses of brain MRIs in patients with traumatic brain injury. *J Neuropsychiatry Clin Neurosci.* 2013;25(1):32–39. https://doi.org/10.1176/appi.neuropsych.11120377. PMID: 23487191; PMCID: PMC7185228.
453. Raji CA, Merrill DA, Barrio JR, Omalu B, Small GW. Progressive focal gray matter volume loss in a former high school football player: A possible magnetic resonance imaging volumetric signature for chronic traumatic encephalopathy. *Am J Geriatr Psychiatry.* 2016;24(10):784–790. https://doi.org/10.1016/j.jagp.2016.07.018. Epub 2016 Jul 28. PMID: 27567184.
454. Mettenburg JM, Branstetter BF, Wiley CA, Lee P, Richardson RM. Improved detection of subtle mesial temporal sclerosis: Validation of a commercially available software for automated segmentation of hippocampal volume. *AJNR Am J Neuroradiol.* 2019;40(3):440–445. https://doi.org/10.3174/ajnr.A5966. Epub 2019 Feb 7. PMID: 30733255; PMCID: PMC7028654.
455. Ross DE, Ochs AL, Seabaugh J, Henshaw T. NeuroQuant® revealed hippocampal atrophy in a patient with traumatic brain injury. *J Neuropsychiatry Clin Neurosci.* 2012;24(1):E33. https://doi.org/10.1176/appi.neuropsych.11020044. PMID: 22450640.
456. Ferrazzano P, Yeske B, Mumford J, et al. Brain magnetic resonance imaging volumetric measures of functional outcome after severe traumatic brain injury in adolescents. *J Neurotrauma.* 2021;38(13):1799–1808. https://doi.org/10.1089/neu.2019.6918. Epub 2021 Feb 24. PMID: 33487126; PMCID: PMC8219192.
457. Wright KL, Hopkins RO, Robertson FE, et al. Assessment of white matter integrity after pediatric traumatic brain injury. *J Neurotrauma.* 2020 October 15;37(20):2188–2197. https://doi.org/10.1089/neu.2019.6691. Epub 2020 May 15. PMID: 32253971; PMCID: PMC7580640.
458. Martindale SL, Shura RD, Rostami R, Taber KH, Rowland JA. Research letter: Blast exposure and brain volume. *J Head Trauma Rehabil.* 2021 November-December 01;36(6):424–428. https://doi.org/10.1097/HTR.0000000000000660. PMID: 33656482.
459. Graham NSN, Jolly A, Zimmerman K, et al. Diffuse axonal injury predicts neurodegeneration after moderate-severe traumatic brain injury. *Brain.* 2020;143(12):3685–3698. https://doi.org/10.1093/brain/awaa316. PMID: 33099608.
460. Grassi DC, Zaninotto AL, Feltrin FS, et al. Dynamic changes in white matter following traumatic brain injury and how diffuse axonal injury relates to cognitive domain. *Brain Inj.* 2021 February 23;35(3):275–284. https://doi.org/10.1080/02699052.2020.1859615. Epub 2021 Jan 28. PMID: 33507820.
461. Sidaros A, Engberg AW, Sidaros K, et al. Diffusion tensor imaging during recovery from severe traumatic brain injury and relation to clinical outcome: A longitudinal study. *Brain.* 2008;131(Pt 2):559–572. https://doi.org/10.1093/brain/awm294. Epub 2007 Dec 14. PMID: 18083753.
462. Shenton ME, Hamoda HM, Schneiderman JS, et al. A review of magnetic resonance imaging and diffusion tensor imaging findings in mild traumatic brain injury. *Brain Imaging Behav.* 2012;6(2):137–192. https://doi.org/10.1007/s11682-012-9156-5. PMID: 22438191; PMCID: PMC3803157.
463. Tollard E, Galanaud D, Perlbarg V et al. Experience of diffusion tensor imaging and 1H spectroscopy for outcome prediction in severe traumatic brain injury: Preliminary results. *Crit Care Med.* 2009;37(4):1448–1455. https://doi.org/10.1097/CCM.0b013e31819cf050. PMID: 19242330.
464. Jang SH, Kim SH, Kwon HG. Diagnostic sensitivity of traumatic axonal injury of the spinothalamic tract in patients with mild traumatic brain injury. *Medicine (Balti- More).* 2022;101(1):e28536. https://doi.org/10.1097/MD.0000000000028536. PMID: 35029922; PMCID: PMC8735717.

465. Jang SH. Diagnostic history of traumatic axonal injury in patients with cerebral concussion and mild traumatic brain injury. *Brain Neurorehabil.* 2016 September;9(2):1–8.
466. Jang SH, Byun DH. Hidden truth in cerebral concussion-traumatic axonal injury: A narrative mini-review. *Healthcare (Basel).* 2022 May 18;10(5):931. https://doi.org/10.3390/healthcare10050931. PMID: 35628068; PMCID: PMC9141295.
467. Jang, SH. traumatic axonal injury in patients with mild traumatic brain injury. In: Gorbunov NV, Long JB, editors. *Traumatic brain injury - pathobiology, advanced diagnostics and acute management [Internet].* London: IntechOpen, 2017 [cited 2022 Oct 02]. Available from: https://www.intechopen.com/chapters/57012. https://doi.org/10.5772/intechopen.70988.
468. Brandstack N, Kurki T, Laalo J, Kauko T, Tenovuo O. Reproducibility of tract-based and region-of-interest DTI analysis of long association tracts. *Clin Neuroradiol.* 2016;26(2):199–208. https://doi.org/10.1007/s00062-014-0349-8. Epub 2014 Oct 5. PMID: 25283182.
469. Reid AT, Camilleri JA, Hoffstaedter F, Eickhoff SB. Tract-specific statistics based on diffusion-weighted probabilistic tractography. *Commun Biol.* 2022 February 17;5(1):138. https://doi.org/10.1038/s42003-022-03073-w. PMID: 35177755; PMCID: PMC8854429.
470. Hanks R, Millis S, Scott S, Gattu R, O'Hara NB, Haacke M, Kou Z. The relation between cognitive dysfunction and diffusion tensor imaging parameters in traumatic brain injury. *Brain Inj.* 2019;33(3):355–363. https://doi.org/10.1080/02699052.2018.1553073. Epub 2018 Dec 19. PMID: 30563361.
471. Toth L, Czigler A, Horvath P, et al. The effect of mild traumatic brain injury on cerebral microbleeds in aging. *Front Aging Neurosci.* 2021 September 30;13:717391. https://doi.org/10.3389/fnagi.2021.717391. PMID: 34658836; PMCID: PMC8514735.
472. Dahl J, Tenovuo O, Posti JP, et al. Cerebral microbleeds and structural white matter integrity in patients with traumatic brain injury-a diffusion tensor imaging study. *Front Neurol.* 2022 May 31;13:888815. https://doi.org/10.3389/fneur.2022.888815. PMID: 35711272; PMCID: PMC9194845.
473. Környei BS, Szabó V, Perlaki G, et al. Cerebral microbleeds May be less detectable by susceptibility weighted imaging MRI from 24 to 72 hours after traumatic brain injury. *Front Neurosci.* 2021 September 30;15:711074. https://doi.org/10.3389/fnins.2021.711074. PMID: 34658762; PMCID: PMC8514822.
474. Hu L, Yang S, Jin B, Wang C. Advanced neuroimaging role in traumatic brain injury: A narrative review. *Front Neurosci.* 2022 April 13;16:872609. https://doi.org/10.3389/fnins.2022.872609. PMID: 35495065; PMCID: PMC9043279.
475. Cosgrove ME, Saadon JR, Mikell CB, et al. Thalamo-prefrontal connectivity correlates with early command-following after severe traumatic brain injury. *Front Neurol.* 2022 February 18;13:826266. https://doi.org/10.3389/fneur.2022.826266. PMID: 35250829; PMCID: PMC8895046.
476. Dailey NS, Smith R, Bajaj S, et al. Elevated aggression and reduced white matter integrity in mild traumatic brain injury: A DTI study. *Front Behav Neurosci.* 2018 June 27;12:118. https://doi.org/10.3389/fnbeh.2018.00118. PMID: 30013466; PMCID: PMC6036267.
477. Dambinova SA, Sowell RL, Maroon JC. Gradual return to play: Potential role of neurotoxicity biomarkers in assessment of concussions severity. *J Mol Biomark Diagn.* 2013;S3:003. https://doi.org/10.4172/2155-9929.S3-003.
478. Patestas MA, Gartner LP. *A textbook of neuroanatomy.* 1st ed. Malden: Blackwell Publishing, 2006.
479. Buyanova IS, Arsalidou M. Cerebral white matter myelination and relations to age, gender, and cognition: A selective review. *Front Hum Neurosci.* 2021;15:662031. https://doi.org/10.3389/fnhum.2021.662031. PMID: 34295229; PMCID: PMC8290169.
480. Donkelaar HJT, Catani M, Domburg PV, Eling PATM, Kusters B, Hori A. The cerebral cortex and complex cerebral functions. In: Donkelaar HTJ, editor. *Clinical neuroanatomy: Brain circuitry and its disorders.* 2nd ed. Switzerland: Springer Nature, 2020; p. 831–952.

481. Gatto RG. Molecular and microstructural biomarkers of neuroplasticity in neurodegenerative disorders through preclinical and diffusion magnetic resonance imaging studies. *J Integr Neurosci.* 2020 September 30;19(3):571–592. https://doi.org/10.31083/j.jin.2020.03.165. PMID: 33070535.
482. Parent A. *Carpenter's human anatomy.* 9th ed. Baltimore, MD: Williams & Wilkins, 1996.
483. Bear MF, Connors BW, Paradiso MA. *Neuroscience: Exploring the brain.* 4th ed. Philadelphia: Wolters Kluwer, 2016.
484. Habib M. Athymhormia and disorders of motivation in basal ganglia disease. *J Neuropsychiatry Clin Neurosci.* 2004; 16(4):509–24. https://doi.org/10.1176/jnp.16.4.509. PMID: 15616180.
485. Podell K, Wisniewski K, Lovell MR. The assessment of echopraxia as a component of executive control deficit in traumatic brain injury. *Brain and Cognition.* 2001 December 1;47(1–2):349–353.
486. Lanfermann H, Raab P, Kretschmann HJ, Weinrich W. *Clinical neuroimaging and clinical neuroanatomy: Atlas of MR imaging and computed tomography.* 4th ed. Stuttgart: Thieme, 2019.
487. Thomsen IV. Evaluation and outcome of aphasia in patients with severe closed head trauma. *J Neurol Neurosurg Psychiatry.* 1975;38(7):713–718. https://doi.org/10.1136/jnnp.38.7.713. PMID: 1159445; PMCID: PMC1083253.
488. Gerstmann's syndrome [Internet]. National Institute of Neurological Disorders and Stroke. U.S. Department of Health and Human Services; [cited 2022 Sep 7]. Available from: https://www.ninds.nih.gov/health-information/disorders/gerstmanns-syndrome
489. Moreira da Silva N, Cowie CJA, Blamire AM, Forsyth R, Taylor PN. Investigating brain network changes and their association with cognitive recovery after traumatic brain injury: A longitudinal analysis. *Front Neurol.* 2020;11:369. https://doi.org/10.3389/fneur.2020.00369. PMID: 32581989; PMCID: PMC7296134.
490. Joy MT, Ben Assayag E, Shabashov-Stone D, et al. CCR5 is a therapeutic target for recovery after stroke and traumatic brain injury. *Cell.* 2019 February 21;176(5):1143–1157.e13. https://doi.org/10.1016/j.cell.2019.01.044. PMID: 30794775; PMCID: PMC7259116.
491. Hofer AS, Schwab ME. Enhancing rehabilitation and functional recovery after brain and spinal cord trauma with electrical neuromodulation. *Curr Opin Neurol.* 2019;32(6):828–835. https://doi.org/10.1097/WCO.0000000000000750. PMID: 31567546; PMCID: PMC6855343.
492. Kononenko O, Watanabe H, Stålhandske L, et al. Focal traumatic brain injury induces neuroplastic molecular responses in lumbar spinal cord. *Restor Neurol Neurosci.* 2019;37(2):87–96. https://doi.org/10.3233/RNN-180882. PMID: 30856132; PMCID: PMC6484246.
493. Kim WS, Lee K, Kim S, Cho S, Paik NJ. Transcranial direct current stimulation for the treatment of motor impairment following traumatic brain injury. *J Neuroeng Rehabil.* 2019 January 25;16(1):14. https://doi.org/10.1186/s12984-019-0489-9. PMID: 30683136; PMCID: PMC6347832.
494. Moisset X, Lefaucheur JP. Non pharmacological treatment for neuropathic pain: Invasive and non-invasive cortical stimulation. *Rev Neurol (Paris).* 2019;175(1–2):51–58. https://doi.org/10.1016/j.neurol.2018.09.014. Epub 2018 Oct 12. PMID: 30322590.
495. Sonmez AI, Camsari DD, Nandakumar AL, et al. Accelerated TMS for depression: A systematic review and meta-analysis. *Psychiatry Res.* 2019;273:770–781. https://doi.org/10.1016/j.psychres.2018.12.041. Epub 2018 Dec 7. PMID: 31207865; PMCID: PMC6582998.
496. Kundu B, Brock AA, Englot DJ, Butson CR, Rolston JD. Deep brain stimulation for the treatment of disorders of consciousness and cognition in traumatic brain injury patients: A review. *Neurosurg Focus.* 2018;45(2):E14. https://doi.org/10.3171/2018.5.FOCUS18168. PMID: 30064315; PMCID: PMC6193266.
497. Zaninotto AL, El-Hagrassy MM, Green JR, et al. Transcranial direct current stimulation (tDCS) effects on traumatic brain injury (TBI) recovery: A systematic review. *Dement Neuropsychol.* 2019;13(2):172–179. https://doi.org/10.1590/1980-57642018dn13-020005. PMID: 31285791; PMCID: PMC6601308.

498. Galgano M, Toshkezi G, Qiu X, Russell T, Chin L, Zhao LR. Traumatic brain injury: Current treatment strategies and future endeavors. *Cell Transplant.* 2017;26(7):1118–1130. https://doi.org/10.1177/0963689717714102. PMID: 28933211; PMCID: PMC5657730.
499. Sanes JR, Jessell TM Repairing the damaged brain. In: Kandel ER, Schwartz JH, Jessell TM, Siegelbaum SA, Hudspeth AJ, editors. *Principles of neural science.* 5th ed. New York: McGraw Hill, 2013; p. 1284–1305.
500. Thakkar P, Thampi SB, Keziah S, Ramanathan S. An unusual case of posttraumatic visual agnosia posing challenges to rehabilitation. *Am J Phys Med Rehabil.* 2021;100(11):e172–e174. https://doi.org/10.1097/PHM.0000000000001792. PMID: 34001836.
501. Ardila A. Gerstmann syndrome. *Curr Neurol Neurosci Rep.* 2020 August 27;20(11):48. https://doi.org/10.1007/s11910-020-01069-9. PMID: 32852667.
502. Ardila A. Some unusual neuropsychological syndromes: Somatoparaphrenia, akinetopsia, reduplicative paramnesia, autotopagnosia. *Arch Clin Neuropsychol.* 2016;31(5):456–64. https://doi.org/10.1093/arclin/acw021. Epub 2016 May 4. PMID: 27193360.
503. Lo Buono V, De Salvo S, Paladina G, et al. Anton's syndrome associated with autotopagnosia. *Appl Neuro-Psychol Adult.* 2020;27(3):294–298. https://doi.org/10.1080/23279095.2018.1538048. Epub 2019 Jan 20. PMID: 30661390.
504. Kale U, el-Naggar M, Hawthorne M. Verbal auditory agnosia with focal EEG abnormality: An unusual case of a child presenting to An ENT surgeon with "deafness". *J Laryngol Otol.* 1995;109(5):431–432. https://doi.org/10.1017/s002221510013035x PMID: 7798001.
505. Turnbull OH, McCarthy RA. When is a view unusual? A single case study of orientation-dependent visual agnosia. *Brain Res Bull.* 1996;40(5–6):497–502.; discussion 502–503. https://doi.org/10.1016/0361-9230(96)00148-7. PMID: 8886380.
506. Balsamo M, Trojano L, Giamundo A, Grossi D. Left hand tactile agnosia after posterior callosal lesion. *Cortex.* 2008;44(8):1030–1036. https://doi.org/10.1016/j.cortex.2008.01.003. Epub 2008 May 23. PMID: 18589409.
507. Saygin AP, Leech R, Dick F. Nonverbal auditory agnosia with lesion to Wernicke's area. *Neuropsychologia.* 2010;48(1):107–113. https://doi.org/10.1016/j.neuropsychologia.2009.08.015. PMID: 19698727; PMCID: PMC2794980.
508. Bosshart H, Capek S. An unusual case of random fire-setting behavior associated with lacunar stroke. *Forensic Sci Int.* 2011 June 15;209(1–3):e8–e10. https://doi.org/10.1016/j.forsciint.2011.03.012. Epub 2011 Apr 13. PMID: 21489732.
509. Albert ML, Reches A, Silverberg R. Hemianopic colour blindness. *J Neurol Neurosurg Psychiatry.* 1975;38(6):546–549. https://doi.org/10.1136/jnnp.38.6.546. PMID: 1080190; PMCID: PMC492025.
510. van der Ham IJM, Martens MAG, Claessen MHG, van den Berg E. landmark agnosia: Evaluating the definition of landmark-based navigation impairment. *Arch Clin Neuropsychol.* 2017;32(4):472–482. https://doi.org/10.1093/arclin/acx013. PMID: 28164221.
511. Lindau M, Bjork R. Anosognosia and anosodiaphoria in mild cognitive impairment and Alzheimer's disease. *Dement Geriatr Cogn Dis Extra.* 2014;4(3):465–480. https://doi.org/10.1159/000369132. PMID: 25759713; PMCID: PMC4282043.
512. Udesen H, Madsen AL. Balint-syndrom–visuel desorientering [Balint's syndrome–visual disorientation]. *Ugeskr Laeger.* 1992 May 18; 154(21):1492–1494. Danish. PMID: 1598720.
513. Sarkar S, Tripathy K. Cortical blindness. 2022 May 29. In: *StatPearls [Internet].* Treasure Island, FL: StatPearls Publishing, 2022 Jan–. PMID: 32809461.
514. Gazzaniga MS. *Human: The science behind what makes us unique.* New York: Harper Collins, 2008.
515. Kim JM, Woo SB, Lee Z, Heo SJ, Park D. Verbal auditory agnosia in a patient with traumatic brain injury: A case report. *Medicine (Baltimore).* 2018;97(11): e0136. https://doi.org/10.1097/MD.0000000000010136. PMID: 29538212; PMCID: PMC5882388.
516. Sacks O. *The man who mistook his wife for a hat and other clinical tales.* New York: Summit Books, 2006, p 8–22.

517. Shah K, Jain SB, Wadhwa R. Capgras syndrome. 2022 June 4. In: *StatPearls [Internet]*. Treasure Island, FL: StatPearls Publishing; 2022. PMID: 34033319.
518. Vallar G, Ronchi R. Somatoparaphrenia: A body delusion. A review of the neuropsychological literature. *Exp Brain Res*. 2009;192(3):533–551. https://doi.org/10.1007/s00221-008-1562-y. Epub 2008 Sep 24. PMID: 18813916.
519. Pugnaghi M, Molinari M, Panzetti P, Nichelli PF, Zamboni G. "My sister's hand is in my bed": A case of somatoparaphrenia. *Neurol Sci*. 2012;33(5):1205–1207. https://doi.org/10.1007/s10072-011-0874-z. Epub 2011 Dec 11. PMID: 22160730.
520. Kandel ER. *In search of memory: The emergence of a new science of mind*. New York: WW Norton & Company, 2006.
521. Sturm VE, Hua AY, Rosen HJ. Self-awareness and frontal lobe networks. In: Miller BL, Cummings JL, editors. *The human frontal lobes: Functions and disorders*. New York: The Guilford Press, 2018. Chapter 11.
522. Pinker S. *How the mind works*. London, England; New York, NY; Victoria, Australia; Ontario Canada; Auckland, New Zealand: Penguin Books, 1997.
523. Van Horn JD, Irimia A, Torgerson CM, Chambers MC, Kikinis R, Toga AW. Mapping connectivity damage in the case of Phineas Gage. *PLoS One*. 2012;7(5):e37454. https://doi.org/10.1371/journal.pone.0037454. Epub 2012 May 16. PMID: 22616011; PMCID: PMC3353935.
524. Destrieux C, Fischl B, Dale A, Halgren E. Automatic parcellation of human cortical gyri and sulci using standard anatomical nomenclature. *Neuroimage*. 2010 October 15;53(1):1–15. https://doi.org/10.1016/j.neuroimage.2010.06.010. Epub 2010 Jun 12. PMID: 20547229; PMCID: PMC2937159.
525. Di Ieva A, Lam T, Alcaide-Leon P, Bharatha A, Montanera W, Cusimano MD. Magnetic resonance susceptibility weighted imaging in neurosurgery: Current applications and future perspectives. *J Neurosurg*. 2015;123(6):1463–1475. https://doi.org/10.3171/2015.1.JNS142349. Epub 2015 Jul 24. PMID: 26207600.
526. Van Essen DC, Drury HA. Structural and functional analyses of human cerebral cortex using a surface-based atlas. *J Neurosci*. 1997 September 15;17(18):7079–7102. https://doi.org/10.1523/JNEUROSCI.17-18-07079.1997. PMID: 9278543; PMCID: PMC6573261.
527. Sporns O, Tononi G, Kötter R. The human connectome: A structural description of the human brain. *PLoS Comput Biol*. 2005;1(4):e42. https://doi.org/10.1371/journal.pcbi.0010042. PMID: 16201007; PMCID: PMC1239902.
528. Hagmann P, Cammoun L, Gigandet X, et al. Mapping the structural core of human cerebral cortex. *PLoS Biol*. 2008;6(7):e159. https://doi.org/10.1371/journal.pbio.0060159. PMID: 18597554; PMCID: PMC2443193.
529. Koch C. *Consciousness: Confessions of a romantic reductionist*. Cambridge: The MIT Press, 2012.
530. Nieuwenhuys R, Voogd J, Huijzen CV. *The human central nervous system*. 4th ed. Berlin: Springer, 2008.
531. Ivanova MV, Zhong A, Turken A, Baldo JV, Dronkers NF. Functional contributions of the arcuate Fasciculus to language processing. *Front Hum Neurosci*. 2021 June 25;15:672665. https://doi.org/10.3389/fnhum.2021.672665. PMID: 34248526; PMCID: PMC8267805.
532. Bubb EJ, Metzler-Baddeley C, Aggleton JP. The cingulum bundle: Anatomy, function, and dysfunction. *Neurosci Biobehav Rev*. 2018;92:104–127. https://doi.org/10.1016/j.neubiorev.2018.05.008. Epub 2018 May 16. PMID: 29753752; PMCID: PMC6090091.
533. Senova S, Fomenko A, Gondard E, Lozano AM. Anatomy and function of the fornix in the context of its potential as a therapeutic target. *J Neurol Neurosurg Psychiatry*. 2020;91(5):547–559. https://doi.org/10.1136/jnnp-2019-322375. Epub 2020 Mar 4. PMID: 32132227; PMCID: PMC7231447.
534. Latini F, Trevisi G, Fahlström M, et al. New insights into the anatomy, connectivity and clinical implications of the middle longitudinal Fasciculus. *Front Neuroanat*. 2021 January 29;14:610324. https://doi.org/10.3389/fnana.2020.610324. PMID: 33584207; PMCID: PMC7878690.

535. Yeatman JD, Weiner KS, Pestilli F, Rokem A, Mezer A, Wandell BA. The vertical occipital fasciculus: A century of controversy resolved by in vivo measurements. *Proc Natl Acad Sci USA*. 2014;111(48):E5214–E5223. https://doi.org/10.1073/pnas.1418503111. Epub 2014 Nov 17. PMID: 25404310; PMCID: PMC4260539.
536. Navarro-Orozco D, Bollu PC. Neuroanatomy, medial lemniscus (Reils band, reils ribbon). 2021 August 11. In: *StatPearls [Internet]*. Treasure Island, FL: StatPearls Publishing, 2022 Jan–. PMID: 30252296.
537. Mehra D, Moshirfar M. Neuroanatomy, optic tract. 2021 July 31. In: *StatPearls [internet]*. Treasure Island, FL: StatPearls Publishing, 2022. PMID: 31751030.
538. Edlow BL, Barra ME, Zhou DW, et al. Personalized connectome mapping to guide targeted therapy and promote recovery of consciousness in the intensive care unit. *Neurocrit Care*. 2020;33(2):364–375. https://doi.org/10.1007/s12028-020-01062-7. Epub 2020 Aug 13. PMID: 32794142; PMCID: PMC8336723.
539. Edlow BL, Haynes RL, Takahashi E, et al. Disconnection of the ascending arousal system in traumatic coma. *J Neuropathol Exp Neurol*. 2013;72(6):505–23. https://doi.org/10.1097/NEN.0b013e3182945bf6. PMID: 23656993; PMCID: PMC3761353.
540. Das M, Mayilsamy K, Mohapatra SS, Mohapatra S. Mesenchymal stem cell therapy for the treatment of traumatic brain injury: Progress and prospects. *Rev Neurosci*. 2019 November 26;30(8):839–855. https://doi.org/10.1515/revneuro-2019-0002. PMID: 31203262.
541. Uddin LQ, Rayman J, Zaidel E. Split-Brain reveals separate but equal self-recognition in the two cerebral hemispheres. *Conscious Cogn*. 2005;14(3):633–640. https://doi.org/10.1016/j.concog.2005.01.008. PMID: 16091274.
542. Kawachi J. Brodmann areas 17, 18, and 19 in the human brain: An overview. *Brain Nerve*. 2017;69(4):397–410. Japanese. https://doi.org/10.11477/mf.1416200756. PMID: 28424394.
543. The Nobel prize in physiology or medicine 1981 [Internet]. NobelPrize.org. [cited 2022 August 22]. Available from: https://www.nobelprize.org/prizes/medicine/1981/sperry/article/
544. Morey RA, Haswell CC, Selgrade ES, et al. Effects of chronic mild traumatic brain injury on white matter integrity in Iraq and Afghanistan war veterans. *Hum Brain Mapp*. 2013;34(11):2986–2999. https://doi.org/10.1002/hbm.22117. Epub 2012 Jun 15. PMID: 22706988; PMCID: PMC3740035.
545. Miller DR, Hayes JP, Lafleche G, Salat DH, Verfaellie M. White matter abnormalities are associated with chronic postconcussion symptoms in blast-related mild traumatic brain injury. *Hum Brain Mapp*. 2016;37(1):220–229. https://doi.org/10.1002/hbm.23022. Epub 2015 Oct 24. PMID: 26497829; PMCID: PMC4760357.
546. Petrie EC, Cross DJ, Yarnykh VL, et al. Neuroimaging, behavioral, and psychological sequelae of repetitive combined blast/impact mild traumatic brain injury in Iraq and Afghanistan war veterans. *J Neurotrauma*. 2014;31(5):425–436. https://doi.org/10.1089/neu.2013.2952. PMID: 24102309; PMCID: PMC3934596.
547. Taber KH, Hurley RA, Haswell CC, Rowland JA, Hurt SD, Lamar CD, Morey RA. White matter compromise in veterans exposed to primary blast forces. *J Head Trauma Rehabil*. 2015;30(1):E15–E25. https://doi.org/10.1097/HTR.0000000000000030. PMID: 24590156; PMCID: PMC4470620.
548. Venkatasubramanian PN, Pina-Crespo JC, Mathews K, et al. Initial biphasic fractional anisotropy response to blast-induced mild traumatic brain injury in a mouse model. *Mil Med*. 2020;185(Suppl 1):243–247. https://doi.org/10.1093/milmed/usz307. PMID: 32074348; PMCID: PMC7029837.
549. Glenn GR, Kuo LW, Chao YP, Lee CY, Helpern JA, Jensen JH. Mapping the orientation of white matter fiber bundles: A comparative study of diffusion tensor imaging, diffusional kurtosis imaging, and diffusion spectrum imaging. *AJNR Am J Neuroradiol*. 2016;37(7):1216–1222. https://doi.org/10.3174/ajnr.A4714. Epub 2016 Mar 3. PMID: 26939628; PMCID: PMC4946981.

550. Wedeen VJ, Wang RP, Schmahmann JD, et al. Diffusion spectrum magnetic resonance imaging (DSI) tractography of crossing fibers. *Neuroimage*. 2008 July 15;41(4):1267–1277. https://doi.org/10.1016/j.neuroimage.2008.03.036. Epub 2008 Apr 8. PMID: 18495497.
551. Meng Y, Zhang X. In vivo diffusion spectrum imaging of non-human primate brain: Initial experience in transcallosal fiber examination. *Quant Imaging Med Surg*. 2014; 4(2):129–135. https://doi.org/10.3978/j.issn.2223-4292.2014.04.05. PMID: 24834425; PMCID: PMC4014874.
552. Wedeen VJ, Hagmann P, Tseng WY, Reese TG, Weisskoff RM. Mapping complex tissue architecture with diffusion spectrum magnetic resonance imaging. *Magn ReSon Med*. 2005;54(6):1377–86. https://doi.org/10.1002/mrm.20642. PMID: 16247738.
553. Fox MD. Mapping symptoms to brain networks with the human connectome. *N Engl J Med*. 2018;379(23):2237–2245. https://doi.org/10.1056/NEJMra1706158. PMID: 30575457.
554. Warren DE, Power JD, Bruss J, et al. Network measures predict neuropsychological outcome after brain injury. *Proc Natl Acad Sci U S A*. 2014 September 30;111(39): 14247–14252. https://doi.org/10.1073/pnas.1322173111. Epub 2014 Sep 15. PMID: 25225403; PMCID: PMC4191760.
555. Laganiere S, Boes AD, Fox MD. Network localization of hemichorea-hemiballismus. *Neurology*. 2016;86(23):2187–95. https://doi.org/10.1212/WNL.0000000000002741. Epub 2016 May 11. PMID: 27170566; PMCID: PMC4898318.
556. Darby RR, Laganiere S, Pascual-Leone A, Prasad S, Fox MD. Finding the imposter: Brain connectivity of lesions causing delusional misidentifications. *Brain*. 2017;140(2): 497–507. https://doi.org/10.1093/brain/aww288. Epub 2017 Jan 12. PMID: 28082298; PMCID: PMC5278302.
557. Fasano A, Laganiere SE, Lam S, Fox MD. Lesions causing freezing of gait localize to a cerebellar functional network. *Ann Neurol*. 2017;81(1):129–141. https://doi.org/10.1002/ana.24845. PMID: 28009063; PMCID: PMC5266642.
558. Darby RR, Horn A, Cushman F, Fox MD. Lesion network localization of criminal behavior. *Proc Natl Acad Sci USA*. 2018 January 16;115(3):601–606. https://doi.org/10.1073/pnas.1706587115. Epub 2017 Dec 18. PMID: 29255017; PMCID: PMC5776958.
559. Obaid S, Qureshi HM, Aljishi A, et al. Child neurology: Functional reorganization mediating supplementary motor area syndrome recovery in agenesis of the corpus callosum. *Neurology*. 2022 May 26;99(4):161–165. https://doi.org/10.1212/WNL.0000000000200772. Epub ahead of print. PMID: 35618432; PMCID: PMC9421776.
560. Ludwig E, Klingler J *Atlas cerebri humani: The inner structure of the brain*. Boston: Little Brown and Company, 1956.
561. Edlow BL, Takahashi E, Wu O, et al. Neuroanatomic connectivity of the human as- cending arousal system critical to consciousness and its disorders. *J Neuropathol Exp Neurol*. 2012;71(6):531–546. https://doi.org/10.1097/NEN.0b013e3182588293. PMID: 22592840; PMCID: PMC3387430.
562. Gulyaeva NV. Molecular mechanisms of neuroplasticity: An expanding universe. *Biochemistry (Mosc)*. 2017;82(3):237–242. https://doi.org/10.1134/S0006297917030014. PMID: 28320264.
563. Sandhu Z, Tanglay O, Young IM, et al. Parcellation-based anatomic modeling of the default mode network. *Brain Behav*. 2021;11(2):e01976. https://doi.org/10.1002/brb3.1976. Epub 2020 Dec 18. PMID: 33337028; PMCID: PMC7882165.
564. Alves PN, Foulon C, Karolis V, et al. An improved neuroanatomical model of the default-mode network reconciles previous neuroimaging and neuropathological findings. *Commun Biol*. 2019 October 10;2:370. https://doi.org/10.1038/s42003-019-0611-3. PMID: 31633061; PMCID: PMC6787009.
565. Buckner RL, Andrews-Hanna JR, Schacter DL. The brain's default network: Anatomy, function, and relevance to disease. *Ann N Y Acad Sci*. 2008;1124:1–38. https://doi.org/10.1196/annals.1440.011. PMID: 18400922.

566. Andrews-Hanna JR, Reidler JS, Sepulcre J, Poulin R, Buckner RL. Functional-anatomic fractionation of the brain's default network. *Neuron*. 2010 February 25;65(4):550–562. https://doi.org/10.1016/j.neuron.2010.02.005. PMID: 20188659; PMCID: PMC2848443.
567. Concepcion M, Otaduy G. Physics of diffusion weighted and diffusion tensor imaging. In: Leite CDC, Castillo M, editors. *Diffusion weighted and diffusion tensor imaging: A clinical guide*. New York: Thieme, 2016; p. 1–18.
568. Ashikaga R, Araki Y, Ishida O. MRI of head injury using FLAIR. *Neuroradiology*. 1997;39(4):239–242. https://doi.org/10.1007/s002340050401. PMID: 9144669.
569. Moe HK, Follestad T, Andelic N, et al. Traumatic axonal injury on clinical MRI: Association with the Glasgow coma scale score at scene of injury or at admission and prolonged posttraumatic amnesia. *J Neurosurg*. 2020;23:1–12. https://doi.org/10.3171/2020.6.JNS20112. Epub ahead of print. PMID: 33096528.
570. Dhollander T, Clemente A, Singh M, et al. Fixel-based analysis of diffusion MRI: Methods, applications, challenges and opportunities. *Neuroimage*. 2021;241:118417. https://doi.org/10.1016/j.neuroimage.2021.118417. Epub 2021 Jul 21. PMID: 34298083.
571. Lu LH, Barrett AM, Cibula JE, Gilmore RL, Fennell EB, Heilman KM. Dissociation of anosognosia and phantom movement during the wada test. *J Neurol Neurosurg Psychiatry*. 2000;69(6):820–823. https://doi.org/10.1136/jnnp.69.6.820. PMID: 11080240; PMCID: PMC1737173.
572. Pearson J, Westbrook F. Phantom perception: Voluntary and involuntary nonretinal vision. *Trends Cogn Sci*. 2015;19(5):278–284. https://doi.org/10.1016/j.tics.2015.03.004. Epub 2015 Apr 8. PMID: 25863415.
573. Ramachandran VS, Hirstein W. The perception of phantom limbs. The d. O. Hebb lecture. *Brain*. 1998;121(Pt 9):1603–1630. https://doi.org/10.1093/brain/121.9.1603. PMID: 9762952.
574. Huang J. Agnosia - neurologic disorders [Internet]. Merck Manuals Professional Edition. Merck Manuals; [cited 2022 September 18]. Available from: https://www.merckmanuals.com/professional/neurologic-disorders/function-and-dysfunction-of-the-cerebral-lobes/agnosia. 2022.
575. Saetta G, Zindel-Geisseler O, Stauffacher F, Serra C, Vannuscorps G, Brugger P. Aso- Matognosia: Structured interview and assessment of visuomotor imagery. *Front Psychol*. 2021 January 14;11:544544. https://doi.org/10.3389/fpsyg.2020.544544. PMID: 33519574; PMCID: PMC7840572.
576. Martinaud O. Visual agnosia and focal brain injury. *Rev Neurol (Paris)*. 2017;173(7–8):451–460. https://doi.org/10.1016/j.neurol.2017.07.009. Epub 2017 Aug 24. PMID: 28843416.
577. Hawryluk GWJ, Rubiano AM, Totten AM, et al. Guidelines for the management of severe traumatic brain injury: 2020 update of the decompressive craniectomy recommendations. *Neurosurgery*. 2020;87(3):427–434. https://doi.org/10.1093/neuros/nyaa278. PMID: 32761068; PMCID: PMC7426189.
578. Liotta EM. Management of cerebral edema, brain compression, and intracranial pressure. *Continuum (Minneap Minn)*. 2021;27(5):1172–1200. https://doi.org/10.1212/CON.0000000000000988. PMID: 34618757.
579. Lewis SR, Evans DJ, Butler AR, Schofield-Robinson OJ, Alderson P. Hypothermia for traumatic brain injury. *Cochrane Database Syst Rev*. 2017 September 21;9(9):CD001048. https://doi.org/10.1002/14651858.CD001048.pub5. PMID: 28933514; PMCID: PMC6483736.
580. Mani K, Cater B, Hudlikar A. Cognition and return to work after mild/moderate traumatic brain injury: A systematic review. *Work*. 2017 September 14;58(1):51–62. https://doi.org/10.3233/WOR-172597. PMID: 28922176.
581. Basso A, Previgliano I, Servadei F. Traumatic brain injuries. In: Aarli JA, Avanzini G, Bertolate JM, et al., editors. *Neurological disorders: Public health challenges*. Switzerland: World Health Organization, 2006; p. 164.

582. Yue JK, Phelps RR, Hemmerle DD, et al., & TRACK-TBI Investigators. Predictors of six-month inability to return to work in previously employed subjects after mild traumatic brain injury: A TRACK-TBI pilot study. *J Concussion*. 2021 January–December;5. https://doi.org/10.1177/20597002211007271. Epub 2021 Apr 6. PMID: 34046212; PMCID: PMC8153496.
583. O'Neill J, Hibbard MR, Brown M, et al. The effect of employment on quality of life and community integration after traumatic brain injury. *J Head Trauma Rehabil*. 1998;13(4):68–79. https://doi.org/10.1097/00001199-199808000-00007. PMID: 9651241.
584. van der Vlegel M, Polinder S, Mikolic A, et al. The center-TBI participants and investigators. The association of post-concussion and post- traumatic stress disorder symptoms with health-related quality of life, health care use and return-to-work after mild traumatic brain injury. *J Clin Med*. 2021;10(11):2473. https://doi.org/10.3390/jcm10112473. PMID: 34199591; PMCID: PMC8199686.
585. Dumke HA Posttraumatic headache and its impact on return to work after mild traumatic brain injury. *J Head Trauma Rehabil*. 2017;32(2):E55–E65. https://doi.org/10.1097/HTR.0000000000000244. PMID: 27323219.
586. Theadom A, Barker-Collo S, Jones K, et al., & BIONIC4you Research Group. Work limitations 4 years after mild traumatic brain injury: A cohort study. *Arch Phys Med Rehabil*. 2017;98(8):1560–1566. https://doi.org/10.1016/j.apmr.2017.01.010. Epub 2017 Feb 8. PMID: 28188778.
587. Lebel C, Deoni S. The development of brain white matter microstructure. *Neuroimage*. 2018 November 15;182:207–218. https://doi.org/10.1016/j.neuroimage.2017.12.097. Epub 2018 Jan 3. PMID: 29305910; PMCID: PMC6030512.
588. Sibilia F, Custer RM, Irimia A, Sepehrband F, Toga AW, Cabeen RP, & TRACK-TBI Investigators. Life after mild traumatic brain injury: Widespread structural brain changes associated with psychological distress revealed with multimodal magnetic resonance imaging. *Biol. Psychiatry Global Open Sci*. 2022:1–12. https://www.medrxiv.org/content/10.1101/2021.11.03.21265823v1
589. Narayana PA. White matter changes in patients with mild traumatic brain injury: MRI perspective. *Concussion*. 2017 March 22;2(2):CNC35. https://doi.org/10.2217/cnc-2016-0028. PMID: 30202576; PMCID: PMC6093760.
590. Feydy A, Carlier R, Roby-Brami A, et al. Longitudinal study of motor recovery after stroke: Recruitment and focusing of brain activation. *Stroke*. 2002;33(6):1610–1617. https://doi.org/10.1161/01.str.0000017100.68294.52. PMID: 12053000.
591. Seitz RJ, Huang Y, Knorr U, Tellmann L, Herzog H, Freund HJ. Large-scale plasticity of the human motor cortex. *Neuroreport*. 1995 March 27;6(5):742–744. https://doi.org/10.1097/00001756-199503270-00009. PMID: 7605938.
592. Marshall RS, Perera GM, Lazar RM, Krakauer JW, Constantine RC, DeLaPaz RL. Evolution of cortical activation during recovery from corticospinal tract infarction. *Stroke*. 2000;31(3):656–661. https://doi.org/10.1161/01.str.31.3.656. PMID: 10700500.
593. Tonti E, Budini M, Vingolo EM. Visuo-acoustic Stimulation's role in synaptic plasticity: A review of the literature. *Int J Mol Sci*. 2021;22(19):10783. https://doi.org/10.3390/ijms221910783. PMID: 34639122; PMCID: PMC8509608.
594. Johnston MV. Plasticity in the developing brain: Implications for rehabilitation. *Dev Disabil Res Rev*. 2009;15(2):94–101. https://doi.org/10.1002/ddrr.64. PMID: 19489084.
595. Dimyan MA, Cohen LG. Neuroplasticity in the context of motor rehabilitation after stroke. *Nat Rev Neurol*. 2011;7(2):76–85. https://doi.org/10.1038/nrneurol.2010.200. Epub 2011 Jan 18. PMID: 21243015; PMCID: PMC4886719.
596. Nowak DA, Grefkes C, Ameli M, Fink GR. Interhemispheric competition after stroke: Brain stimulation to enhance recovery of function of the affected hand. *Neurorehabil Neural Repair*. 2009;23(7):641–656. https://doi.org/10.1177/1545968309336661. Epub 2009 Jun 16. PMID: 19531606.

597. Desmurget M, Bonnetblanc F, Duffau H. Contrasting acute and slow-growing lesions: A new door to brain plasticity. *Brain*. 2007;130(Pt 4):898–914. https://doi.org/10.1093/brain/awl300. Epub 2006 Nov 21. PMID: 17121742.
598. Floel A, Cohen LG. Recovery of function in humans: Cortical stimulation and pharmacological treatments after stroke. *Neurobiol Dis*. 2010;37(2):243–2451. https://doi.org/10.1016/j.nbd.2009.05.027. Epub 2009 Jun 9. PMID: 19520165; PMCID: PMC4886709.
599. Saur D, Lange R, Baumgaertner A, et al. Dynamics of language reorganization after stroke. *Brain*. 2006;129(Pt 6):1371–1384. https://doi.org/10.1093/brain/awl090. Epub 2006 Apr 25. PMID: 16638796.
600. Kujala T, Alho K, Näätänen R. Cross-modal reorganization of human cortical functions. *Trends Neurosci*. 2000;23(3):115–120. https://doi.org/10.1016/s0166-2236(99)01504-0. PMID: 10675915.
601. Bashir S, Mizrahi I, Weaver K, Fregni F, Pascual-Leone A. Assessment and modulation of neural plasticity in rehabilitation with transcranial magnetic stimulation. *PM R*. 2010;2(12 Suppl 2):S253–S268. https://doi.org/10.1016/j.pmrj.2010.10.015. PMID: 21172687; PMCID: PMC3951769.
602. Rauschecker JP. Compensatory plasticity and sensory substitution in the cerebral cortex. *Trends Neurosci*. 1995;18(1):36–43. https://doi.org/10.1016/0166-2236(95)93948-w. PMID: 7535489.
603. Pascual-Leone A, Torres F. Plasticity of the sensorimotor cortex representation of the reading finger in braille readers. *Brain*. 1993;116(Pt 1):39–52. https://doi.org/10.1093/brain/116.1.39. PMID: 8453464.
604. Ewall G, Parkins S, Lin A, Jaoui Y, Lee HK. Cortical and subcortical circuits for cross-modal plasticity induced by loss of vision. *Front Neural Circuits*. 2021 May 25;15:665009. https://doi.org/10.3389/fncir.2021.665009. PMID: 34113240; PMCID: PMC8185208.
605. Froudist-Walsh S, Browning PG, Young JJ, Murphy KL, Mars RB, Fleysher L, Croxson PL, Macro-connectomics and microstructure predict dynamic plasticity patterns in the non-human primate brain. *Elife*. 2018 November 21;7:e34354. https://doi.org/10.7554/eLife.34354. PMID: 30462609; PMCID: PMC6249000.
606. Schaefers AT, Teuchert-Noodt G. Developmental neuroplasticity and the origin of neurodegenerative diseases. *World J Biol Psychiatry*. 2016;17(8):587–599. https://doi.org/10.3109/15622975.2013.797104. Epub 2013 May 24. PMID: 23705632.
607. Moreno-Jiménez EP, Flor-García M, Terreros-Roncal J, et al. Adult hippocampal neurogenesis is abundant in neurologically healthy subjects and drops sharply in patients with Alzheimer's disease. *Nat Med*. 2019;25(4):554–560. https://doi.org/10.1038/s41591-019-0375-9. Epub 2019 Mar 25. PMID: 30911133.
608. Weerasinghe-Mudiyanselage PDE, Ang MJ, Kang S, Kim JS, Moon C. Structural plasticity of the hippocampus in neurodegenerative diseases. *Int J Mol Sci*. 2022 March 20;23(6):3349. https://doi.org/10.3390/ijms23063349. PMID: 35328770; PMCID: PMC8955928.
609. Lai KO, Ip NY. Structural plasticity of dendritic spines: The underlying mechanisms and its dysregulation in brain disorders. *Biochim Biophys Acta*. 2013;1832(12):2257–2263. https://doi.org/10.1016/j.bbadis.2013.08.012. Epub 2013 Sep 6. PMID: 24012719.
610. Hogan MK, Hamilton GF, Horner PJ. Neural stimulation and molecular mechanisms of plasticity and regeneration: A review. *Front Cell Neurosci*. 2020 October 14;14:271. https://doi.org/10.3389/fncel.2020.00271. PMID: 33173465; PMCID: PMC7591397.
611. Naeve GS, Ramakrishnan M, Kramer R, Hevroni D, Citri Y, Theill LE. Neuritin: A Gene induced by neural activity and neurotrophins that promotes neuritogenesis. *Proc Natl Acad Sci U S A*. 1997 March 18;94(6):2648–2653. https://doi.org/10.1073/pnas.94.6.2648. PMID: 9122250; PMCID: PMC20143.
612. Flavell SW, Greenberg ME Signaling mechanisms linking neuronal activity to gene expression and plasticity of the nervous system. *Annu Rev Neurosci*. 2008;31:563–590. https://doi.org/10.1146/annurev.neuro.31.060407.125631. PMID: 18558867; PMCID: PMC2728073.

613. Crenn P, Hamchaoui S, Bourget-Massari A, Hanachi M, Melchior JC, Azouvi P. Changes in weight after traumatic brain injury in adult patients: A longitudinal study. *Clin Nutr.* 2014;33(2):348–353. https://doi.org/10.1016/j.clnu.2013.06.003. Epub 2013 Jun 10. PMID: 23810396.
614. Cope EC, Gould E. Adult neurogenesis, glia, and the extracellular matrix. *Cell Stem Cell.* 2019;24(5):690–705. https://doi.org/10.1016/j.stem.2019.03.023. PMID: 31051133; PMCID: PMC7961263.
615. Smith AC, Scofield MD, Kalivas PW. The tetrapartite synapse: Extracellular matrix remodeling contributes to corticoaccumbens plasticity underlying drug addiction. *Brain Res.* 2015;1628(Pt A):29–39. https://doi.org/10.1016/j.brainres.2015.03.027. Epub 2015 Mar 30. PMID: 25838241; PMCID: PMC4589426.
616. Chancey JH, Adlaf EW, Sapp MC, Pugh PC, Wadiche JI, Overstreet-Wadiche LS. GABA depolarization is required for experience-dependent synapse unsilencing in adult-born neurons. *J Neurosci.* 2013 April 10;33(15):6614–6622. https://doi.org/10.1523/JNEUROSCI.0781-13.2013. PMID: 23575858; PMCID: PMC3657840.
617. Carulli D, Verhaagen J. An extracellular perspective on CNS maturation: Perineuronal nets and the control of plasticity. *Int J Mol Sci.* 2021 February 28;22(5):2434. https://doi.org/10.3390/ijms22052434. PMID: 33670945; PMCID: PMC7957817.
618. Sims RE, Butcher JB, Parri HR, Glazewski S. Astrocyte and neuronal plasticity in the somatosensory system. *Neural Plast.* 2015;2015:732014. https://doi.org/10.1155/2015/732014. Epub 2015 Aug 4. PMID: 26345481; PMCID: PMC4539490.
619. Liu HH, McClatchy DB, Schiapparelli L, Shen W, Yates JR 3rd, Cline HT. Role of the visual experience-dependent nascent proteome in neuronal plasticity. *Elife.* 2018;7:e33420. https://doi.org/10.7554/eLife.33420. PMID: 29412139; PMCID: PMC5815848.
620. Bonfanti L, Charvet CJ. Brain plasticity in humans and model systems: Advances, challenges, and future directions. *Int J Mol Sci.* 2021 August 28;22(17):9358. https://doi.org/10.3390/ijms22179358. PMID: 34502267; PMCID: PMC8431131.
621. Bao H, Song J. Treating brain disorders by targeting adult neural stem cells. *Trends Mol Med.* 2018;24(12):991–1006. https://doi.org/10.1016/j.molmed.2018.10.001. Epub 2018 Nov 14. PMID: 30447904; PMCID: PMC6351137.
622. Consalez GG, Goldowitz D, Casoni F, Hawkes R. Origins, development, and compartmentation of the granule cells of the cerebellum. *Front Neural Circuits.* 2021 January 15;14:611841. https://doi.org/10.3389/fncir.2020.611841. PMID: 33519389; PMCID: PMC7843939.
623. Qiu MG, Zhang JN, Zhang Y, Li QY, Xie B, Wang J. Diffusion tensor imaging-based research on human white matter anatomy. *ScientificWorldJournal.* 2012;2012:530432. https://doi.org/10.1100/2012/530432. Epub 2012 Nov 25. PMID: 23226983; PMCID: PMC3512272.
624. Rader MA, Ellis DW. The Sensory Stimulation Assessment Measure (SSAM): A tool for early evaluation of severely brain-injured patients. *Brain Inj.* 1994 May-Jun;8(4):309–321. https://doi.org/10.3109/02699059409150982. PMID: 8081346.
625. Hernandez F, Giordano C, Goubran M, et al. Lateral impacts correlate with falx cerebri displacement and corpus callosum trauma in sports-related concussions. *Biomech Model Mechanobiol.* 2019 Jun;18(3):631–649. https://doi.org/10.1007/s10237-018-01106-0. Epub 2019 Mar 12. PMID: 30859404.
626. Omalu BI, DeKosky ST, Minster RL, Kamboh MI, Hamilton RL, Wecht CH. Chronic traumatic encephalopathy in a National Football League player. *Neurosurgery.* 2005 Jul;57(1):128–134; discussion 128–134. https://doi.org/10.1227/01.neu.0000163407.92769.ed. PMID: 15987548.
627. Omalu B. Chronic traumatic encephalopathy. *Prog Neurol Surg.* 2014;28:38–49. https://doi.org/10.1159/000358761. Epub 2014 Jun 6. PMID: 24923391.

628. Panikkath R, Panikkath D, Mojumder D, Nugent K. The alien hand syndrome. *Proc (Bayl Univ Med Cent)*. 2014 Jul;27(3): 219–220. https://doi.org/10.1080/08998280.2014.11929115. PMID: 24982566; PMCID: PMC4059570.
629. Campbell WW. Disorders of speech and language. In: *DeJong's the neurologic examination*. 7th ed. Wolters Kluwer and Lippincott Williams & Wilkins, 2013; p. 87–112.
630. Morell AA, Eichberg DG, Shah AH, et al. Using machine learning to evaluate large-scale brain networks in patients with brain tumors: Traditional and non-traditional eloquent areas. *Neurooncol Adv*. 2022 Sep 19;4(1):vdac142. https://doi.org/10.1093/noajnl/vdac142. PMID: 36299797; PMCID: PMC9586213.
631. Seeley WW. The salience network: A neural system for perceiving and responding to homeostatic demands. *J Neurosci*. 2019 Dec 11;39(50):9878–9882. https://doi.org/10.1523/JNEUROSCI.1138-17.2019. Epub 2019 Nov 1. PMID: 31676604; PMCID: PMC6978945.
632. Menon V, Uddin LQ. Saliency, switching, attention and control: A network model of insula function. *Brain Struct Funct*. 2010 Jun;214(5–6):655–667. https://doi.org/10.1007/s00429-010-0262-0. Epub 2010 May 29. PMID: 20512370; PMCID: PMC2899886.
633. Heinonen J, Numminen J, Hlushchuk Y, Antell H, Taatila V, Suomala J. Default mode and executive networks areas: Association with the serial order in divergent thinking. *PLoS One*. 2016 Sep 14;11(9):e0162234. https://doi.org/10.1371/journal.pone.0162234. PMID: 27627760; PMCID: PMC5023093.
634. Vossel S, Geng JJ, Fink GR. Dorsal and ventral attention systems: Distinct neural circuits but collaborative roles. *Neuroscientist*. 2014 Apr;20(2):150–159. https://doi.org/10.1177/1073858413494269. Epub 2013 Jul 8. PMID: 23835449; PMCID: PMC4107817.
635. Mallas EJ, De Simoni S, Scott G, et al. Abnormal dorsal attention network activation in memory impairment after traumatic brain injury. *Brain*. 2021 Feb 12;144(1): 114–127. https://doi.org/10.1093/brain/awaa380. PMID: 33367761.
636. Corbetta M, Shulman GL. Spatial neglect and attention networks. *Annu Rev Neurosci*. 2011;34:569–599. https://doi.org/10.1146/annurev-neuro-061010-113731. PMID: 21692662; PMCID: PMC3790661.
637. Bateman JR, Filley CM, Ross ED, et al. Aprosodia and prosoplegia with right frontal neurodegeneration. *Neurocase*. 2019 Oct;25(5):187–194. https://doi.org/10.1080/13554794.2019.1646291. Epub 2019 Jul 23. PMID: 31335278; PMCID: PMC7510567.
638. Dieguez S. Cotard syndrome. *Front Neurol Neurosci*. 2018;42:23–34. https://doi.org/10.1159/000475679. Epub 2017 Nov 17. PMID: 29151088.
639. Hayashi R, Yamaguchi S, Narimatsu T, Miyata H, Katsumata Y, Mimura M. Statokinetic dissociation (Riddoch Phenomenon) in a patient with homonymous hemianopsia as the first sign of posterior cortical atrophy. *Case Rep Neurol*. 2017 Nov 10;9(3):256–260. https://doi.org/10.1159/000481304. PMID: 29422846; PMCID: PMC5803707.
640. Zeki S, Ffytche DH. The Riddoch syndrome: Insights into the neurobiology of conscious vision. *Brain*. 1998 Jan;121(Pt 1):25–45. https://doi.org/10.1093/brain/121.1.25. PMID: 9549486.
641. Thakur T, Gupta V. Auditory hallucinations. 2022 May 2. In: *StatPearls [Internet]*. Treasure Island, FL: StatPearls Publishing, 2022 Jan–. PMID: 32491565.
642. Pysick H, Dexter D, Lindsay C. Verbal amnesia secondary to unilateral infarct of the mediodorsal thalamic nucleus. *WMJ*. 2021 Oct;120(3):247–249. PMID: 34710312.
643. Covell T, Siddiqui W. Korsakoff syndrome. 2022 Jul 20. In: *StatPearls [Internet]*. Treasure Island, FL: StatPearls Publishing, 2022 Jan–. PMID: 30969676.
644. Gennaro RJ. Synesthesia, hallucination, and autism. *Front Biosci (Landmark Ed)*. 2021 Jan 1;26(4):797–809. https://doi.org/10.2741/4918. PMID: 33049694.

645. Chen P, Hartman AJ, Priscilla Galarza C, DeLuca J. Global processing training to improve visuospatial memory deficits after right-brain stroke. *Arch Clin Neuropsychol.* 2012 Dec;27(8):891–905. https://doi.org/10.1093/arclin/acs089. Epub 2012 Oct 15. PMID: 23070314; PMCID: PMC3589919.
646. Kertesz A, Jesso S, Harciarek M, Blair M, McMonagle P. What is semantic dementia?: A cohort study of diagnostic features and clinical boundaries. *Arch Neurol.* 2010 Apr;67(4):483–489. https://doi.org/10.1001/archneurol.2010.55. PMID: 20385916.
647. Kurowski K, Blumstein SE. Phonetic basis of phonemic paraphasias in aphasia: Evidence for cascading activation. *Cortex.* 2016 Feb;75:193–203. https://doi.org/10.1016/j.cortex.2015.12.005. Epub 2015 Dec 31. PMID: 26808838; PMCID: PMC4754157.
648. Milner AD. Is visual processing in the dorsal stream accessible to consciousness? *Proc Biol Sci.* 2012 Jun 22;279(1737):2289–2298. https://doi.org/10.1098/rspb.2011.2663. Epub 2012 Mar 28. PMID: 22456882; PMCID: PMC3350678.
649. Yagmurlu K, Middlebrooks EH, Tanriover N, Rhoton AL Jr. Fiber tracts of the dorsal language stream in the human brain. *J Neurosurg.* 2016 May;124(5):1396–1405. https://doi.org/10.3171/2015.5.JNS15455. Epub 2015 Nov 20. PMID: 26587654.
650. Weiller C, Reisert M, Peto I, et al. The ventral pathway of the human brain: A continuous association tract system. *Neuroimage.* 2021 Jul 1;234:117977. https://doi.org/10.1016/j.neuroimage.2021.117977. Epub 2021 Mar 21. PMID: 33757905.
651. Blom JD. Leroy's elusive little people: A systematic review on lilliputian hallucinations. *Neurosci Biobehav Rev.* 2021 Jun;125:627–636. https://doi.org/10.1016/j.neubiorev.2021.03.002. Epub 2021 Mar 4. PMID: 33676962.
652. Szczotka J, Wierzchoń M. Splitting the unity of bodily self: Toward a comprehensive review of phenomenology and psychopathology of heautoscopy. *Psychopathology.* 2022 Nov 4;1–9. https://doi.org/10.1159/000526869. Epub ahead of print. PMID: 36349795.
653. Sato Y, Berrios GE. Extracampine hallucinations. *Lancet.* 2003 Apr 26;361(9367):1479–1480. https://doi.org/10.1016/s0140-6736(03)13128-5. PMID: 12727431.
654. Watanabe K. [Paroxysmal perceptual alteration in comparison with hallucination—a review of its clinical reports and discussion of its pathophysiological mechanism in the present day, when second generation antipsychotics are widely used]. *Seishin Shinkeigaku Zasshi.* 2009;111(2):127–136. Japanese. PMID: 19378769.
655. Choi SH, Kim YB, Paek SH, Cho ZH. Papez circuit observed by in vivo human brain with 7.0T MRI super-resolution track density imaging and track tracing. *Front Neuroanat.* 2019 Feb 18;13:17. https://doi.org/10.3389/fnana.2019.00017. PMID: 30833891; PMCID: PMC6387901.
656. Aggleton JP, Nelson AJD, O'Mara SM. Time to retire the serial Papez circuit: Implications for space, memory, and attention. *Neurosci Biobehav Rev.* 2022 Sep;140:104813. https://doi.org/10.1016/j.neubiorev.2022.104813. Epub 2022 Aug 5. PMID: 35940310.
657. O'Neill TJ, Davenport EM, Murugesan G, Montillo A, Maldjian JA. Applications of resting state functional MR imaging to traumatic brain injury. *Neuroimaging Clin N Am.* 2017 Nov;27(4):685–696. https://doi.org/10.1016/j.nic.2017.06.006. Epub 2017 Aug 18. PMID: 28985937; PMCID: PMC5708891.
658. Lee RR, Huang M. Magnetoencephalography in the diagnosis of concussion. *Prog Neurol Surg.* 2014;28:94–111. https://doi.org/10.1159/000358768. Epub 2014 Jun 6. PMID: 24923396.
659. Raji CA, Henderson TA. PET and single-photon emission computed tomography in brain concussion. *Neuroimaging Clin N Am.* 2018 Feb;28(1):67–82. https://doi.org/10.1016/j.nic.2017.09.003. PMID: 29157854.
660. Amen DG, Willeumier K, Omalu B, Newberg A, Raghavendra C, Raji CA. Perfusion neuroimaging abnormalities alone distinguish National Football League players from a healthy population. *J Alzheimers Dis.* 2016 Apr 25;53(1):237–241. https://doi.org/10.3233/JAD-160207. PMID: 27128374; PMCID: PMC4942725.

661. https://www.merriam-webster.com/dictionary/mild. (Accessed January 27, 2023)
662. Dwyer B, Katz DI. Postconcussion syndrome. *Handb Clin Neurol.* 2018;158:163–178. https://doi.org/10.1016/B978-0-444-63954-7.00017-3. PMID: 30482344.
663. Mac Donald CL, Barber J, Andre J, et al. 5-Year imaging sequelae of concussive blast injury and relation to early clinical outcome. *Neuroimage Clin.* 2017 Feb 9; 14:371–378. https://doi.org/10.1016/j.nicl.2017.02.005. PMID: 28243574; PMCID: PMC5320067.
664. Nicolas S, Nicolas D. Triptans. 2022 Aug 25. In: *StatPearls [internet].* Treasure Island, FL: StatPearls Publishing, 2022. PMID: 32119394.
665. Jackson JL, Shimeall W, Sessums L, et al. Tricyclic antidepressants and headaches: Systematic review and meta-analysis. *BMJ.* 2010 Oct 20;341:c5222. https://doi.org/10.1136/bmj.c5222. PMID: 20961988; PMCID: PMC2958257.
666. Hu C, Zhang Y, Tan G. Advances in topiramate as prophylactic treatment for migraine. *Brain Behav.* 2021 Oct;11(10):e2290. https://doi.org/10.1002/brb3.2290. Epub 2021 Sep 2. PMID: 34472696; PMCID: PMC8553310.
667. Schneider J, Patterson M, Jimenez XF. Beyond depression: Other uses for tricyclic antidepressants. *Cleve Clin J Med.* 2019 Dec;86(12):807–814. https://doi.org/10.3949/ccjm.86a.19005. PMID: 31821138.
668. Edvinsson L. CGRP and migraine: From bench to bedside. *Rev Neurol (Paris).* 2021 Sep;177(7):785–790. https://doi.org/10.1016/j.neurol.2021.06.003. Epub 2021 Jul 15. PMID: 34275653.
669. Taylor RL, Wise KJ, Taylor D, Chaudhary S, Thorne PR. Patterns of vestibular dysfunction in chronic traumatic brain injury. *Front Neurol.* 2022 Dec 1;13:942349. https://doi.org/10.3389/fneur.2022.942349. PMID: 36530624; PMCID: PMC9751886.
670. Falls C. Videonystagmography and posturography. *Adv Otorhinolaryngol.* 2019;82:32–38. https://doi.org/10.1159/000490269. Epub 2019 Jan 15. PMID: 30947200.
671. Ganança MM, Caovilla HH, Ganança FF. Electronystagmography versus videonystagmography. *Braz J Otorhinolaryngol.* 2010 May-Jun;76(3):399–403. https://doi.org/10.1590/S1808-86942010000300021. PMID: 20658023; PMCID: PMC9442181.
672. Cary D Alberstone, Edward C Benzel, Imad M Najm, Michael P Steinmetz. Vestibular system. *Anatomic basis of neurologic diagnosis.* New York, Stuttgart: Thieme, 2009; p. 411–421.
673. Nochi M. "Loss of self" in the narratives of people with traumatic brain injuries: A qualitative analysis. *Soc Sci Med.* 1998 Apr;46(7):869–878. https://doi.org/10.1016/s0277-9536(97)00211-6. PMID: 9541072.
674. Galeno E, Pullano E, Mourad F, Galeoto G, Frontani F. Effectiveness of vestibular rehabilitation after concussion: A systematic review of randomised controlled trial. Healthcare *(Basel).* 2022 Dec 28;11(1):90. https://doi.org/10.3390/healthcare11010090. PMID: 36611549; PMCID: PMC9819464.
675. Sinnott AM, Elbin RJ, Collins MW, Reeves VL, Holland CL, Kontos AP. Persistent vestibular-ocular impairment following concussion in adolescents. *J Sci Med Sport.* 2019 Dec;22(12):1292–1297. https://doi.org/10.1016/j.jsams.2019.08.004. Epub 2019 Aug 8. PMID: 31521485; PMCID: PMC6825555.
676. Hunt DL, Oldham J, Aaron SE, Tan CO, Meehan WP 3rd, Howell DR. Dizziness, psychosocial function, and postural stability following sport-related concussion. *Clin J Sport Med.* 2022 Jul 1;32(4):361–367. https://doi.org/10.1097/JSM.0000000000000923. Epub 2021 Mar 9. PMID: 34009789; PMCID: PMC8426409.
677. Mucha A, Fedor S, DeMarco D. Vestibular dysfunction and concussion. *Handb Clin Neurol.* 2018;158:135–144. https://doi.org/10.1016/B978-0-444-63954-7.00014-8. PMID: 30482341.
678. Alashram AR, Annino G, Raju M, Padua E. Effects of physical therapy interventions on balance ability in people with traumatic brain injury: A systematic review. *NeuroRehabilitation.* 2020;46(4):455–466. https://doi.org/10.3233/NRE-203047. PMID: 32508337.

679. Kleffelgaard I, Soberg HL, Tamber AL, et al. The effects of vestibular rehabilitation on dizziness and balance problems in patients after traumatic brain injury: A randomized controlled trial. *Clin Rehabil.* 2019 Jan;33(1):74–84. https://doi.org/10.1177/0269215518791274. Epub 2018 Jul 30. PMID: 30056743.
680. Martínez-Molina N, Siponkoski ST, Särkämö T. Cognitive efficacy and neural mechanisms of music-based neurological rehabilitation for traumatic brain injury. *Ann NY Acad Sci.* 2022 Sep;1515(1):20–32. https://doi.org/10.1111/nyas.14800. Epub 2022 Jun 8. PMID: 35676218; PMCID: PMC9796942.
681. Chen Y, Wang L, You W, et al. Hyperbaric oxygen therapy promotes consciousness, cognitive function, and prognosis recovery in patients following traumatic brain injury through various pathways. *Front Neurol.* 2022 Aug 10;13:929386. https://doi.org/10.3389/fneur.2022.929386. PMID: 36034283; PMCID: PMC9402226.
682. Lu Y, Zhou X, Cheng J, Ma Q. Early intensified rehabilitation training with hyperbaric oxygen therapy improves functional disorders and prognosis of patients with traumatic brain injury. *Adv Wound Care (New Rochelle).* 2021 Dec;10(12):663–670. https://doi.org/10.1089/wound.2018.0876. Epub 2019 Mar 15. PMID: 34546088; PMCID: PMC8568788.
683. Bremer B, Wu Q, Mora Álvarez MG, et al. Mindfulness meditation increases default mode, salience, and central executive network connectivity. *Sci Rep.* 2022 Aug 2;12(1):13219. https://doi.org/10.1038/s41598-022-17325-6. PMID: 35918449; PMCID: PMC9346127.
684. Galetto V, Sacco K. Neuroplastic changes induced by cognitive rehabilitation in traumatic brain injury: A review. *Neurorehabil Neural Repair.* 2017 Sep;31(9):800–813. https://doi.org/10.1177/1545968317723748. Epub 2017 Aug 8. PMID: 28786307.
685. Nowell C, Downing M, Bragge P, Ponsford J. Current practice of cognitive rehabilitation following traumatic brain injury: An international survey. *Neuropsychol Rehabil.* 2020 Dec;30(10):1976–1995. https://doi.org/10.1080/09602011.2019.1623823. Epub 2019 Jun 5. PMID: 31164047.
686. Maggio MG, De Luca R, Molonia F, et al. Cognitive rehabilitation in patients with traumatic brain injury: A narrative review on the emerging use of virtual reality. *J Clin Neurosci.* 2019 Mar;61:1–4. https://doi.org/10.1016/j.jocn.2018.12.020. Epub 2019 Jan 4. PMID: 30616874.
687. Lee SY, Amatya B, Judson R, et al. Clinical practice guidelines for rehabilitation in traumatic brain injury: A critical appraisal. *Brain Inj.* 2019;33(10):1263–1271. https://doi.org/10.1080/02699052.2019.1641747. Epub 2019 Jul 17. PMID: 31314607.
688. TBI (Traumatic Brain Injury). https://clinicaltrials.gov/ct2/results?cond=TBI+%28Traumatic+Brain+Injury%29&term=&cntry=&state=&city=&dist=. (Accessed on January 28, 2023).
689. Guideline Development Panel for the Treatment of PTSD in Adults, American Psychological Association. Summary of the clinical practice guideline for the treatment of posttraumatic stress disorder (PTSD) in adults. *Am Psychol.* 2019 Jul-Aug;74(5):596–607. https://doi.org/10.1037/amp0000473. PMID: 31305099.
690. Palacios EM, Yuh EL, Mac Donald CL, et al. Diffusion tensor imaging reveals elevated diffusivity of white matter microstructure that is independently associated with long-term outcome after mild traumatic brain injury: A TRACK-TBI study. *J Neurotrauma.* 2022 Oct;39(19–20):1318–1328. https://doi.org/10.1089/neu.2021.0408. Epub 2022 Jul 18. PMID: 35579949; PMCID: PMC9529303.
691. Liston C, Chen AC, Zebley BD, et al. Default mode network mechanisms of transcranial magnetic stimulation in depression. *Biol Psychiatry.* 2014 Oct 1;76(7):517–526. https://doi.org/10.1016/j.biopsych.2014.01.023. Epub 2014 Feb 5. PMID: 24629537; PMCID: PMC4209727.
692. Lindsey A, Ellison RL, Herrold AA, et al. rTMS/iTBS and cognitive rehabilitation for deficits associated with TBI and PTSD: A theoretical framework and review. *J Neuropsychiatry Clin Neurosci.* 2023 Winter;35(1):28–38. https://doi.org/10.1176/appi.neuropsych.21090227. Epub 2022 Jul 25. PMID: 35872613.

693. Mez J, Daneshvar DH, Kiernan PT, et al. Clinicopathological evaluation of chronic traumatic encephalopathy in players of American football. *JAMA*. 2017 Jul 25;318(4):360–370. https://doi.org/10.1001/jama.2017.8334. PMID: 28742910; PMCID: PMC5807097.

694. Cary D Alberstone, Edward C Benzel, Imad M Najm, Michael P Steinmetz. Visual system. *Anatomic basis of neurologic diagnosis*. New York; Stuttgart: Thieme, 2009; p. 384–397.

695. Cary D Alberstone, Edward C Benzel, Imad M Najm, Michael P Steinmetz. Oculomotor system. *Anatomic basis of neurologic diagnosis*. New York; Stuttgart: Thieme, 2009; p 422–469.

696. Hui X, Haider AH, Hashmi ZG, et al. Increased risk of pneumonia among ventilated patients with traumatic brain injury: Every day counts! *J Surg Res*. 2013 Sep;184(1):438–443. https://doi.org/10.1016/j.jss.2013.05.072. Epub 2013 Jun 13. PMID: 23816243.

697. Kreitzer N, Rath K, Kurowski BG, et al. Rehabilitation practices in patients with moderate and severe traumatic brain injury. *J Head Trauma Rehabil*. 2019 Sep/Oct;34(5):E66–E72. https://doi.org/10.1097/HTR.0000000000000477. PMID: 30829824; PMCID: PMC8730801.

698. O'Brien KH, Wallace T, Kemp AM, Pei Y. Cognitive-communication complaints and referrals for speech-language pathology services following concussion. *Am J Speech Lang Pathol*. 2022 Mar 10;31(2):790–807. https://doi.org/10.1044/2021_AJSLP-21-00254. Epub 2022 Jan 18. PMID: 35041792.

699. Pietsch K, Lyon T, Dhillon VK. Speech language pathology rehabilitation. *Med Clin North Am*. 2018 Nov;102(6):1121–1134. https://doi.org/10.1016/j.mcna.2018.06.010. Epub 2018 Sep 20. PMID: 30342613.

700. Iaccarino MA, Bhatnagar S, Zafonte R. Rehabilitation after traumatic brain injury. *Handb Clin Neurol*. 2015;127:411–422. https://doi.org/10.1016/B978-0-444-52892-6.00026-X. PMID: 25702231.

701. Marklund N, Bellander BM, Godbolt AK, Levin H, McCrory P, Thelin EP. Treatments and rehabilitation in the acute and chronic state of traumatic brain injury. *J Intern Med*. 2019 Jun;285(6):608–623. https://doi.org/10.1111/joim.12900. PMID: 30883980; PMCID: PMC6527474.

702. Elkbuli A, Fanfan D, Sutherland M, et al. The association between early versus late physical therapy initiation and outcomes of trauma patients with and without traumatic brain injuries. *J Surg Res*. 2022 May;273:34–43. https://doi.org/10.1016/j.jss.2021.11.011. Epub 2022 Jan 10. PMID: 35026443.

703. 2014 Report of the Texas Traumatic Brain Injury Advisory Council Presented to the Governor of Texas, the Lieutenant Governor, The Speaker of the Texas House of Representatives, and The Texas Legislature.

704. Brooks CA, Lindstrom J, McCray J, Whiteneck GG. Cost of medical care for a population-based sample of persons surviving traumatic brain injury. *J Head Trauma Rehabil*. 1995 August;10(4):1–13.

705. Humphreys I, Wood RL, Phillips CJ, Macey S. The costs of traumatic brain injury: A literature review. *Clinicoecon Outcomes Res*. 2013 Jun 26;5:281–287. https://doi.org/10.2147/CEOR.S44625. PMID: 23836998; PMCID: PMC3699059.

706. Borghol A, Aucoin M, Onor I, Jamero D, Hawawini F. Modafinil for the improvement of patient outcomes following traumatic brain injury. *Innov Clin Neurosci*. 2018 Apr 1;15(3–4):17–23. PMID: 29707422; PMCID: PMC5906085.

707. van Dijck JTJM, Dijkman MD, Ophuis RH, Ruiter GCW. In-hospital costs after severe traumatic brain injury: A systematic review and quality assessment. *PLoS One*. 2019 May;14(5):e0216743.

708. Schneier AJ, Shields BJ, Hostetler SG, Xiang H, Smith GA. Incidence of pediatric traumatic brain injury and associated hospital resource utilization in the United States. *Pediatrics*. 2006 Aug;118(2):483–492. https://doi.org/10.1542/peds.2005-2588. PMID: 16882799.

709. Dismuke CE, Walker RJ, Egede LE. Utilization and cost of health services in individuals with traumatic brain injury. *Glob J Health Sci*. 2015 Apr 19;7(6):156–169. https://doi.org/10.5539/gjhs.v7n6p156. PMID: 26153156; PMCID: PMC4803849.

710. Turner-Stokes L, Dzingina M, Shavelle R, Bill A, Williams H, Sephton K. Estimated life-time savings in the cost of ongoing care following specialist rehabilitation for severe traumatic brain linjury in the United Kingdom. *J Head Trauma Rehabil.* 2019 Jul/Aug;34(4):205–214. https://doi.org/10.1097/HTR.0000000000000473. PMID: 30801440; PMCID: PMC6687405.
711. Miller GF, DePadilla L, Xu L. Costs of nonfatal traumatic brain injury in the United States, 2016. *Med Care.* 2021 May 1;59(5):451–455. https://doi.org/10.1097/MLR.0000000000001511. PMID: 33528230; PMCID: PMC8026675.
712. Zasler ND, Ameis A, Riddick-Grisham SN. Life care planning after traumatic brain injury. *Phys Med Rehabil Clin N Am.* 2013 Aug;24(3):445–465. https://doi.org/10.1016/j.pmr.2013.03.009. Epub 2013 May 11. PMID: 23910485.
713. Sharp DJ, Scott G, Leech R. Network dysfunction after traumatic brain injury. *Nat Rev Neurol.* 2014 Mar;10(3):156–166. https://doi.org/10.1038/nrneurol.2014.15. Epub 2014 Feb 11. PMID: 24514870.
714. https://health.mil/Reference-Center/Publications/2015/12/01/Traumatic-Brain-Injury, (Accessed on February 8, 2023).
715. https://www.health.mil/Reference-Center/Policies/2015/04/06/Traumatic-Brain-Injury-Updated-Definition-and-Reporting, (Accessed on February 9, 2023).
716. Newsome MR, Mayer AR, Lin X, Troyanskaya M, Jackson GR, Scheibel RS, Walder A, Sathiyaraj A, Wilde EA, Mukhi S, Taylor BA, Levin HS. Chronic Effects of Blast-Related TBI on Subcortical Functional Connectivity in Veterans. J Int Neuropsychol Soc. 2016 Jul;22(6):631-42. doi: 10.1017/S1355617716000448. Epub 2016 Jun 6. Erratum in: J Int Neuropsychol Soc. 2016 Aug;22(7):790-2. PMID: 27264731.
717. Xu L, Ware JB, Kim JJ, Shahim P, Silverman E, Magdamo B, Dabrowski C, Wesley L, Le MD, Morrison J, Zamore H, Lynch CE, Petrov D, Chen HI, Schuster J, Diaz-Arrastia R, Sandsmark DK. Arterial Spin Labeling Reveals Elevated Cerebral Blood Flow with Distinct Clusters of Hypo- and Hyperperfusion after Traumatic Brain Injury. J Neurotrauma. 2021 Sep 15;38(18):2538-2548. doi: 10.1089/neu.2020.7553. Epub 2021 Jun 10. PMID: 34115539; PMCID: PMC8403182.
718. Iutaka T, de Freitas MB, Omar SS, Scortegagna FA, Nael K, Nunes RH, Pacheco FT, Maia Júnior ACM, do Amaral LLF, da Rocha AJ. Arterial Spin Labeling: Techniques, Clinical Applications, and Interpretation. Radiographics. 2023 Jan;43(1):e220088. doi: 10.1148/rg.220088. PMID: 36367822.
719. Rashid A, Manghi A. Calcitonin Gene-Related Peptide Receptor. 2022 Jul 12. In: StatPearls [Internet]. Treasure Island (FL): StatPearls Publishing; 2023 Jan–. PMID: 32809483.

Index

Note: - Page numbers with *italics* denote the figure and **bold** for the tables.

D

E

F

G

M

N

U

V

W